HEALTH
A CONCERN FOR EVERY AMERICAN

HEALTH
A CONCERN FOR EVERY AMERICAN

Hannah Nordhaus

INFORMATION PLUS® REFERENCE SERIES
Formerly published by Information Plus, Wylie, Texas

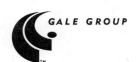

GALE GROUP

Detroit
New York
San Francisco
London
Boston
Woodbridge, CT

HEALTH: A CONCERN FOR EVERY AMERICAN
Hannah Nordhaus, *Author*
John Riddle, *Researcher*

The Gale Group Staff:

Editorial: John F. McCoy, *Project Manager and Series Editor*; Andrew Claps, *Series Associate Editor*; Jason M. Everett, *Series Associate Editor*; Michael T. Reade, *Series Associate Editor*; Rita Runchock, *Managing Editor*; Luann Brennan, *Editor*

Image and Multimedia Content: Barbara J. Yarrow, *Manager, Imaging and Multimedia Content*; Robyn Young, *Project Manager, Imaging and Multimedia Content*

Indexing: Lynne Maday, *Indexing Specialist*; Amy Suchowski, *Indexing Specialist*

Permissions: Ryan Thomason, *Permissions Specialist*; Maria Franklin, *Permissions Manager*

Product Design: Michelle DiMercurio, *Senior Art Director*; Kenn Zorn, *Product Design Manager*

Production: Evi Seoud, *Assistant Manager, Composition Purchasing and Electronic Prepress*; NeKita McKee, *Buyer*; Dorothy Maki, *Manufacturing Manager*

ISBN 0-7876-5103-6 (set)
ISBN 0-7876-5395-0 (this volume)
ISSN 1534-1623 (this volume)
Printed in the United States of America
10 9 8 7 6 5 4 3 2 1

TABLE OF CONTENTS

A primary indicator of the well-being of a nation is the health of its people and the availability of health care. Many factors can affect a person's health: heredity, race/ethnicity, gender, income, education, geography, violent crime, environmental agents, exposure to infectious diseases, and access to health care. This chapter provides an overview of vital health statistics and the health status of Americans.

Americans are spending an increasing amount of money on health care, with the money coming from both private and public funds. This chapter explores the types of services that Americans pay for; the reasons for cost increases; and what can be done about controlling skyrocketing costs. Programs such as Medicare, Medicaid, and long-term health care are also discussed.

This chapter begins with a comparison of monetary issues concerning health care. It concludes with comparisons of the health care systems in the United States, Germany, Canada, United Kingdom, France, and Japan.

Many factors affect the availability of health insurance, including employment, income, and age. Sources of health insurance—for those who can afford it or are eligible to receive it—are private insurance, Medicare, and Medicaid. Although many Americans, including millions of children, are uninsured, government programs and legislation have been designed to reverse this strain on American society.

Modern health care treatment requires that its practitioners have a great deal of training and skill. This chapter examines the training, working conditions, earnings, and related issues pertaining to health care professionals. Alternative forms of health care, such as acupuncture and herbalism, are also discussed.

There are many different types of health care institutions in the United States, including hospitals, hospices, nursing homes, home health care, and mental health facilities, and each is profiled here. Among the issues discussed are the plight of public hospitals and the rapid rise of home health care agencies.

Chronic diseases are prolonged illnesses that do not resolve spontaneously and are rarely cured completely. This chapter examines the causes, treatment, and prevention of cardiovascular disease, cancer, respiratory diseases, and diabetes.

Degenerative diseases are noninfectious disorders where the victim becomes progressively disabled. This chapter looks at the prevalence, causes, and treatment of arthritis, osteoporosis, multiple sclerosis, Parkinson's disease, and Alzheimer's disease.

Genetic diseases are conditions caused by changes or mutations to the victim's genes, which are then passed from one generation to the next. This chapter examines the prevalence, causes, and treatment of muscular dystrophy, Huntington's disease, cystic fibrosis, sickle-cell disease, and Tay-Sachs disease.

Infectious diseases are those caused by viruses or bacteria transmitted from one person to another through casual contact or through bodily fluids. The most frequently reported diseases are discussed. This chapter also contains more in-depth examinations of the prevalence, causes, and treatment of influenza, tuberculosis, AIDS, and Lyme disease.

Millions of Americans suffer from mental illness. This chapter presents the findings of two studies on the nation's mental health. Schizophrenia, depression, anxiety disorders, eating disorders, and suicide are also defined and discussed.

PREFACE

Health: A Concern for Every American is the latest volume in the ever-growing *Information Plus Reference Series*. Previously published by the Information Plus company of Wylie, Texas, the *Information Plus Reference Series* (and its companion set, the *Information Plus Compact Series*) became a Gale Group product when Gale and Information Plus merged in early 2000. Those of you familiar with the series as published by Information Plus will notice a few changes from the 1999 edition. Gale has adopted a new layout and style that we hope you will find easy to use. Other improvements include greatly expanded indexes in each book, and more descriptive tables of contents.

While some changes have been made to the design, the purpose of the *Information Plus Reference Series* remains the same. Each volume of the series presents the latest facts on a topic of pressing concern in modern American life. These topics include today's most controversial and most studied social issues: abortion, capital punishment, care for the elderly, crime, health care, the environment, immigration, minorities, social welfare, women, youth, and many more. Although written especially for the high school and undergraduate student, this series is an excellent resource for anyone in need of factual information on current affairs.

By presenting the facts, it is Gale's intention to provide its readers with everything they need to reach an informed opinion on current issues. To that end, there is a particular emphasis in this series on the presentation of scientific studies, surveys, and statistics. This data is generally presented in the form of tables, charts, and other graphics placed within the text of each book. Every graphic is directly referred to and carefully explained in the text. The source of each graphic is presented within the graphic itself. The data used in these graphics is drawn from the most reputable and reliable sources, in particular from the various branches of the U.S. government and from major independent polling organizations. Every effort was made to secure the most recent information available. The reader should bear in mind that many major studies take years to conduct, and that additional years often pass before the data from these studies is made available to the public. Therefore, in many cases the most recent information available in 2001 dated from 1998 or 1999. Older statistics are sometimes presented as well, if they are of particular interest and no more-recent information exists.

Although statistics are a major focus of the *Information Plus Reference Series* they are by no means its only content. Each book also presents the widely held positions and important ideas that shape how the book's subject is discussed in the United States. These positions are explained in detail and, where possible, in the words of those who support them. Some of the other material to be found in these books includes: historical background; descriptions of major events related to the subject; relevant laws and court cases; and examples of how these issues play out in American life. Some books also feature primary documents, or have pro and con debate sections giving the words and opinions of prominent Americans on both sides of a controversial topic. All material is presented in an even-handed and unbiased manner; the reader will never be encouraged to accept one view of an issue over another.

HOW TO USE THIS BOOK

Americans are among the world's healthiest people. Thanks to the great wealth of the United States, its health care system is among the world's foremost. Thanks to the tremendous advances in medicine and technology that have taken place throughout the twentieth century, that system is capable of healing many people whose conditions would have been irreversible even a few decades earlier. Yet at the beginning of the twenty-first century health and health care remains one of the most heavily debated topics in American society. Many Americans are concerned about the increasing cost of health care, the possibility of declines in quality, the failure of the health care system to treat everyone equally, and the continued threat to their health posed by incurable disorders such as cancer and AIDS. This book presents the latest information available on the U.S. health care system and the health of those who are served by it. Trends in the cost of health care over time are examined, as are trends in the quality of care received by those of different races or income levels. The nature of the most serious health problems facing Americans today are explored.

Health: A Concern for Every American consists of thirteen chapters and three appendixes. Each chapter covers a major issue related to the health of Americans; for a summary of the information covered in each chapter, please see the synopses provided in the Table of Contents at the front of the book. Chapters generally begin with an overview of the basic facts and background information on the chapter's topic, then proceed to examine sub-topics of particular interest. For example, Chapter 6: Health Care Institutions begins with a brief history of hospitals in the United States, and describes the basic types of hospitals that can be found in America today. The section on hospitals continues with statistics on why people are admitted to hospitals and how long they are likely to stay there. It concludes with an examination of the organ transplant system. The chapter then moves on to discuss other types of health care institutions and organizations, namely: urgent care centers, nursing homes, hospices, managed care organizations, professional home health care, and mental health treatment centers. Each of these health care organizations is described and its role in the overall American health care system is discussed, with a special emphasis on the problems and controversies faced by different types of health care institutions. Readers can find their way through a chapter by looking for the section and sub-section headings, which are clearly set off from the text. Or, they can refer to the book's extensive index, if they already know what they are looking for.

Statistical Information

The tables and figures featured throughout *Health: A Concern for Every American* will be of particular use to the reader in learning about this topic. These tables and figures represent an extensive collection of the most recent and valuable statistics on the health of Americans

and the health care system that serves them; for example: the life expectancy of Americans, the rate at which they are hospitalized compared with other developed nations, the number of them who suffer from various serious disorders, and their level of satisfaction with the American health care system. Gale believes that making this information available to the reader is the most important way in which we fulfill the goal of this book: To help readers understand the topic of health and health care in the United States and reach their own conclusions about controversial issues related to it.

Each table or figure has a unique identifier appearing above it, for ease of identification and reference. Titles for the tables and figures explain their purpose. At the end of each table or figure, the original source of the data is provided.

In order to help readers understand these often complicated statistics, all tables and figures are explained in the text. References in the text direct the reader to the relevant statistics. Furthermore, the contents of all tables and figures are fully indexed. Please see the opening section of the index at the back of this volume for a description of how to find tables and figures within it.

In addition to the main body text and images, *Health: A Concern for Every American* has three appendices. The first is the Important Names and Addresses directory. Here the reader will find contact information for a number of organizations that study health. The second appendix is the Resources section, which is provided to assist the reader in conducting his or her own research. In this section, the author and editors of *Health: A Concern for Every American* describe some of the sources that were most useful during the compilation of this book. The final appendix is this book's index. It has been greatly expanded from previous editions, and should make it even easier to find specific topics in this book.

COMMENTS AND SUGGESTIONS

The editor of the *Information Plus Reference Series* welcomes your feedback on *Health: A Concern for Every American*. Please direct all correspondence to:

Editor
Information Plus Reference Series
27500 Drake Rd.
Farmington Hills, MI, 48331-3535

ACKNOWLEDGEMENTS

The editors wish to thank the copyright holders of the excerpted material included in this volume and the permissions managers of many book and magazine publishing companies for assisting us in securing reproduction rights. We are also grateful to the staffs of the Detroit Public Library, the Library of Congress, the University of Detroit Mercy Library, Wayne State University Purdy/Kresge Library Complex, and the University of Michigan Libraries for making their resources available to us. Following is a list of the copyright holders who have granted us permission to reproduce material in this volume of Health: A Concern for Every American. *Every effort has been made to trace copyright, but if omissions have been made, please let us know.*

COPYRIGHTED MATERIAL IN HEALTH: A CONCERN FOR EVERY AMERICAN WAS REPRODUCED FROM THE FOLLOWING PERIODICALS:

From *Advance Data from Vital and Health Statistics,* 1998, illustration. National Center for Health Statistics, 1998. Reproduced by permission.

From *Cancer Facts and Figures,* 1998, 2000, illustrations. Copyright © 1998 and 2000 by the American Cancer Society. Both reproduced by permission.

From a study *1998 Data Compendium,* illustration. Health Care Financing Administration. Reproduced by permission.

Health Affairs, 1997 and Jan/Feb, 1998 illustrations. Copyright © 1997 and 1998 by Project-Hope. All reproduced by permission.

Health Care Financing Review, Spring and Fall, 1997, 2000, illustrations. All reproduced by permission of the Health Care Financing Review.

From a study *1999 and 2000 Healthy Confidence Survey,* illustrations. Copyright © 1999 and 2000 by the Employee Benefit Research Institute. All reproduced by permission of the Employee Benefit Research Institute.

Health, United States, 1998 and 2000, illustrations. All reproduced by permission of the National Center for Health Statistics.

From *2001 Heart and Stroke Statistical Update,* 2000, illustrations. Copyright © 2000 by the American Heart Association. Both reproduced by permission of the American Heart Association.

From *Heart and Stroke Facts: 1998 Statistical Supplement,* 1998, illustration. Copyright © 1998 by the American Heart Association. Reproduced by permission.

From a study in *Mental Health,* United States, 1994, illustration. Center for Mental Health, 1994. Reproduced by permission.

From *Morbidity and Morality Weekly Report,* November, 1996, illustration. Courtesy of the Centers for Disease Control.

The Gallup Poll Monthly, October 6–9, September 11–13, 2000, illustrations. Copyright copy; 2000 by The Gallup Organization. Reproduced by permission of The Gallup Organization.

CHAPTER 1
INDICATORS OF THE NATION'S HEALTH STATUS

A primary indicator of the well-being of a nation is the health of its people and the availability of health care. Many factors can affect a person's health: heredity, race/ethnicity, gender, income, education, geography, violent crime, environmental agents, exposure to infectious diseases, and access to health care. This chapter provides an overview of vital health statistics and the health status of Americans.

BIRTHRATES AND FERTILITY RATES

The birthrate is the number of live births per 1,000 women. The fertility rate, on the other hand, is the number of live births per 1,000 women between 15 and 44 years of age, generally considered a woman's prime childbearing years.

The National Center for Health Statistics (NCHS) estimated that there were almost 4 million live births in the United States in 1998, or a birthrate of 14.6 births per 1,000 women. That was a slight increase over the 1997 rate (14.5 per 1,000 women), the lowest since birthrates began to decline in the second half of the 20th century (24.1 births per 1,000 women in 1950).

The birthrates for women ages 30–34 (87.4 births per 1,000 women in 1998) and 35–39 (37.4 births per 1,000 women) have increased dramatically since 1980. The birthrates for teenagers 15–19 (51.1 births per 1,000 women) were about the same as in 1980, but were down somewhat from a high of 60 births per 100,000 in the early 1990s. Women ages 20–29 continued to have the highest birthrates. In 1985, however, birthrates among women 25–29 years old surpassed those in the 20–24 age group, a trend that continued through 1998. (See Table 1.1.)

Fertility rates focus on live births to mothers in the primary childbearing age group, 15–44. In 1998 the fertility rate for American women was 65.6 births per 1,000

women, again an increase over 1997 (65 per 1,000). Hispanic women (101.1 per 1,000) had significantly higher fertility rates than non-Hispanic women. The rates for non-Hispanic black women (73 per 1,000) and Asian/Pacific Islander (API) mothers (64 per 1,000) were somewhat higher than for non-Hispanic white women (57.7 per 1,000). (See Table 1.1.)

Factors other than age, race, and ethnicity can have dramatic effects on fertility rates. For example, women who are currently married and living with their husbands have much higher fertility rates than those who are separated, widowed, divorced, or have never married.

Prenatal Care and Low Birthweight

Early prenatal care can detect, and often correct, many potential health problems early in pregnancy. Regular visits to a physician or clinic usually give the mother-to-be information and encouragement about eating properly, exercising regularly, taking vitamins, and avoiding harmful substances such as alcohol, drugs, and tobacco. The benefits of these preventive measures can literally make a lifetime of difference for a newborn.

Sophisticated procedures, such as obstetric ultrasound scans and amniocentesis, can be performed to detect possible birth defects and other prenatal problems. The ultrasound uses high-frequency sound waves to compose a picture of the fetus and is used to detect and assess fetal development and any malformations in the fetus. During amniocentesis, a physician inserts a needle through the abdominal wall into the uterus to obtain a small sample of the amniotic fluid surrounding the fetus. When tested in a laboratory, this fluid can reveal chromosomal abnormalities, metabolic disorders, and physical abnormalities. Pregnant women over the age of 35 are often advised to undergo this procedure, because they are at somewhat greater risk than younger women of giving birth to babies with chromosomal abnormalities.

TABLE 1.1

Crude birth rates, fertility rates, and birth rates by age of mother, according to detailed race and Hispanic origin: selected years 1950–98

Race, Hispanic origin, and year	Crude birth rate[1]	Fertility rate[2]	10–14 years	15–19 years Total	15–17 years	18–19 years	20–24 years	25–29 years	30–34 years	35–39 years	40–44 years	45–54 years[3]
All races					Live births per 1,000 women							
1950	24.1	106.2	1.0	81.6	40.7	132.7	196.6	166.1	103.7	52.9	15.1	1.2
1960	23.7	118.0	0.8	89.1	43.9	166.7	258.1	197.4	112.7	56.2	15.5	0.9
1970	18.4	87.9	1.2	68.3	38.8	114.7	167.8	145.1	73.3	31.7	8.1	0.5
1980	15.9	68.4	1.1	53.0	32.5	82.1	115.1	112.9	61.9	19.8	3.9	0.2
1985	15.8	66.3	1.2	51.0	31.0	79.6	108.3	111.0	69.1	24.0	4.0	0.2
1990	16.7	70.9	1.4	59.9	37.5	88.6	116.5	120.2	80.8	31.7	5.5	0.2
1994	15.2	66.7	1.4	58.9	37.6	91.5	111.1	113.9	81.5	33.7	6.4	0.3
1995	14.8	65.6	1.3	56.8	36.0	89.1	109.8	112.2	82.5	34.3	6.6	0.3
1996	14.7	65.3	1.2	54.4	33.8	86.0	110.4	113.1	83.9	35.3	6.8	0.3
1997	14.5	65.0	1.1	52.3	32.1	83.6	110.4	113.8	85.3	36.1	7.1	0.4
1998	14.6	65.6	1.0	51.1	30.4	82.0	111.2	115.9	87.4	37.4	7.3	0.4
Race of child:[4] White												
1950	23.0	102.3	0.4	70.0	31.3	120.5	190.4	165.1	102.6	51.4	14.5	1.0
1960	22.7	113.2	0.4	79.4	35.5	154.6	252.8	194.9	109.6	54.0	14.7	0.8
1970	17.4	84.1	0.5	57.4	29.2	101.5	163.4	145.9	71.9	30.0	7.5	0.4
1980	14.9	64.7	0.6	44.7	25.2	72.1	109.5	112.4	60.4	18.5	3.4	0.2
Race of mother:[5] White												
1980	15.1	65.6	0.6	45.4	25.5	73.2	111.1	113.8	61.2	18.8	3.5	0.2
1985	15.0	64.1	0.6	43.3	24.4	70.4	104.1	112.3	69.9	23.3	3.7	0.2
1990	15.8	68.3	0.7	50.8	29.5	78.0	109.8	120.7	81.7	31.5	5.2	0.2
1994	14.4	64.9	0.8	51.1	30.7	82.1	106.2	115.5	83.2	33.7	6.2	0.3
1995	14.2	64.4	0.8	50.1	30.0	81.2	106.3	114.8	84.6	34.5	6.4	0.3
1996	14.1	64.3	0.8	48.1	28.4	78.4	107.2	116.1	86.3	35.6	6.7	0.3
1997	13.9	63.9	0.7	46.3	27.1	75.9	106.7	116.6	87.8	36.4	6.9	0.4
1998	14.0	64.6	0.6	45.4	25.9	74.6	107.2	119.1	90.5	37.8	7.2	0.4
Race of child:[4] Black												
1960	31.9	153.5	4.3	156.1	—	—	295.4	218.6	137.1	73.9	21.9	1.1
1970	25.3	115.4	5.2	140.7	101.4	204.9	202.7	136.3	79.6	41.9	12.5	1.0
1980	22.1	88.1	4.3	100.0	73.6	138.8	146.3	109.1	62.9	24.5	5.8	0.3
Race of mother:[5] Black												
1980	21.3	84.9	4.3	97.8	72.5	135.1	140.0	103.9	59.9	23.5	5.6	0.3
1985	20.4	78.8	4.5	95.4	69.3	132.4	135.0	100.2	57.9	23.9	4.6	0.3
1990	22.4	86.8	4.9	112.8	82.3	152.9	160.2	115.5	68.7	28.1	5.5	0.3
1994	19.5	76.9	4.6	104.5	76.3	148.3	146.0	104.0	65.8	28.9	5.9	0.3
1995	18.2	72.3	4.2	96.1	69.7	137.1	137.1	98.6	64.0	28.7	6.0	0.3
1996	17.8	70.7	3.6	91.4	64.7	132.5	136.8	98.2	63.3	29.1	6.1	0.3
1997	17.7	70.7	3.3	88.2	60.8	130.1	139.0	99.5	64.3	29.7	6.5	0.3
1998	17.7	71.0	2.9	85.4	56.8	126.9	141.9	101.8	64.7	30.5	6.7	0.3
American Indian or Alaska Native mothers[5]												
1980	20.7	82.7	1.9	82.2	51.5	129.5	143.7	106.6	61.8	28.1	8.2	*
1985	19.8	78.6	1.7	79.2	47.7	124.1	139.1	109.6	62.6	27.4	6.0	*
1990	18.9	76.2	1.6	81.1	48.5	129.3	148.7	110.3	61.5	27.5	5.9	*
1994	17.1	70.9	1.9	80.8	51.3	130.3	134.2	104.1	61.2	27.5	5.9	0.4
1995	16.6	69.1	1.8	78.0	47.8	130.7	132.5	98.4	62.2	27.7	6.1	*
1996	16.6	68.7	1.7	73.9	46.4	122.3	133.9	98.5	63.2	28.5	6.3	*
1997	16.6	69.1	1.7	71.8	45.3	117.6	134.9	100.8	64.2	29.3	6.4	0.4
1998	17.1	70.7	1.6	72.1	44.4	118.4	139.3	102.2	66.3	30.2	6.4	*
Asian or Pacific Islander mothers[5]												
1980	19.9	73.2	0.3	26.2	12.0	46.2	93.3	127.4	96.0	38.3	8.5	0.7
1985	18.7	68.4	0.4	23.8	12.5	40.8	83.6	123.0	93.6	42.7	8.7	1.2
1990	19.0	69.6	0.7	26.4	16.0	40.2	79.2	126.3	106.5	49.6	10.7	1.1
1994	17.5	66.8	0.7	27.1	16.1	44.1	73.1	118.6	105.2	51.3	11.6	1.0
1995	17.3	66.4	0.7	26.1	15.4	43.4	72.4	113.4	106.9	52.4	12.1	0.8
1996	17.0	65.9	0.6	24.6	14.9	40.4	70.7	111.2	109.2	52.2	12.2	0.8
1997	16.9	66.3	0.5	23.7	14.3	39.3	70.5	113.2	110.3	54.1	11.9	0.9
1998	16.4	64.0	0.4	23.1	13.8	38.3	68.8	110.4	105.1	52.8	12.0	0.9

Ideally, every woman should receive prenatal care, and the NCHS reported that the United States is capable of supplying prenatal care to 90 percent of pregnant women during the first trimester (three months) of pregnancy. Not all mothers-to-be, however, see a doctor for early prenatal care.

Maternal education level has been found to be strongly associated with the likelihood of receiving prenatal care. Between 1980 and 1996, rates of early prenatal care were higher for women with more education. (See Figure 1.1.) While approximately 90 percent of white mothers

TABLE 1.1

Crude birth rates, fertility rates, and birth rates by age of mother, according to detailed race and Hispanic origin: selected years 1950–98
[CONTINUED]

Race, Hispanic origin, and year	Crude birth rate[1]	Fertility rate[2]	Age of mother									
			10–14 years	15–19 years			20–24 years	25–29 years	30–34 years	35–39 years	40–44 years	45–54 years[3]
				Total	15–17 years	18–19 years						
				Live births per 1,000 women								
Hispanic mothers[5,6,7]												
1980	23.5	95.4	1.7	82.2	52.1	126.9	156.4	132.1	83.2	39.9	10.6	0.7
1990	26.7	107.7	2.4	100.3	65.9	147.7	181.0	153.0	98.3	45.3	10.9	0.7
1994	25.5	105.6	2.7	107.7	74.0	158.0	188.2	153.2	95.4	44.3	10.7	0.6
1995	25.2	105.0	2.7	106.7	72.9	157.9	188.5	153.8	95.9	44.9	10.8	0.6
1996	24.8	104.9	2.6	101.8	69.0	151.1	189.5	161.0	98.1	45.1	10.8	0.6
1997	24.2	102.8	2.3	97.4	66.3	144.3	184.2	161.7	97.9	45.0	10.8	0.6
1998	24.3	101.1	2.1	93.6	62.3	140.1	178.4	160.2	98.9	44.9	10.8	0.6
White, non-Hispanic mothers[5,6,7]												
1980	14.2	62.4	0.4	41.2	22.4	67.7	105.5	110.6	59.9	17.7	3.0	0.1
1990	14.4	62.8	0.5	42.5	23.2	66.6	97.5	115.3	79.4	30.0	4.7	0.2
1994	12.8	58.3	0.5	40.4	22.8	67.4	90.9	107.9	80.7	32.1	5.7	0.2
1995	12.6	57.6	0.4	39.3	22.0	66.1	90.0	106.5	82.0	32.9	5.9	0.3
1996	12.4	57.3	0.4	37.6	20.6	63.7	90.1	107.0	83.5	34.0	6.2	0.3
1997	12.2	57.0	0.4	36.0	19.4	61.9	89.8	107.2	85.2	34.9	6.4	0.3
1998	12.3	57.7	0.3	35.2	18.4	60.6	90.7	109.7	88.0	36.4	6.7	0.4
Black, non-Hispanic mothers[5,6,7]												
1980	22.9	90.7	4.6	105.1	77.2	146.5	152.2	111.7	65.2	25.8	5.8	0.3
1990	23.0	89.0	5.0	116.2	84.9	157.5	165.1	118.4	70.2	28.7	5.6	0.3
1994	20.0	79.0	4.7	107.7	78.6	152.9	150.3	107.0	67.5	29.5	6.0	0.3
1995	18.8	74.5	4.3	99.3	72.1	141.9	141.7	102.0	65.9	29.4	6.1	0.3
1996	18.3	72.5	3.8	94.2	66.6	136.6	140.9	100.8	64.9	29.7	6.2	0.3
1997	18.1	72.4	3.4	90.8	62.6	134.0	143.0	101.9	65.8	30.3	6.6	0.3
1998	18.2	73.0	3.0	88.2	58.8	130.9	146.4	104.6	66.6	31.2	6.8	0.3

— Data not available.
* Based on fewer than 20 births.
[1] Live births per 1,000 population.
[2] Total number of live births regardless of age of mother per 1,000 women 15–44 years of age.
[3] Prior to 1997 data are for live births to mothers 45–49 years of age per 1,000 women 45–49 years of age. Starting in 1997 data are for live births to mothers 45–54 years of age per 1,000 women 45–49 years of age.
[4] Live births are tabulated by race of child.
[5] Live births are tabulated by race and/or Hispanic origin of mother.
[6] Trend data for Hispanics and non-Hispanics are affected by expansion of the reporting area for an Hispanic-origin item on the birth certificate and by immigration. These two factors affect numbers of events, composition of the Hispanic population, and maternal and infant health characteristics. The number of States in the reporting area increased from 22 in 1980, to 23 and the District of Columbia (DC) in 1983–87, 30 and DC in 1988, 47 and DC in 1989, 48 and DC in 1990, 49 and DC in 1991–92, and 50 and DC in 1993 and later years.
[7] Rates in 1985 were not calculated because estimates for the Hispanic and non-Hispanic populations were not available.

Notes: Data are based on births adjusted for underregistration for 1950 and on registered births for all other years. Beginning in 1970, births to persons who were not residents of the 50 States and the District of Columbia are excluded. The race groups, white, black, American Indian or Alaska Native, and Asian or Pacific Islander, include persons of Hispanic and non-Hispanic origin. Conversely, persons of Hispanic origin may be of any race.

SOURCE: *Health, United States, 2000,* National Center for Health Statistics, Hyattsville, MD, 2000

with 13 years or more of education obtained prenatal care between 1980 and 1996, rates were less stable for those with less education. Use of prenatal care among white women with less than 12 years of education declined steadily from 1980 (66 percent) to 1989 (59 percent), and then rose to near 70 percent in 1996. Prenatal care rates for black women in each educational group were lower than those of white women, but rates for black women rose significantly during the 1990s.

The most educated white, Hispanic, and API women were approximately 1.3 times as likely to have early prenatal care as the least educated. Among black and American Indian/Alaska Native women, the most educated were 1.5 times as likely to receive early care as the least educated. (See Figure 1.2.)

Early prenatal care can prevent or reduce the risk of low birthweight, or babies weighing less than 2,500 grams (5.5 pounds) at birth. Premature infants and those with low birthweights are at the greatest risk of death and disability. About 80 percent of women at risk for delivering a low-birthweight infant can be identified in the first prenatal visit. Between 1985 and 1998, the proportion of newborn babies weighing less than 2,500 grams increased from 6.8 percent to 7.6 percent.

Black mothers were about twice as likely as white and Hispanic women to give birth to low-birthweight infants. In 1998, 13.2 percent of non-Hispanic black mothers, 7.4 percent of API mothers, 6.8 percent of American Indian/Alaska Native mothers, 6.5 percent of white mothers, and 6.4 percent of Hispanic mothers delivered

FIGURE 1.1

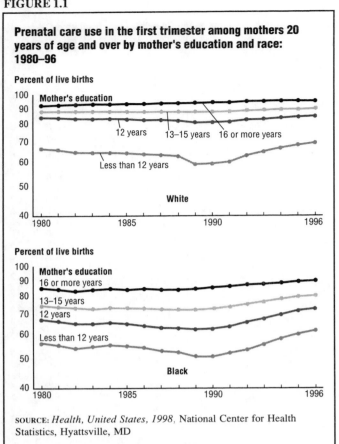

Prenatal care use in the first trimester among mothers 20 years of age and over by mother's education and race: 1980–96

Percent of live births

White

Percent of live births

Black

SOURCE: *Health, United States, 1998*, National Center for Health Statistics, Hyattsville, MD

low-birthweight babies. (See Table 1.2.) Mothers-to-be who smoked cigarettes were almost twice as likely to deliver low-birthweight babies (12 percent) as were non-smokers (7.2 percent). (See Table 1.2.)

Infant Mortality

In 1998 the infant mortality rate—deaths of infants under one year old—stood at 7.2 per 1,000 live births. (See Table 1.3.) Although the mortality rate for black infants dropped to 14.1 deaths per 1,000 live births, it was still more than twice the rate for whites and Hispanics (6 per 1,000 live births). Table 1.4 shows the U.S. infant mortality rate as compared with those of other industrialized nations. The United States had higher infant mortality rates than 24 other countries in 1994—almost twice as many deaths as those nations with the lowest infant mortality rates.

In 1998 congenital anomalies (irregularities the child was born with) were the most frequent cause of death among infants. Short gestation (being born before complete development can occur) and sudden infant death syndrome were the next most common causes, followed by respiratory distress syndrome and maternal complications of pregnancy. (See Table 1.5.)

LIFE EXPECTANCY

In 1998 the U.S. Bureau of the Census estimated that the average life expectancy at birth had reached a record-high of 76.7 years. Life expectancy for females (79.5 years) outstripped that of males (73.8 years) by nearly six

FIGURE 1.2

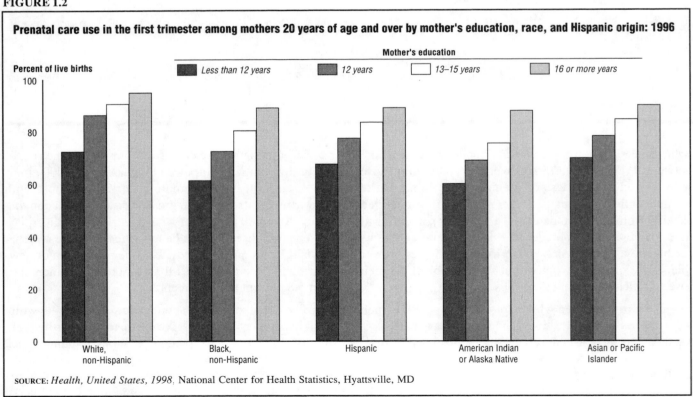

Prenatal care use in the first trimester among mothers 20 years of age and over by mother's education, race, and Hispanic origin: 1996

Mother's education

Percent of live births

Less than 12 years | 12 years | 13–15 years | 16 or more years

White, non-Hispanic | Black, non-Hispanic | Hispanic | American Indian or Alaska Native | Asian or Pacific Islander

SOURCE: *Health, United States, 1998*, National Center for Health Statistics, Hyattsville, MD

TABLE 1.2

Low-birthweight live births, according to mother's detailed race, Hispanic origin, and smoking status: selected years 1970–98

Birthweight, race of mother, Hispanic origin of mother, and smoking status of mother	1970	1975	1980	1985	1990	1992	1993	1994	1995	1996	1997	1998
Low birthweight (less than 2,500 grams)					Percent of live births[1]							
All races	7.93	7.38	6.84	6.75	6.97	7.08	7.22	7.28	7.32	7.39	7.51	7.57
White	6.85	6.27	5.72	5.65	5.70	5.80	5.98	6.11	6.22	6.34	6.46	6.52
Black	13.90	13.19	12.69	12.65	13.25	13.31	13.34	13.24	13.13	13.01	13.01	13.05
American Indian or Alaska Native	7.97	6.41	6.44	5.86	6.11	6.22	6.42	6.45	6.61	6.49	6.75	6.81
Asian or Pacific Islander	—	—	6.68	6.16	6.45	6.57	6.55	6.81	6.90	7.07	7.23	7.42
Chinese	6.67	5.29	5.21	4.98	4.69	4.98	4.91	4.76	5.29	5.03	5.06	5.34
Japanese	9.03	7.47	6.60	6.21	6.16	7.00	6.53	6.91	7.26	7.27	6.82	7.50
Filipino	10.02	8.08	7.40	6.95	7.30	7.43	6.99	7.77	7.83	7.92	8.33	8.23
Hawaiian and part Hawaiian	—	—	7.23	6.49	7.24	6.89	6.76	7.20	6.84	6.77	7.20	7.15
Other Asian or Pacific Islander	—	—	6.83	6.19	6.65	6.68	6.89	7.06	7.05	7.42	7.54	7.76
Hispanic origin (selected States)[2,3]	—	—	6.12	6.16	6.06	6.10	6.24	6.25	6.29	6.28	6.42	6.44
Mexican	—	—	5.62	5.77	5.55	5.61	5.77	5.80	5.81	5.86	5.97	5.97
Puerto Rican	—	—	8.95	8.69	8.99	9.19	9.23	9.13	9.41	9.24	9.39	9.68
Cuban	—	—	5.62	6.02	5.67	6.10	6.18	6.27	6.50	6.46	6.78	6.50
Central and South American	—	—	5.76	5.68	5.84	5.77	5.94	6.02	6.20	6.03	6.26	6.47
Other and unknown Hispanic	—	—	6.96	6.83	6.87	7.24	7.51	7.54	7.55	7.68	7.93	7.59
White, non-Hispanic (selected States)[2]	—	—	5.67	5.60	5.61	5.73	5.92	6.06	6.20	6.36	6.47	6.55
Black, non-Hispanic (selected States)[2]	—	—	12.71	12.61	13.32	13.40	13.43	13.34	13.21	13.12	13.11	13.17
Cigarette smoker[4]	—	—	—	—	11.25	11.49	11.84	12.28	12.18	12.13	12.06	12.01
Nonsmoker[4]	—	—	—	—	6.14	6.35	6.56	6.71	6.79	6.91	7.07	7.18
Very low birthweight (less than 1,500 grams)												
All races	1.17	1.16	1.15	1.21	1.27	1.29	1.33	1.33	1.35	1.37	1.42	1.45
White	0.95	0.92	0.90	0.94	0.95	0.96	1.01	1.02	1.06	1.09	1.13	1.15
Black	2.40	2.40	2.48	2.71	2.92	2.96	2.96	2.96	2.97	2.99	3.04	3.08
American Indian or Alaska Native	0.98	0.95	0.92	1.01	1.01	0.95	1.05	1.10	1.10	1.21	1.19	1.24
Asian or Pacific Islander	—	—	0.92	0.85	0.87	0.91	0.86	0.93	0.91	0.99	1.05	1.10
Chinese	0.80	0.52	0.66	0.57	0.51	0.67	0.63	0.58	0.67	0.64	0.74	0.75
Japanese	1.48	0.89	0.94	0.84	0.73	0.85	0.74	0.92	0.87	0.81	0.78	0.84
Filipino	1.08	0.93	0.99	0.86	1.05	1.05	0.95	1.19	1.13	1.20	1.29	1.35
Hawaiian and part Hawaiian	—	—	1.05	1.03	0.97	1.02	1.14	1.20	0.94	0.97	1.41	1.53
Other Asian or Pacific Islander	—	—	0.96	0.91	0.92	0.93	0.89	0.93	0.91	1.04	1.07	1.12
Hispanic origin (selected States)[2,3]	—	—	0.98	1.01	1.03	1.04	1.06	1.08	1.11	1.12	1.13	1.15
Mexican	—	—	0.92	0.97	0.92	0.94	0.97	0.99	1.01	1.01	1.02	1.02
Puerto Rican	—	—	1.29	1.30	1.62	1.70	1.66	1.63	1.79	1.70	1.85	1.86
Cuban	—	—	1.02	1.18	1.20	1.24	1.23	1.31	1.19	1.35	1.36	1.33
Central and South American	—	—	0.99	1.01	1.05	1.02	1.02	1.06	1.13	1.14	1.17	1.23
Other and unknown Hispanic	—	—	1.01	0.96	1.09	1.10	1.23	1.29	1.28	1.48	1.35	1.38
White, non-Hispanic (selected States)[2]	—	—	0.86	0.90	0.93	0.94	1.00	1.01	1.04	1.08	1.12	1.15
Black, non-Hispanic (selected States)[2]	—	—	2.46	2.66	2.93	2.97	2.99	2.99	2.98	3.02	3.05	3.11
Cigarette smoker[4]	—	—	—	—	1.73	1.74	1.77	1.81	1.85	1.85	1.83	1.87
Nonsmoker[4]	—	—	—	—	1.18	1.22	1.28	1.30	1.31	1.35	1.40	1.44

— Data not available.

[1] Excludes live births with unknown birthweight. Percent based on live births with known birthweight.

[2] Trend data for Hispanics and non-Hispanics are affected by expansion of the reporting area for an Hispanic-origin item on the birth certificate and by immigration. These two factors affect numbers of events, composition of the Hispanic population, and maternal and infant health characteristics. The number of States in the reporting area increased from 22 in 1980, to 23 and the District of Columbia (DC) in 1983–87, 30 and DC in 1988, 47 and DC in 1989, 48 and DC in 1990, 49 and DC i n 1991–92, and 50 and DC in 1993 and later years.

[3] Includes mothers of all races.

[4] Percent based on live births with known smoking status of mother and known birthweight. Includes data for 43 States and the District of Columbia (DC) in 1989, 45 States and DC in 1990, 46 States and DC in 1991–93, and 46 States, DC, and New York City (NYC) in 1994–98. Excludes data for California, Indiana, New York (but includes NYC in 1994–98), and South Dakota (1989–98), Oklahoma (1989–90), and Louisiana and Nebraska (1989), which did not require the reporting of mother's tobacco use during pregnancy on the birth certificate.

Notes: The race groups, white, black, American Indian or Alaska Native, and Asian or Pacific Islander, include persons of Hispanic and non-Hispanic origin. Conversely, persons of Hispanic origin may be of any race.

SOURCE: *Health, United States, 2000*, National Center for Health Statistics, Hyattsville, MD, 2000

years. White females had the longest life expectancy, 80 years, compared with 74.8 years for black females, 74.5 years for white males, and 67.6 years for black males. (See Table 1.6.)

Many factors may contribute to the significantly lower life expectancy for black men. In addition to issues of access to health care, some observers suggest that black males must deal with greater stress, leaving them more

TABLE 1.3

Infant deaths and infant mortality rates, by age and race and Hispanic origin: final 1997 and preliminary 1998

[Data are based on a continuous file of records received from the States. Rates per 1,000 live births. Figures for 1998 are based on weighted data rounded to the nearest individual, so categories may not add to totals. Rates for Hispanic origin should be interpreted with caution because of inconsistencies between reporting Hispanic origin on birth and death certificates]

Age and race/Hispanic origin	1998 Number	1998 Rate	1997 Number	1997 Rate
All races [1]				
Under 1 year	28,486	7.2	28,045	7.2
Under 28 days	18,832	4.8	18,524	4.8
28 days-11 months	9,654	2.4	9,521	2.5
White, total [2]				
Under 1 year	18,795	6.0	18,539	6.0
Under 28 days	12,479	4.0	12,269	4.0
28 days-11 months	6,316	2.0	6,270	2.0
White, non-Hispanic				
Under 1 year	14,299	6.0	14,170	6.1
Under 28 days	9,390	4.0	9,340	4.0
28 days-11 months	4,908	2.1	4,830	2.1
Black, total [2]				
Under 1 year	8,579	14.1	8,496	14.2
Under 28 days	5,661	9.3	5,637	9.4
28 days-11 months	2,918	4.8	2,859	4.8
Hispanic [3]				
Under 1 year	4,397	6.0	4,240	6.0
Under 28 days	2,965	4.0	2,785	3.9
28 days-11 months	1,432	1.9	1,455	2.0

[1] Includes races other than white and black.
[2] Race and Hispanic origin are reported separately on both the birth and death certificates. Data for persons of Hispanic origin are included in the data for each race group, according to the decedent's reported race.
[3] Includes all persons of Hispanic origin of any race.
Note: Data are subject to sampling and/or random variation.

SOURCE: Joyce A. Martin et al., "Births and Deaths: Preliminary Data for 1998," *National Vital Statistics Report,* vol. 47, no. 25, October 5, 1999

susceptible to various diseases. Among black males in 1998, the observed number of deaths due to homicides, human immunodeficiency virus/acquired immunodeficiency syndrome (HIV/AIDS), and cardiovascular disease was much higher than would be expected based on their proportion in the overall population. (See Table 1.7 for comparative causes of death between black males and other populations.)

MORTALITY

Years of Potential Life Lost

"Years of potential life lost" (YPLL) is a term used by medical and public health officials to describe the number of years deceased persons might have lived if they had not died prematurely (before their life expectancy). In 1998 most YPLL resulted from malignant neoplasms (cancers), heart diseases, and unintentional injuries (accidents).

The increase in life expectancy in the 20th century has meant a decrease in the YPLL rate. In 1980 a total of 10,267.6 years per 100,000 population were lost to persons under age 75; by 1998 that number had declined to 7,733.3 total years lost. Although heart disease remains the number-one killer in the United States, it has been responsible for a smaller proportion of YPLL since 1980 (2,065.3 in 1980; 1,343.2 in 1998). Similarly, years lost to cerebrovascular diseases (e.g., strokes), liver diseases, pneumonia, and motor-vehicle accidents have also declined since 1980. And after increasing dramatically between 1980 and the mid-1990s, years lost to HIV infection dropped by more than half between 1996 and 1998. On the other hand, YPLL rates for diabetes and pulmonary diseases (diseases of the lungs) rose over this same period. (See Table 1.8.)

With the exception of suicide, the YPLL for black males were significantly higher than for white males. In 1998, for all causes, black males lost 15,998.7 years of potential life per 100,000 population, compared with 8,972.8 years for white males. Black males lost considerably more years of life to heart disease, cerebrovascular diseases, cancers, HIV, and homicide and legal intervention than did white males. (See Table 1.8.)

Leading Causes of Death

RACIAL DIFFERENCES. Heart disease was the leading cause of death among Americans in 1998. Cancer (malignant neoplasm) was the second-leading cause for all groups except American Indian/Alaska Native males and API females. There were significant racial and ethnic

TABLE 1.4

Infant mortality rates, feto-infant mortality rates, and postneonatal mortality rates, and average annual percent change: selected countries, 1989 and 1994

[Data are based on reporting by countries]

Country[4]	Infant mortality rate[1]			Feto-infant mortality rate[2]			Postneonatal mortality rate[3]		
	1989[5]	1994[6]	Average annual percent change	1989[7]	1994[8]	Average annual percent change	1989[9]	1994[10]	Average annual percent change
Japan	4.59	4.25	-1.5	8.65	7.52	-2.8	2.01	1.92	-0.9
Singapore	6.61	4.34	-8.1	10.97	7.71	-6.8	2.01	1.88	-1.3
Hong Kong	7.43	4.43	-9.8	11.99	9.14	-5.3	2.64	1.79	-7.5
Sweden	5.77	4.45	-5.1	9.42	7.54	-4.4	2.03	1.46	-6.4
Finland	6.03	4.72	-4.8	10.57	7.08	-7.7	1.91	1.24	-6.3
Switzerland	7.34	5.12	-7.0	11.43	8.57	-5.6	2.91	1.85	-8.7
Norway	7.72	5.23	-7.5	12.65	9.77	-5.0	3.96	1.65	-16.1
Denmark	7.95	5.45	-7.3	13.07	9.90	-5.4	3.31	1.45	-15.2
Germany	- - -	5.60	- - -	- - -	9.64	- - -	- - -	2.38	- - -
Netherlands	6.78	5.64	-3.6	12.60	11.04	-2.6	2.20	1.63	-5.8
Ireland	7.55	5.93	-4.7	13.92	11.87	-3.9	3.21	1.96	-9.4
Australia	8.46	6.05	-6.5	12.80	9.53	-5.7	3.45	1.95	-10.8
Northern Ireland	6.90	6.05	-2.6	12.00	11.28	-1.2	2.91	1.89	-8.3
England and Wales	8.45	6.20	-6.0	13.15	10.58	-4.3	3.69	2.06	-11.0
Scotland	8.73	6.20	-6.6	13.75	10.75	-4.8	4.00	2.21	-11.2
Austria	8.31	6.25	-5.5	12.18	9.58	-4.7	3.45	2.39	-7.1
Canada	7.13	6.30	-3.0	11.28	10.16	-2.6	2.47	2.15	-3.4
France	7.54	6.47	-3.8	13.75	11.48	-4.4	3.70	3.32	-2.7
Italy	8.77	6.63	-5.4	14.72	11.59	-5.8	1.94	2.06	1.5
Spain	7.78	6.69	-3.0	12.19	11.09	-2.3	2.67	2.44	-1.8
New Zealand	10.32	7.24	-8.5	14.92	10.26	-8.9	5.78	3.53	-11.6
Israel	10.06	7.80	-6.2	15.01	11.13	-7.2	3.47	3.09	-2.9
Greece	9.78	7.93	4.1	17.88	13.70	-4.3	3.15	2.33	-5.9
Czech Republic	9.97	7.95	4.4	14.10	11.10	-4.7	3.02	3.21	1.2
United States	9.81	8.02	-3.9	14.13	11.76	-3.6	3.59	2.90	-4.2
Portugal	12.18	8.06	-7.9	20.16	16.30	-5.2	4.12	3.25	-4.6
Belgium	8.53	8.20	-1.3	14.44	13.42	-1.5	3.87	4.01	1.2
Cuba	11.08	9.40	4.0	22.94	21.10	-2.7	3.91	4.13	2.8
Slovakia	13.46	11.19	-3.6	18.02	15.32	-3.2	4.24	3.84	-2.0
Puerto Rico	14.27	11.47	4.3	23.57	21.51	-1.8	3.09	2.83	-1.7
Hungary	15.74	11.55	-6.0	21.04	15.08	-6.4	4.05	3.60	-2.3
Chile	17.06	11.99	-6.8	23.51	18.34	4.0	7.96	5.15	-8.3
Kuwait	17.33	12.68	-4.4	25.39	21.51	-2.1	5.22	3.34	-6.2
Costa Rica	13.90	13.71	-0.3	23.20	21.99	-2.6	5.32	5.20	-0.8
Poland	15.96	15.13	-1.1	21.49	20.77	-0.7	4.44	3.84	-2.9
Bulgaria	14.37	16.31	2.6	20.33	22.51	2.1	7.05	7.54	1.4
Russian Federation	18.06	18.58	0.6	27.14	26.46	-0.5	7.34	6.74	-1.7
Romania	26.90	23.89	-2.3	35.16	30.47	-2.8	19.95	14.84	-5.7

- - - Data not available.
[1] Number of deaths of infants under 1 year per 1,000 live births.
[2] Number of late fetal deaths plus infant deaths under 1 year per 1,000 live births plus late fetal deaths.
[3] Number of postneonatal deaths per 1,000 live births.
[4] Refers to countries, territories, cities, or geographic areas.
[5] Data for Spain are for 1988, and data for Kuwait are for 1987. As German unification did not take place until 1990, no data are available for prior years.
[6] Data for Canada, Cuba, France, Israel, New Zealand, and Spain are for 1993. Data for Belgium are for 1992.
[7] Data for Greece and Spain are for 1988, data for Belgium are for 1987, and data for Kuwait are for 1986.
[8] Data for Canada, Chile, France, Ireland, Israel, Italy, New Zealand, and Portugal are for 1993. Data for Belgium, Cuba, and Spain are for 1992. Data for Costa Rica are for 1991.
[9] Data for Costa Rica and Italy are for 1988 and data for Kuwait and Spain are for 1987.
[10] Data for Canada, France, Israel, and New Zealand are for 1993. Data for Belgium, Italy, and Spain are for 1992. Data for Costa Rica and Cuba are for 1991.

Notes: Rankings are from lowest to highest infant mortality rates based on the latest data available for countries or geographic areas with at least 1 million population and with "complete" counts of live births and infant deaths as indicated in the United Nations Demographic Yearbook, 1995 edition. Some of the international variation in infant mortality rates (IMR) is due to differences among countries in distinguishing between fetal and infant deaths. The feto-infant mortality rate (FIMR) is an alternative measure of pregnancy outcome that reduces the effect of international differences in distinguishing between fetal and infant deaths. The United States ranks 25th on the IMR, 23rd on the FIMR, and 22nd on the postneonatal mortality rate.

World Health Organization: World Health Statistics Annuals. Vols. 1990-1995. Geneva; United Nations: Demographic Yearbook 1990 and 1995. New York; Centers for Disease Control and Prevention, National Center for Health Statistics. Vital statistics of the United States, 1989 and 1994, vol II, mortality, part A. Washington: Public Health Service. 1993 and unpublished.

SOURCE: *Health, United States, 1998*, National Center for Health Statistics, Hyattsville, MD, 1998

variations in the 10 leading causes of death. (See Table 1.7.) In 1998 chronic liver disease and cirrhosis were listed as the 10th-leading cause of death for all Americans; they were not, however, listed as a leading cause of death among blacks, APIs, or white women. In contrast, violent deaths (homicide and legal intervention) were the fifth-leading cause of death for black and Hispanic men; ninth for API men; and 10th for American Indian/Alaska Native men. Homicide and legal intervention did not rank as a top cause of death for white men.

TABLE 1.5

Infant deaths and infant mortality rates for the 10 leading causes of infant death, by race and Hispanic origin: preliminary 1998

[Data are based on a continuous file of records received from the States. Rates per 100,000 live births. Figures are based on weighted data rounded to the nearest individual, so categories may not add to totals. Rates for Hispanic origin should be interpreted with caution because of inconsistencies between reporting Hispanic origin on birth and death certificates]

Rank [1]	Cause of death and race (Based on the Ninth Revision, International Classification of Diseases, 1975)	Number	Rate
All races [2]			
...	All causes	28,488	722.3
1	Congenital anomalies	6,266	158.9
2	Disorders relating to short gestation and unspecified low birthweight	4,011	101.7
3	Sudden infant death syndrome	2,529	64.1
4	Respiratory distress syndrome	1,328	33.7
4	Newborn affected by maternal complications of pregnancy	1,328	33.7
6	Newborn affected by complications of placenta, cord, and membranes	932	23.6
7	Infections specific to the perinatal period	815	20.7
8	Accidents and adverse effects	726	18.4
9	Intrauterine hypoxia and birth asphyxia	459	11.6
10	Pneumonia and influenza	400	10.1
...	All other causes (Residual)	9,694	245.8
White, total [3]			
...	All causes	18,838	603.3
1	Congenital anomalies	4,868	155.9
2	Disorders relating to short gestation and unspecified low birthweight	2,221	71.1
3	Sudden infant death syndrome	1,645	52.7
4	Respiratory distress syndrome	863	27.6
5	Newborn affected by maternal complications of pregnancy	826	26.5
6	Newborn affected by complications of placenta, cord, and membranes	616	19.7
7	Infections specific to the perinatal period	548	17.6
8	Accidents and adverse effects	498	15.9
9	Intrauterine hypoxia and birth asphyxia	322	10.3
10	Pneumonia and influenza	245	7.8
...	All other causes (Residual)	6,186	198.1
White, non-Hispanic			
...	All causes	14,351	606.8
1	Congenital anomalies	3,740	158.1
2	Disorders relating to short gestation and unspecified low birthweight	1,622	68.6
3	Sudden infant death syndrome	1,407	59.5
4	Newborn affected by maternal complications of pregnancy	637	26.9
5	Respiratory distress syndrome	625	26.4
6	Newborn affected by complications of placenta, cord, and membranes	482	20.4
7	Infections specific to the perinatal period	411	17.4
8	Accidents and adverse effects	384	16.2
9	Intrauterine hypoxia and birth asphyxia	260	11.0
10	Neonatal hemorrhage	175	7.4
...	All other causes (Residual)	4,608	194.8
Black, total [3]			
...	All causes	8,545	1,400.4
1	Disorders relating to short gestation and unspecified low birthweight	1,656	271.4
2	Congenital anomalies	1,121	183.7
3	Sudden infant death syndrome	782	128.2
4	Newborn affected by maternal complications of pregnancy	451	73.9
5	Respiratory distress syndrome	432	70.8
6	Newborn affected by complications of placenta, cord, and membranes	286	46.9
7	Infections specific to the perinatal period	248	40.6
8	Accidents and adverse effects	210	34.4
9	Intrauterine hypoxia and birth asphyxia	122	20.0
10	Pneumonia and influenza	121	19.8
...	All other causes (Residual)	3,116	510.6

[1] Rank based on number of deaths.
[2] Includes races other than white and black.
[3] Race and Hispanic origin are reported separately on both the birth and death certificate. Data for persons of Hispanic origin are included in the data for each race group, according to the decedent's reported race.

Note: Data are subject to sampling and/or random variation.

SOURCE: Joyce A. Martin et al., "Births and Deaths: Preliminary Data for 1998," *National Vital Statistics Report,* vol. 47, no. 25, October 5, 1999

AGE DIFFERENCES. In 1998, as would be expected, death rates were highest for persons aged 85 and older (15,177 per 100,000 population). From age 55 on, death rates more than doubled with each additional decade of life. (See Table 1.9.)

The 10 leading causes of death in 1998 for all ages are shown in Table 1.10. Accidents and adverse effects were the leading cause of death for children 1–4 years of age, followed by congenital anomalies and homicide and legal intervention. While children 5–14 years old were

TABLE 1.6

Life expectancy at birth, at 65 years of age, and at 75 years of age, according to race and sex: selected years 1900–98

Specified age and year	All races Both sexes	Male	Female	White Both sexes	Male	Female	Black Both sexes	Male	Female
At birth				Remaining life expectancy in years					
1900[1,2]	47.3	46.3	48.3	47.6	46.6	48.7	[3]33.0	[3]32.5	[3]33.5
1950[2]	68.2	65.6	71.1	69.1	66.5	72.2	60.7	58.9	62.7
1960[2]	69.7	66.6	73.1	70.6	67.4	74.1	63.2	60.7	65.9
1970	70.8	67.1	74.7	71.7	68.0	75.6	64.1	60.0	68.3
1980	73.7	70.0	77.4	74.4	70.7	78.1	68.1	63.8	72.5
1985	74.7	71.1	78.2	75.3	71.8	78.7	69.3	65.0	73.4
1986	74.7	71.2	78.2	75.4	71.9	78.8	69.1	64.8	73.4
1987	74.9	71.4	78.3	75.6	72.1	78.9	69.1	64.7	73.4
1988	74.9	71.4	78.3	75.6	72.2	78.9	68.9	64.4	73.2
1989	75.1	71.7	78.5	75.9	72.5	79.2	68.8	64.3	73.3
1990	75.4	71.8	78.8	76.1	72.7	79.4	69.1	64.5	73.6
1991	75.5	72.0	78.9	76.3	72.9	79.6	69.3	64.6	73.8
1992	75.8	72.3	79.1	76.5	73.2	79.8	69.6	65.0	73.9
1993	75.5	72.2	78.8	76.3	73.1	79.5	69.2	64.6	73.7
1994	75.7	72.4	79.0	76.5	73.3	79.6	69.5	64.9	73.9
1995	75.8	72.5	78.9	76.5	73.4	79.6	69.6	65.2	73.9
1996	76.1	73.1	79.1	76.8	73.9	79.7	70.2	66.1	74.2
1997	76.5	73.6	79.4	77.1	74.3	79.9	71.1	67.2	74.7
1998	76.7	73.8	79.5	77.3	74.5	80.0	71.3	67.6	74.8
At 65 years									
1900–1902[1,2]	11.9	11.5	12.2	—	11.5	12.2	—	10.4	11.4
1950[2]	13.9	12.8	15.0	—	12.8	15.1	13.9	12.9	14.9
1960[2]	14.3	12.8	15.8	14.4	12.9	15.9	13.9	12.7	15.1
1970	15.2	13.1	17.0	15.2	13.1	17.1	14.2	12.5	15.7
1980	16.4	14.1	18.3	16.5	14.2	18.4	15.1	13.0	16.8
1985	16.7	14.5	18.5	16.8	14.5	18.7	15.2	13.0	16.9
1986	16.8	14.6	18.6	16.9	14.7	18.7	15.2	13.0	17.0
1987	16.9	14.7	18.7	17.0	14.8	18.8	15.2	13.0	17.0
1988	16.9	14.7	18.6	17.0	14.8	18.7	15.1	12.9	16.9
1989	17.1	15.0	18.8	17.2	15.1	18.9	15.2	13.0	16.9
1990	17.2	15.1	18.9	17.3	15.2	19.1	15.4	13.2	17.2
1991	17.4	15.3	19.1	17.5	15.4	19.2	15.5	13.4	17.2
1992	17.5	15.4	19.2	17.6	15.5	19.3	15.7	13.5	17.4
1993	17.3	15.3	18.9	17.4	15.4	19.0	15.5	13.4	17.1
1994	17.4	15.5	19.0	17.5	15.6	19.1	15.7	13.6	17.2
1995	17.4	15.6	18.9	17.6	15.7	19.1	15.6	13.6	17.1
1996	17.5	15.7	19.0	17.6	15.8	19.1	15.8	13.9	17.2
1997	17.7	15.9	19.2	17.8	16.0	19.3	16.1	14.2	17.6
1998	17.8	16.0	19.2	17.8	16.1	19.3	16.1	14.3	17.4
At 75 years									
1980	10.4	8.8	11.5	10.4	8.8	11.5	9.7	8.3	10.7
1985	10.6	9.0	11.7	10.6	9.0	11.7	10.1	8.7	11.1
1986	10.7	9.1	11.7	10.7	9.1	11.8	10.1	8.6	11.1
1987	10.7	9.1	11.8	10.7	9.1	11.8	10.1	8.6	11.1
1988	10.6	9.1	11.7	10.7	9.1	11.7	10.0	8.5	11.0
1989	10.9	9.3	11.9	10.9	9.3	11.9	10.1	8.6	11.0
1990	10.9	9.4	12.0	11.0	9.4	12.0	10.2	8.6	11.2
1991	11.1	9.5	12.1	11.1	9.5	12.1	10.2	8.7	11.2
1992	11.2	9.6	12.2	11.2	9.6	12.2	10.4	8.9	11.4
1993	10.9	9.5	11.9	11.0	9.5	12.0	10.2	8.7	11.1
1994	11.0	9.6	12.0	11.1	9.6	12.0	10.3	8.9	11.2
1995	11.0	9.7	11.9	11.1	9.7	12.0	10.2	8.8	11.1
1996	11.1	9.8	12.0	11.1	9.8	12.0	10.3	9.0	11.2
1997	11.2	9.9	12.1	11.2	9.9	12.1	10.7	9.3	11.5
1998	11.3	10.0	12.2	11.3	10.0	12.2	10.5	9.2	11.3

— Data not available.

[1] Death registration area only. The death registration area increased from 10 States and the District of Columbia in 1900 to the coterminous United States in 1933.
[2] Includes deaths of persons who were not residents of the 50 States and the District of Columbia.
[3] Figure is for the all other population.

Notes: Beginning in 1997 life table methodology was revised to construct complete life tables by single years of age that extend to age 100. (Anderson RN. Method for Constructing Complete Annual U.S. Life Tables. National Center for Health Statistics. Vital Health Stat 2(129). 1999.) Previously abridged life tables were constructed for five-year age groups ending with the age group 85 years and over.

SOURCE: *Health, United States, 2000*, National Center for Health Statistics, Hyattsville, MD, 2000

TABLE 1.7

Leading causes of death and numbers of deaths, according to sex, detailed race, and Hispanic origin: 1980 and 1998

Sex, race, Hispanic origin, and rank order	1980		1998	
	Cause of death	Deaths	Cause of death	Deaths
All persons				
...	All causes	1,989,841	All causes	2,337,256
1	Diseases of heart	761,085	Diseases of heart	724,859
2	Malignant neoplasms	416,509	Malignant neoplasms	541,532
3	Cerebrovascular diseases	170,225	Cerebrovascular diseases	158,448
4	Unintentional injuries	105,718	Chronic obstructive pulmonary diseases	112,584
5	Chronic obstructive pulmonary diseases	56,050	Unintentional injuries	97,835
6	Pneumonia and influenza	54,619	Pneumonia and influenza	91,871
7	Diabetes mellitus	34,851	Diabetes mellitus	64,751
8	Chronic liver disease and cirrhosis	30,583	Suicide	30,575
9	Atherosclerosis	29,449	Nephritis, nephrotic syndrome, and nephrosis	26,182
10	Suicide	26,869	Chronic liver disease and cirrhosis	25,192
Male				
...	All causes	1,075,078	All causes	1,157,260
1	Diseases of heart	405,661	Diseases of heart	353,897
2	Malignant neoplasms	225,948	Malignant neoplasms	282,065
3	Unintentional injuries	74,180	Unintentional injuries	63,042
4	Cerebrovascular diseases	69,973	Cerebrovascular diseases	61,145
5	Chronic obstructive pulmonary diseases	38,625	Chronic obstructive pulmonary diseases	57,018
6	Pneumonia and influenza	27,574	Pneumonia and influenza	40,979
7	Suicide	20,505	Diabetes mellitus	29,584
8	Chronic liver disease and cirrhosis	19,768	Suicide	24,538
9	Homicide and legal intervention	19,088	Chronic liver disease and cirrhosis	16,343
10	Diabetes mellitus	14,325	Homicide and legal intervention	14,023
Female				
...	All causes	914,763	All causes	1,179,996
1	Diseases of heart	355,424	Diseases of heart	370,962
2	Malignant neoplasms	190,561	Malignant neoplasms	259,467
3	Cerebrovascular diseases	100,252	Cerebrovascular diseases	97,303
4	Unintentional injuries	31,538	Chronic obstructive pulmonary diseases	55,566
5	Pneumonia and influenza	27,045	Pneumonia and influenza	50,892
6	Diabetes mellitus	20,526	Diabetes mellitus	35,167
7	Atherosclerosis	17,848	Unintentional injuries	34,793
8	Chronic obstructive pulmonary diseases	17,425	Alzheimer's disease	15,671
9	Chronic liver disease and cirrhosis	10,815	Nephritis, nephrotic syndrome, and nephrosis	13,621
10	Certain conditions originating in the perinatal period	9,815	Septicemia	13,506
White				
...	All causes	1,738,607	All causes	2,015,984
1	Diseases of heart	683,347	Diseases of heart	635,549
2	Malignant neoplasms	368,162	Malignant neoplasms	470,139
3	Cerebrovascular diseases	148,734	Cerebrovascular diseases	136,855
4	Unintentional injuries	90,122	Chronic obstructive pulmonary diseases	104,061
5	Chronic obstructive pulmonary diseases	52,375	Unintentional injuries	82,178
6	Pneumonia and influenza	48,369	Pneumonia and influenza	81,659
7	Diabetes mellitus	28,868	Diabetes mellitus	51,706
8	Atherosclerosis	27,069	Suicide	27,648
9	Chronic liver disease and cirrhosis	25,240	Chronic liver disease and cirrhosis	21,771
10	Suicide	24,829	Nephritis, nephrotic syndrome, and nephrosis	21,369
Black				
...	All causes	233,135	All causes	278,440
1	Diseases of heart	72,956	Diseases of heart	78,294
2	Malignant neoplasms	45,037	Malignant neoplasms	61,193
3	Cerebrovascular diseases	20,135	Cerebrovascular diseases	18,237
4	Unintentional injuries	13,480	Unintentional injuries	12,801
5	Homicide and legal intervention	10,283	Diabetes mellitus	11,378
6	Certain conditions originating in the perinatal period	6,961	Homicide and legal intervention	8,420
7	Pneumonia and influenza	5,648	Pneumonia and influenza	8,326
8	Diabetes mellitus	5,544	Chronic obstructive pulmonary diseases	7,205
9	Chronic liver disease and cirrhosis	4,790	Human immunodeficiency virus infection	7,180
10	Nephritis, nephrotic syndrome, and nephrosis	3,416	Certain conditions originating in the perinatal period	4,841

TABLE 1.7

Leading causes of death and numbers of deaths, according to sex, detailed race, and Hispanic origin: 1980 and 1998 [CONTINUED]

Sex, race, Hispanic origin, and rank order	1980		1998	
	Cause of death	Deaths	Cause of death	Deaths
American Indian or Alaska Native				
...	All causes	6,923	All causes	10,845
1	Diseases of heart	1,494	Diseases of heart	2,383
2	Unintentional injuries	1,290	Malignant neoplasms	1,834
3	Malignant neoplasms	770	Unintentional injuries	1,292
4	Chronic liver disease and cirrhosis	410	Diabetes mellitus	645
5	Cerebrovascular diseases	322	Cerebrovascular diseases	497
6	Pneumonia and influenza	257	Chronic liver disease and cirrhosis	467
7	Homicide and legal intervention	219	Pneumonia and influenza	389
8	Diabetes mellitus	210	Chronic obstructive pulmonary diseases	369
9	Certain conditions originating in the perinatal period	199	Suicide	310
10	Suicide	181	Homicide and legal intervention	228
Asian or Pacific Islander				
...	All causes	11,071	All causes	31,987
1	Diseases of heart	3,265	Diseases of heart	8,633
2	Malignant neoplasms	2,522	Malignant neoplasms	8,366
3	Cerebrovascular diseases	1,028	Cerebrovascular diseases	2,859
4	Unintentional injuries	810	Unintentional injuries	1,564
5	Pneumonia and influenza	342	Pneumonia and influenza	1,497
6	Suicide	249	Diabetes mellitus	1,022
7	Certain conditions originating in the perinatal period	246	Chronic obstructive pulmonary diseases	949
8	Diabetes mellitus	227	Suicide	640
9	Homicide and legal intervention	211	Homicide and legal intervention	383
10	Chronic obstructive pulmonary diseases	207	Nephritis, nephrotic syndrome, and nephrosis	335
Hispanic				
...	—	—	All causes	98,406
1	—	—	Diseases of heart	24,596
2	—	—	Malignant neoplasms	19,528
3	—	—	Unintentional injuries	8,248
4	—	—	Cerebrovascular diseases	5,587
5	—	—	Diabetes mellitus	4,741
6	—	—	Pneumonia and influenza	3,277
7	—	—	Homicide and legal intervention	2,978
8	—	—	Chronic liver disease and cirrhosis	2,845
9	—	—	Chronic obstructive pulmonary diseases	2,528
10	—	—	Certain conditions originating in the perinatal period	1,987
White male				
...	All causes	933,878	All causes	990,190
1	Diseases of heart	364,679	Diseases of heart	309,952
2	Malignant neoplasms	198,188	Malignant neoplasms	244,109
3	Unintentional injuries	62,963	Unintentional injuries	52,398
4	Cerebrovascular diseases	60,095	Chronic obstructive pulmonary diseases	52,172
5	Chronic obstructive pulmonary diseases	35,977	Cerebrovascular diseases	51,766
6	Pneumonia and influenza	23,810	Pneumonia and influenza	35,795
7	Suicide	18,901	Diabetes mellitus	24,249
8	Chronic liver disease and cirrhosis	16,407	Suicide	22,174
9	Diabetes mellitus	12,125	Chronic liver disease and cirrhosis	14,096
10	Atherosclerosis	10,543	Nephritis, nephrotic syndrome, and nephrosis	10,406
Black male				
...	All causes	130,138	All causes	143,417
1	Diseases of heart	37,877	Diseases of heart	37,662
2	Malignant neoplasms	25,861	Malignant neoplasms	32,523
3	Unintentional injuries	9,701	Unintentional injuries	8,788
4	Cerebrovascular diseases	9,194	Cerebrovascular diseases	7,765
5	Homicide and legal intervention	8,385	Homicide and legal intervention	6,873
6	Certain conditions originating in the perinatal period	3,869	Human immunodeficiency virus infection	4,994
7	Pneumonia and influenza	3,386	Diabetes mellitus	4,511
8	Chronic liver disease and cirrhosis	3,020	Pneumonia and influenza	4,178
9	Chronic obstructive pulmonary diseases	2,429	Chronic obstructive pulmonary diseases	4,039
10	Diabetes mellitus	2,010	Certain conditions originating in the perinatal period	2,732

TABLE 1.7

Leading causes of death and numbers of deaths, according to sex, detailed race, and Hispanic origin: 1980 and 1998 [CONTINUED]

Sex, race, Hispanic origin, and rank order	1980 Cause of death	Deaths	1998 Cause of death	Deaths
American Indian or Alaska Native male				
...	All causes	4,193	All causes	5,994
1	Unintentional injuries	946	Diseases of heart	1,322
2	Diseases of heart	917	Malignant neoplasms	941
3	Malignant neoplasms	408	Unintentional injuries	867
4	Chronic liver disease and cirrhosis	239	Diabetes mellitus	308
5	Homicide and legal intervention	164	Chronic liver disease and cirrhosis	278
6	Cerebrovascular diseases	163	Suicide	246
7	Pneumonia and influenza	148	Chronic obstructive pulmonary diseases	207
8	Suicide	147	Pneumonia and influenza	197
9	Certain conditions originating in the perinatal period	107	Cerebrovascular diseases	194
10	Diabetes mellitus	86	Homicide and legal intervention	170
Asian or Pacific Islander male				
...	All causes	6,809	All causes	17,659
1	Diseases of heart	2,174	Diseases of heart	4,961
2	Malignant neoplasms	1,485	Malignant neoplasms	4,492
3	Unintentional injuries	556	Cerebrovascular diseases	1,420
4	Cerebrovascular diseases	521	Unintentional injuries	989
5	Pneumonia and influenza	227	Pneumonia and influenza	809
6	Suicide	159	Chronic obstructive pulmonary diseases	600
7	Chronic obstructive pulmonary diseases	158	Diabetes mellitus	516
8	Homicide and legal intervention	151	Suicide	459
9	Certain conditions originating in the perinatal period	128	Homicide and legal intervention	273
10	Diabetes mellitus	103	Certain conditions originating in the perinatal period	172
Hispanic male				
...	—	—	All causes	55,821
1	—	—	Diseases of heart	12,932
2	—	—	Malignant neoplasms	10,465
3	—	—	Unintentional injuries	6,229
4	—	—	Cerebrovascular diseases	2,646
5	—	—	Homicide and legal intervention	2,544
6	—	—	Diabetes mellitus	2,203
7	—	—	Chronic liver disease and cirrhosis	2,096
8	—	—	Pneumonia and influenza	1,657
9	—	—	Suicide	1,429
10	—	—	Chronic obstructive pulmonary diseases	1,422
White female				
...	All causes	804,729	All causes	1,025,794
1	Diseases of heart	318,668	Diseases of heart	325,597
2	Malignant neoplasms	169,974	Malignant neoplasms	226,030
3	Cerebrovascular diseases	88,639	Cerebrovascular diseases	85,089
4	Unintentional injuries	27,159	Chronic obstructive pulmonary diseases	51,889
5	Pneumonia and influenza	24,559	Pneumonia and influenza	45,864
6	Diabetes mellitus	16,743	Unintentional injuries	29,780
7	Atherosclerosis	16,526	Diabetes mellitus	27,457
8	Chronic obstructive pulmonary diseases	16,398	Alzheimer's disease	14,723
9	Chronic liver disease and cirrhosis	8,833	Nephritis, nephrotic syndrome, and nephrosis	10,963
10	Certain conditions originating in the perinatal period	6,512	Septicemia	10,741
Black female				
...	All causes	102,997	All causes	135,023
1	Diseases of heart	35,079	Diseases of heart	40,632
2	Malignant neoplasms	19,176	Malignant neoplasms	28,670
3	Cerebrovascular diseases	10,941	Cerebrovascular diseases	10,472
4	Unintentional injuries	3,779	Diabetes mellitus	6,867
5	Diabetes mellitus	3,534	Pneumonia and influenza	4,148
6	Certain conditions originating in the perinatal period	3,092	Unintentional injuries	4,013
7	Pneumonia and influenza	2,262	Chronic obstructive pulmonary diseases	3,166
8	Homicide and legal intervention	1,898	Septicemia	2,564
9	Chronic liver disease and cirrhosis	1,770	Nephritis, nephrotic syndrome, and nephrosis	2,400
10	Nephritis, nephrotic syndrome, and nephrosis	1,722	Human immunodeficiency virus infection	2,186

TABLE 1.7

Leading causes of death and numbers of deaths, according to sex, detailed race, and Hispanic origin: 1980 and 1998 [CONTINUED]

Sex, race, Hispanic origin, and rank order	1980		1998	
	Cause of death	Deaths	Cause of death	Deaths
American Indian or Alaska Native female				
. . .	All causes	2,730	All causes	4,851
1	Diseases of heart	577	Diseases of heart	1,061
2	Malignant neoplasms	362	Malignant neoplasms	893
3	Unintentional injuries	344	Unintentional injuries	425
4	Chronic liver disease and cirrhosis	171	Diabetes mellitus	337
5	Cerebrovascular diseases	159	Cerebrovascular diseases	303
6	Diabetes mellitus	124	Pneumonia and influenza	192
7	Pneumonia and influenza	109	Chronic liver disease and cirrhosis	189
8	Certain conditions originating in the perinatal period	92	Chronic obstructive pulmonary diseases	162
9	Nephritis, nephrotic syndrome, and nephrosis	56	Nephritis, nephrotic syndrome, and nephrosis	86
10	Homicide and legal intervention	55	Septicemia	68
Asian or Pacific Islander female				
. . .	All causes	4,262	All causes	14,328
1	Diseases of heart	1,091	Malignant neoplasms	3,874
2	Malignant neoplasms	1,037	Diseases of heart	3,672
3	Cerebrovascular diseases	507	Cerebrovascular diseases	1,439
4	Unintentional injuries	254	Pneumonia and influenza	688
5	Diabetes mellitus	124	Unintentional injuries	575
6	Certain conditions originating in the perinatal period	118	Diabetes mellitus	506
7	Pneumonia and influenza	115	Chronic obstructive pulmonary diseases	349
8	Congenital anomalies	104	Suicide	181
9	Suicide	90	Nephritis, nephrotic syndrome, and nephrosis	172
10	Homicide and legal intervention	60	Certain conditions originating in the perinatal period	156
Hispanic female				
. . .	—	—	All causes	42,585
1	—	—	Diseases of heart	11,664
2	—	—	Malignant neoplasms	9,063
3	—	—	Cerebrovascular diseases	2,941
4	—	—	Diabetes mellitus	2,538
5	—	—	Unintentional injuries	2,019
6	—	—	Pneumonia and influenza	1,620
7	—	—	Chronic obstructive pulmonary diseases	1,106
8	—	—	Certain conditions originating in the perinatal period	864
9	—	—	Chronic liver disease and cirrhosis	749
10	—	—	Congenital anomalies	722

. . . Category not applicable.
— Data not available.

SOURCE: *Health, United States, 2000*, National Center for Health Statistics, Hyattsville, MD, 2000

also most likely to die from accidents, cancer was the second-most prevalent cause of death, followed by homicide and legal intervention, congenital anomalies, and suicide.

Unintentional injuries were the leading cause of death for young people ages 15–24. Homicide was the second-leading cause of death, followed by suicide. Cancer was the fourth-leading cause of death among this age group.

Among adults ages 25–44 in 1998, accidents were the most frequent cause of death, and cancer was second. Heart disease and suicide were the third- and fourth-leading causes, respectively, followed by HIV and homicide.

Among adults 45–64 years old, cancer and heart disease were ranked the first- and second-leading causes of deaths, respectively. Among those aged 65 and over, these two categories were reversed.

SELF-ASSESSED HEALTH STATUS

The NCHS asked respondents to household interviews to evaluate their health status by considering several factors. The researchers asked respondents whether or not they thought themselves to be in fair or poor health. Table 1.11 shows that, in 1998, only a small percentage of people considered their health to be fair or poor (9.1 percent). Older persons, those with lower incomes, and black Americans most often rated their health status as fair or poor.

TABLE 1.8

Years of potential life lost before age 75 for selected causes of death, according to sex, detailed race, and Hispanic origin: selected years 1980–98

Sex, race, Hispanic origin, and cause of death	Crude			Age adjusted[1]				
	1980	1990	1998	1980	1990	1996	1997	1998
All persons	Years lost before age 75 per 100,000 population under 75 years of age							
All causes	10,267.6	8,997.0	7,733.3	9,813.5	8,518.3	7,748.0	7,398.4	7,229.4
Diseases of heart	2,065.3	1,517.6	1,343.2	1,877.5	1,363.0	1,222.6	1,190.2	1,155.5
Ischemic heart disease	1,454.3	942.1	757.5	1,307.4	834.8	704.9	670.2	637.4
Cerebrovascular diseases	332.9	246.2	233.0	302.9	221.1	210.2	207.1	201.2
Malignant neoplasms	1,932.4	1,863.4	1,715.9	1,815.2	1,713.9	1,554.2	1,523.5	1,490.0
Trachea, bronchus, and lung	496.8	516.7	457.8	456.9	466.7	406.2	393.6	385.6
Colorectal	175.8	153.4	142.9	158.5	137.3	123.5	123.3	121.8
Prostate[2]	78.8	89.5	67.6	67.2	76.6	64.6	59.7	57.4
Breast[3]	408.5	416.5	357.5	393.0	381.9	324.3	314.3	301.8
Chronic obstructive pulmonary diseases	164.5	182.5	187.5	141.4	156.9	161.1	158.9	158.1
Pneumonia and influenza	156.4	139.9	122.8	149.1	128.5	114.5	112.6	110.8
Chronic liver disease and cirrhosis	254.1	178.4	159.2	259.1	168.8	145.7	141.7	138.1
Diabetes mellitus	124.6	147.0	174.1	115.1	133.0	153.5	149.9	150.3
Human immunodeficiency virus infection	—	391.2	177.2	—	366.2	401.9	208.7	163.6
Unintentional injuries	1,688.7	1,221.2	1,051.6	1,688.3	1,263.0	1,136.5	1,115.2	1,103.4
Motor vehicle-related injuries	1,017.6	752.4	596.4	1,010.8	788.8	680.8	661.1	646.3
Suicide	401.6	404.8	365.4	402.8	405.9	387.8	378.0	371.5
Homicide and legal intervention	459.5	452.3	307.1	460.9	466.4	394.7	368.9	337.2
White male								
All causes	12,454.3	10,629.4	8,972.8	11,877.4	10,064.6	8,980.1	8,533.2	8,352.0
Diseases of heart	2,907.1	2,058.7	1,782.0	2,681.9	1,856.8	1,623.5	1,576.7	1,517.1
Ischemic heart disease	2,241.0	1,416.9	1,121.0	2,060.2	1,269.3	1,044.7	990.1	939.5
Cerebrovascular diseases	309.0	222.9	216.5	280.2	198.6	194.4	189.8	185.9
Malignant neoplasms	2,087.1	1,970.9	1,803.9	1,939.8	1,793.9	1,620.7	1,576.4	1,553.6
Trachea, bronchus, and lung	709.2	669.7	560.3	647.9	600.0	501.0	479.8	467.9
Colorectal	194.2	174.7	160.9	176.2	155.7	138.8	137.5	135.9
Prostate	72.6	85.0	61.9	59.1	68.3	56.3	51.5	49.4
Chronic obstructive pulmonary diseases	219.3	208.9	199.9	187.1	177.2	167.5	169.3	166.0
Pneumonia and influenza	156.0	143.3	124.4	147.4	130.5	115.1	116.1	110.3
Chronic liver disease and cirrhosis	306.4	233.5	229.7	307.9	219.1	205.1	200.8	196.9
Diabetes mellitus	114.7	141.0	173.9	107.4	127.5	153.0	143.4	148.6
Human immunodeficiency virus infection	—	589.3	164.8	—	544.3	448.0	200.7	149.1
Unintentional injuries	2,553.8	1,766.9	1,484.5	2,523.6	1,821.5	1,591.5	1,561.2	1,560.2
Motor vehicle-related injuries	1,579.9	1,085.4	816.9	1,549.8	1,134.9	933.1	897.1	889.3
Suicide	663.0	694.0	630.3	656.4	692.2	665.7	644.7	638.9
Homicide and legal intervention	455.2	384.7	264.4	452.6	391.6	327.7	314.5	287.7
Black male								
All causes	21,081.4	20,744.8	15,998.7	22,338.5	21,250.2	18,994.6	17,373.4	16,626.0
Diseases of heart	3,383.9	2,769.2	2,564.4	4,179.5	3,338.2	2,969.9	2,918.1	2,856.2
Ischemic heart disease	1,805.9	1,249.8	1,088.3	2,283.2	1,561.4	1,326.2	1,308.8	1,241.0
Cerebrovascular diseases	714.1	546.4	495.1	870.2	655.6	583.0	578.8	547.2
Malignant neoplasms	2,495.1	2,444.5	2,137.0	3,070.6	3,021.7	2,576.8	2,517.0	2,438.9
Trachea, bronchus, and lung	853.7	842.5	660.9	1,087.0	1,077.4	849.2	800.4	775.3
Colorectal	176.1	188.6	193.7	215.9	234.0	225.6	229.1	221.1
Prostate	136.9	143.7	124.0	159.1	177.6	160.2	154.6	149.2
Chronic obstructive pulmonary diseases	223.3	241.4	237.5	258.7	278.7	266.7	250.8	260.4
Pneumonia and influenza	467.1	399.2	273.4	492.6	416.8	328.4	291.7	285.6
Chronic liver disease and cirrhosis	610.1	390.5	234.9	791.8	461.4	293.5	265.3	254.3
Diabetes mellitus	199.8	263.0	330.0	245.5	317.8	357.4	380.2	369.3
Human immunodeficiency virus infection	—	1,622.4	1,027.0	—	1,625.8	2,270.3	1,288.0	1,017.0
Unintentional injuries	2,934.4	2,308.7	1,935.4	2,931.3	2,265.6	1,983.7	1,925.4	1,930.9
Motor vehicle-related injuries.	1,289.2	1,163.1	980.2	1,281.2	1,143.1	997.1	987.6	984.1
Suicide	415.7	482.3	406.4	428.1	478.0	465.6	443.1	414.8
Homicide and legal intervention	2,872.4	3,197.7	1,969.7	2,939.9	3,096.6	2,448.4	2,251.2	2,000.0

TABLE 1.8

Years of potential life lost before age 75 for selected causes of death, according to sex, detailed race, and Hispanic origin: selected years 1980–98 [CONTINUED]

Sex, race, Hispanic origin, and cause of death	Crude			Age adjusted[1]				
	1980	1990	1998	1980	1990	1996	1997	1998
White female								
All causes	6,655.6	5,740.0	5,320.2	6,185.7	5,225.3	4,899.9	4,821.5	4,750.6
Diseases of heart	1,142.1	864.1	769.5	915.3	689.3	637.1	626.2	610.0
Ischemic heart disease	758.1	521.1	420.3	584.8	399.6	352.2	332.0	318.5
Cerebrovascular diseases	275.0	200.1	185.6	231.4	165.4	157.3	153.2	149.0
Malignant neoplasms	1,774.6	1,760.8	1,634.2	1,595.5	1,528.7	1,403.1	1,379.3	1,336.8
Trachea, bronchus, and lung.	295.3	382.7	380.3	258.1	319.2	304.6	298.7	295.4
Colorectal	165.1	133.2	120.9	137.5	109.5	96.8	97.6	95.6
Breast	418.8	420.7	349.3	390.0	373.0	308.5	298.9	285.5
Chronic obstructive pulmonary diseases	117.4	164.6	182.6	94.8	128.9	142.0	140.1	138.8
Pneumonia and influenza	103.6	92.3	92.8	97.0	81.8	79.8	79.0	80.1
Chronic liver disease and cirrhosis	145.2	95.5	90.9	138.7	84.6	77.1	76.3	74.8
Diabetes mellitus	108.0	121.8	134.7	91.4	101.0	110.9	111.1	108.4
Human immunodeficiency virus infection	—	43.4	30.6	—	41.8	73.2	38.5	29.0
Unintentional injuries	793.0	610.1	576.7	816.8	654.1	634.9	627.6	621.0
Motor vehicle-related injuries	525.0	426.7	368.4	539.1	464.8	434.7	428.0	411.4
Suicide	193.0	166.1	154.4	196.1	165.3	153.6	155.3	152.7
Homicide and legal intervention	132.0	117.2	93.5	136.1	123.5	111.1	101.2	101.6
Black female								
All causes	11,795.1	10,966.0	9,429.8	11,863.1	10,662.7	10,012.6	9,475.2	9,282.7
Diseases of heart	2,020.0	1,665.2	1,563.4	2,189.5	1,756.0	1,636.2	1,534.8	1,541.3
Ischemic heart disease	987.7	711.9	618.9	1,078.5	762.1	682.3	636.6	611.6
Cerebrovascular diseases	600.9	458.3	421.4	656.7	481.2	422.9	419.4	411.2
Malignant neoplasms	1,855.8	1,893.9	1,844.9	2,085.5	2,041.9	1,845.0	1,837.9	1,818.3
Trachea, bronchus, and lung	260.3	328.7	331.8	300.2	364.3	323.1	331.8	330.7
Colorectal	162.6	164.4	160.7	179.2	178.3	160.8	153.2	159.1
Breast	382.8	465.4	468.8	448.6	505.6	484.0	472.7	455.0
Chronic obstructive pulmonary diseases	109.0	149.0	184.6	116.3	157.4	187.4	172.2	182.8
Pneumonia and influenza	252.3	214.2	178.4	245.2	206.1	177.2	177.9	175.2
Chronic liver disease and cirrhosis	323.8	193.2	102.8	378.0	203.4	119.8	113.2	98.8
Diabetes mellitus	248.3	279.1	315.3	271.6	299.0	329.5	318.3	314.3
Human immunodeficiency virus infection	—	427.1	454.5	—	402.5	757.5	492.1	432.1
Unintentional injuries	898.9	767.7	694.3	876.0	748.3	751.9	734.6	690.0
Motor vehicle-related injuries	362.9	381.2	364.4	354.7	376.7	396.9	400.4	368.5
Suicide	88.3	90.0	69.1	91.2	89.0	74.7	74.5	70.0
Homicide and legal intervention	605.3	619.7	395.2	593.1	596.5	470.5	422.2	400.8

— Data not available.
[1] Rates are age adjusted to the 1940 U.S. standard million population.
[2] Male only.
[3] Female only.

SOURCE: *Health, United States, 2000,* National Center for Health Statistics, Hyattsville, MD, 2000

TABLE 1.9

Deaths and death rates, by age, sex, and race and Hispanic origin and age-adjusted death rates, by sex, and race and Hispanic origin: final 1997 and preliminary 1998

[Data are based on a continuous file of records received from the States. Age-specific rates per 100,000 population in specified group; age-adjusted rates per 100,000 U.S. standard population. The number of deaths and death rates for Hispanic origin and specified races other than white and black should be interpreted with caution because of inconsistencies between reporting Hispanic origin and race on death certificates and censuses and surveys. Figures for 1998 are based on weighted data rounded to the nearest individual, so categories may not add to totals]

Age, race, and sex	1998		1997	
	Number	Rate	Number	Rate
All races, both sexes				
All ages	2,338,070	865.0	2,314,245	864.7
Under 1 year [1]	28,486	754.3	28,045	738.7
1-4 years	5,224	34.4	5,501	35.8
5-14 years	7,750	19.8	8,061	20.8
15-24 years	30,286	81.4	31,544	86.2
25-34 years	42,031	108.4	45,538	115.0
35-44 years	87,833	197.3	89,408	203.2
45-54 years	145,354	420.3	144,882	430.8
55-64 years	233,116	1,028.0	231,993	1,063.6
65-74 years	458,763	2,493.9	464,274	2,509.8
75-84 years	683,553	5,719.1	670,530	5,728.2
85 years and over	615,223	15,177.0	594,068	15,345.2
Not stated	453	. . .	401	. . .
Age-adjusted rate	. . .	470.8	. . .	479.1
All races, male				
All ages	1,156,040	875.5	1,154,039	880.8
Under 1 year [1]	15,851	821.6	15,788	812.8
1-4 years	2,909	37.5	3,121	39.7
5-14 years	4,617	23.0	4,763	24.0
15-24 years	22,451	117.9	23,312	124.0
25-34 years	28,835	149.8	31,707	160.1
35-44 years	56,477	255.5	58,141	265.7
45-54 years	91,014	538.5	90,587	550.5
55-64 years	139,754	1,293.3	138,876	1,336.6
65-74 years	258,879	3,138.1	263,875	3,191.2
75-84 years	335,103	7,037.9	329,391	7,116.1
85 years and over	199,808	16,826.5	194,161	17,461.9
Not stated	342	. . .	317	. . .
Age-adjusted rate	. . .	587.9	. . .	602.8
All races, female				
All ages	1,182,031	855.0	1,160,206	849.2
Under 1 year [1]	12,634	684.0	12,257	661.1
1-4 years	2,316	31.2	2,380	31.8
5-14 years	3,133	16.4	3,298	17.4
15-24 years	7,835	43.1	8,232	46.3
25-34 years	13,196	67.6	13,831	69.9
35-44 years	31,357	139.9	31,267	141.4
45-54 years	54,340	307.3	54,295	316.1
55-64 years	93,361	786.5	93,117	815.2
65-74 years	199,883	1,970.1	200,399	1,959.0
75-84 years	348,450	4,845.8	341,139	4,820.5
85 years and over	415,414	14,493.6	399,907	14,492.3
Not stated	111	. . .	84	. . .
Age-adjusted rate	. . .	372.3	. . .	375.7

. . . Category not applicable.

[1] Death rates are based on population estimates; they differ from infant mortality rates, which are based on live births and are shown separately for "Under 1 year."

Note: Data are subject to sampling and/or random variation.

SOURCE: Joyce A. Martin et al., "Births and Deaths: Preliminary Data for 1998," *National Vital Statistics Report*, vol. 47, no. 25, October 5, 1999

TABLE 1.10

Deaths and death rates for the 10 leading causes of death in specified age groups: preliminary 1998

[Data are based on a continuous file of records received from the States. Rates per 100,000 population in specified group. Figures are based on weighted data rounded to the nearest individual, so categories may not add to totals]

Rank [1]	Cause of death and age (Based on Ninth Revision, International Classification of Diseases, 1975)	Number	Rate
All ages [2]			
...	All causes	2,338,075	865.0
1	Diseases of heart	724,269	268.0
2	Malignant neoplasms, including neoplasms of lymphatic and hematopoietic tissues	538,947	199.4
3	Cerebrovascular diseases	158,060	58.5
4	Chronic obstructive pulmonary diseases and allied conditions	114,381	42.3
5	Pneumonia and influenza	94,828	35.1
6	Accidents and adverse effects	93,207	34.5
...	Motor vehicle accidents	41,826	15.5
...	All other accidents and adverse effects	51,382	19.0
7	Diabetes mellitus	64,574	23.9
8	Suicide	29,264	10.8
9	Nephritis, nephrotic syndrome, and nephrosis	26,295	9.7
10	Chronic liver disease and cirrhosis	24,936	9.2
...	All other causes	469,314	173.6
1-4 years			
...	All causes	5,195	34.2
1	Accidents and adverse effects	1,881	12.4
...	Motor vehicle accidents	750	4.9
...	All other accidents and adverse effects	1,131	7.4
2	Congenital anomalies	531	3.5
3	Homicide and legal intervention	368	2.4
4	Malignant neoplasms, including neoplasms of lymphatic and hematopoietic tissues	355	2.3
5	Diseases of heart	198	1.3
6	Pneumonia and influenza	133	0.9
7	Septicemia	81	0.5
8	Certain conditions originating in the perinatal period	75	0.5
9	Cerebrovascular diseases	54	0.4
10	Benign neoplasms, carcinoma in situ, and neoplasms of uncertain behavior and of unspecified nature	50	0.3
...	All other causes	1,469	9.7
5-14 years			
...	All causes	7,700	19.7
1	Accidents and adverse effects	3,115	8.0
...	Motor vehicle accidents	1,773	4.5
...	All other accidents and adverse effects	1,342	3.4
2	Malignant neoplasms, including neoplasms of lymphatic and hematopoietic tissues	1,025	2.6
3	Homicide and legal intervention	423	1.1
4	Congenital anomalies	355	0.9
5	Suicide	318	0.8
6	Diseases of heart	304	0.8
7	Chronic obstructive pulmonary diseases and allied conditions	145	0.4
8	Pneumonia and influenza	125	0.3
9	Benign neoplasms, carcinoma in situ, and neoplasms of uncertain behavior and of unspecified nature	80	0.2
10	Cerebrovascular diseases	76	0.2
...	All other causes	1,734	4.4
15-24 years			
...	All causes	30,211	81.2
1	Accidents and adverse effects	12,752	34.3
...	Motor vehicle accidents	9,635	25.9
...	All other accidents and adverse effects	3,117	8.4
2	Homicide and legal intervention	5,233	14.1
3	Suicide	4,003	10.8
4	Malignant neoplasms, including neoplasms of lymphatic and hematopoietic tissues	1,670	4.5
5	Diseases of heart	961	2.6
6	Congenital anomalies	429	1.2
7	Chronic obstructive pulmonary diseases and allied conditions	224	0.6
8	Pneumonia and influenza	211	0.6
9	Human immunodeficiency virus infection	208	0.6
10	Cerebrovascular diseases	182	0.5
...	All other causes	4,338	11.7

TABLE 1.10

Deaths and death rates for the 10 leading causes of death in specified age groups: preliminary 1998 [CONTINUED]

[Data are based on a continuous file of records received from the States. Rates per 100,000 population in specified group. Figures are based on weighted data rounded to the nearest individual, so categories may not add to totals]

Rank [1]	Cause of death and age (Based on Ninth Revision, International Classification of Diseases, 1975)	Number	Rate
25-44 years			
...	All causes	129,309	155.2
1	Accidents and adverse effects	25,153	30.2
...	Motor vehicle accidents	13,585	16.3
...	All other accidents and adverse effects	11,568	13.9
2	Malignant neoplasms, including neoplasms of lymphatic and hematopoietic tissues	21,130	25.4
3	Diseases of heart	16,022	19.2
4	Suicide	11,602	13.9
5	Human immunodeficiency virus infection	8,529	10.2
6	Homicide and legal intervention	7,743	9.3
7	Chronic liver disease and cirrhosis	3,785	4.5
8	Cerebrovascular diseases	3,219	3.9
9	Diabetes mellitus	2,432	2.9
10	Pneumonia and influenza	1,913	2.3
...	All other causes	27,781	33.4
45-64 years			
...	All causes	378,197	660.5
1	Malignant neoplasms, including neoplasms of lymphatic and hematopoietic tissues	132,197	230.9
2	Diseases of heart	98,700	172.4
3	Accidents and adverse effects	17,141	29.9
...	Motor vehicle accidents	8,112	14.2
...	All other accidents and adverse effects	9,029	15.8
4	Cerebrovascular diseases	15,319	26.8
5	Chronic obstructive pulmonary diseases and allied conditions	13,102	22.9
6	Diabetes mellitus	13,062	22.8
7	Chronic liver disease and cirrhosis	10,829	18.9
8	Pneumonia and influenza	6,130	10.7
10	Human immunodeficiency virus infection	3,994	7.0
...	All other causes	60,005	104.8
65 years and over			
...	All causes	1,758,530	5,111.8
1	Diseases of heart	607,422	1,765.7
2	Malignant neoplasms, including neoplasms of lymphatic and hematopoietic tissues	382,468	1,111.8
3	Cerebrovascular diseases	138,891	403.7
4	Chronic obstructive pulmonary diseases and allied conditions	99,697	289.8
5	Pneumonia and influenza	85,909	249.7
6	Diabetes mellitus	48,917	142.2
7	Accidents and adverse effects	32,343	94.0
...	Motor vehicle accidents	7,788	22.6
...	All other accidents and adverse effects	24,555	71.4
8	Nephritis, nephrotic syndrome, and nephrosis	22,749	66.1
9	Alzheimer's disease	22,510	65.4
10	Septicemia	19,024	55.3
...	All other causes	298,600	868.0

... Category not applicable.
[1] Rank based on number of deaths.
[2] Includes deaths under 1 year of age.
Note: Data are subject to sampling and/or random variation.

SOURCE: Joyce A. Martin et al., "Births and Deaths: Preliminary Data for 1998," *National Vital Statistics Report,* vol. 47, no. 25, October 5, 1999

TABLE 1.11

Respondent-assessed health status according to selected characteristics, 1991, 1995, 1997, 1998

Characteristic	Percent with fair or poor health[1]			
	1991	1995	1997[2]	1998[2]
Total[3,4]	10.4	10.6	9.2	9.1
Age				
Under 18 years	2.6	2.6	2.1	1.8
Under 6 years	2.7	2.7	1.9	1.5
6–17 years	2.6	2.5	2.1	1.9
18–44 years	6.1	6.6	5.3	5.3
18–24 years	4.8	4.5	3.4	3.2
25–44 years	6.4	7.2	5.9	5.9
45–54 years	13.4	13.4	11.7	11.6
55–64 years	20.7	21.4	18.2	18.0
65 years and over	29.0	28.3	26.7	26.7
65–74 years	26.0	25.6	23.1	23.9
75 years and over	33.6	32.2	31.5	30.4
Sex[3]				
Male	10.0	10.1	8.8	8.8
Female	10.8	11.1	9.7	9.4
Race[3,5]				
White	9.6	9.7	8.3	8.2
Black	16.8	17.2	15.8	15.7
American Indian or Alaska Native	18.3	18.7	17.3	17.6
Asian or Pacific Islander.	7.8	9.3	7.8	7.1
Race and Hispanic origin[3]				
White, non-Hispanic	9.1	9.1	8.0	7.8
Black, non-Hispanic	16.8	17.3	15.8	15.8
Hispanic[5]	15.6	15.1	13.0	13.1
Mexican[5]	17.0	16.7	13.1	13.5
Poverty status[3,6]				
Poor	22.8	23.7	21.4	22.2
Near poor	14.7	15.5	14.6	15.6
Nonpoor	6.8	6.7	6.1	5.7
Race and Hispanic origin and poverty status[3,6]				
White, non-Hispanic:				
Poor	21.9	22.8	20.6	21.3
Near poor	14.0	14.8	14.1	15.3
Nonpoor	6.4	6.2	5.7	5.3
Black, non-Hispanic:				
Poor	25.8	27.7	25.6	26.3
Near poor	17.0	19.3	19.5	19.3
Nonpoor	10.9	9.9	9.6	9.0
Hispanic:[5]				
Poor	23.6	22.7	19.8	21.7
Near poor	18.0	16.9	14.0	15.3
Nonpoor	9.3	8.7	8.8	7.9

TABLE 1.11

Respondent-assessed health status according to selected characteristics, 1991, 1995, 1997, 1998 [CONTINUED]

Characteristic	Percent with fair or poor health[1]			
	1991	1995	1997[2]	1998[2]
Geographic region[3]				
Northeast	8.3	9.1	8.0	7.9
Midwest	9.1	9.7	8.1	8.0
South	13.1	12.3	10.8	10.9
West	9.7	10.1	8.8	8.4
Location of residence[3]				
Within MSA[7]	9.9	10.1	8.7	8.5
Outside MSA[7]	11.9	12.6	11.1	11.4

[1] As assessed by respondent.
[2] Data starting in 1997 are not strictly comparable with data for earlier years due to the 1997 questionnaire redesign.
[3] Estimates are age adjusted to the year 2000 standard using six age groups: Under 18 years, 18–44 years, 45–54 years, 55–64 years, 65–74 years, and 75 years and over.
[4] Includes all other races not shown separately and unknown poverty status.
[5] The race groups white, black, American Indian or Alaska Native, and Asian or Pacific Islander include persons of Hispanic and non-Hispanic origin; persons of Hispanic origin may be of any race.
[6] Prior to 1997 poverty status is based on family income and family size using Bureau of the Census poverty thresholds. Beginning in 1997 poverty status is based on family income, family size, number of children in the family, and for families with two or fewer adults the age of the adults in the family. Poor persons are defined as below the poverty threshold. Near poor persons have incomes of 100 percent to less than 200 percent of poverty threshold. Nonpoor persons have incomes of 200 percent or greater than the poverty threshold. Missing family income data were imputed for 16–18 percent of persons in 1991 and 1995. Poverty status was unknown for 20 percent of persons in the sample in 1997 and 25 percent in 1998.
[7] MSA is metropolitan statistical area.

SOURCE: *Health, United States, 2000,* National Center for Health Statistics, Hyattsville, MD, 2000

CHAPTER 2

THE INCREASING COST OF HEALTH CARE

HOW MUCH DOES HEALTH CARE COST?

American society places a high value on human life, and generally wants—and expects—high-quality medical care. But quality care has an increasingly high cost. In 1970 the United States spent a little more than 7 percent of its gross domestic product (GDP; the value of all the goods and services produced by the nation) on health care. By 1998 health care had risen to 13.5 percent ($1,149 trillion) of the GDP. (See Table 2.1.) Figure 2.1 compares the growth in health care expenditures with the growth in the GDP.

For many years, the consumer price index (CPI; a measure of the average change in prices paid by consumers) increased at a greater rate for medical care than for any other commodity. From 1980 to 1990, the average annual increase in the overall CPI was 4.7 percent, while the average annual increase in the medical care index stood at 8.1 percent. By 1998–99, the average annual growth in the medical care index had fallen to 3.5 percent. This figure still outpaced the overall CPI (2.2 percent), but the discrepancy was far less remarkable than it had been a decade before. (See Table 2.2.)

In 1994 the Health Care Financing Administration (HCFA), an agency of the U.S. Department of Health and Human Services (HHS), projected that the national health expenditure would grow to $2.17 trillion by 2005, an 88.9 percent increase over 1998. (See Table 2.3. Note that the numbers in Table 2.3 are projections, and therefore differ from the actual numbers presented in some other tables and figures in this chapter.) Medicare was projected to reach $450.9 billion by 2005, making up 20.7 percent of all health care expenditures. By 2005 health expenditures were projected to account for 17.9 percent of the U.S. GDP.

Generally, projections are most accurate for the near future and least accurate for the distant future. For example, predictions for 2030 should be viewed more cautious-

ly than predictions for 2005. Because it is very unlikely that the conditions on which the projections were based will remain the same, the HCFA warned that those projections should not be seen as predictions for the future. Rather, they should provide a basis for policymakers to

FIGURE 2.1

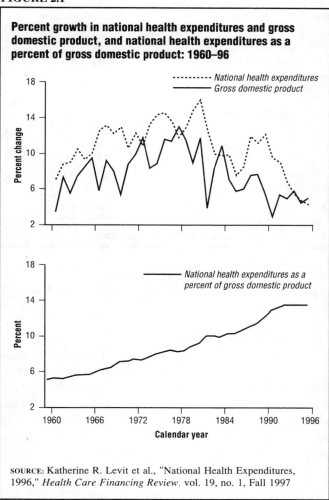

Percent growth in national health expenditures and gross domestic product, and national health expenditures as a percent of gross domestic product: 1960–96

SOURCE: Katherine R. Levit et al., "National Health Expenditures, 1996," *Health Care Financing Review*, vol. 19, no. 1, Fall 1997

TABLE 2.1

National health expenditures, aggregate and per capita amounts, percent distribution, and average annual percent growth by source of funds: selected calendar years 1960–98

Item	1960	1970	1980	1985	1990	1991	1992	1993	1994	1995	1996	1997	1998
							Amount in Billions						
National Health Expenditures	$26.9	$73.2	$247.3	$428.7	$699.4	$766.8	$836.5	$898.5	$947.7	$993.3	$1,039.4	$1,088.2	$1,149.1
Private	20.2	45.5	142.5	254.5	416.2	448.9	483.6	513.2	524.7	537.3	559.0	586.0	626.4
Public	6.6	27.7	104.8	174.2	283.2	317.9	353.0	385.3	423.0	456.0	480.4	502.2	522.7
Federal	2.9	17.8	72.0	123.2	195.2	222.5	251.8	275.4	301.2	326.1	347.3	363.0	376.9
State and Local	3.7	9.9	32.8	51.0	88.0	95.4	101.2	110.0	121.8	129.8	133.1	139.2	145.8
							Number in Millions						
U.S. Population [1]	190	215	235	247	260	263	266	268	271	273	276	278	281
							Amount in Billions						
Gross Domestic Product	$527	$1,036	$2,784	$4,181	$5,744	$5,917	$6,244	$6,558	$6,947	$7,270	$7,662	$8,111	$8,511
							Per Capita Amount						
National Health Expenditures	$141	$341	$1,052	$1,734	$2,689	$2,918	$3,151	$3,351	$3,501	$3,637	$3,772	$3,912	$4,094
Private	106	212	606	1,030	1,600	1,708	1,821	1,914	1,938	1,967	2,028	2,107	2,232
Public	35	129	446	705	1,089	1,210	1,329	1,437	1,563	1,669	1,743	1,806	1,862
Federal	15	83	306	498	750	847	948	1,027	1,113	1,194	1,260	1,305	1,343
State and Local	20	46	140	206	338	363	381	410	450	475	483	500	520
							Percent Distribution						
National Health Expenditures	100.0	100.0	100.0	100.0	100.0	100.0	100.0	100.0	100.0	100.0	100.0	100.0	100.0
Private	75.2	62.2	58	59.4	59.5	58.5	57.8	57.1	55.4	54.1	53.8	53.8	54.5
Public	25	38	42	40.6	40.5	41.5	42.2	42.9	44.6	45.9	46.2	46.2	45.5
Federal	11	24	29	28.7	27.9	29.0	30.1	30.6	31.8	32.8	33.4	33.4	32.8
State and Local	14	14	13	11.9	12.6	12.4	12.1	12.2	12.9	13.1	12.8	12.8	12.7
							Percent of Gross Domestic Product						
National Health Expenditures	5.1	7.1	8.9	10.3	12.2	13.0	13.4	13.7	13.6	13.7	13.6	13.4	13.5
							Average Annual Percent Growth from Previous Year Shown						
National Health Expenditures	—	10.6	12.9	11.6	11.0	9.6	9.1	7.4	5.5	4.8	4.6	4.7	5.6
Private	—	8.5	12.1	12.3	11.3	7.9	7.7	6.1	2.3	2.4	4.0	4.8	6.9
Public	—	15.3	14.2	10.7	10.5	12.3	11.0	9.2	9.8	7.8	5.4	4.5	4.1
Federal	—	19.8	15.0	11.3	10.5	14.0	13.1	9.4	9.4	8.3	6.5	4.5	3.8
State and Local	—	10.2	12.7	9.2	10.4	8.4	6.1	8.6	10.8	6.6	2.5	4.6	4.7
U.S. Population	—	1.2	0.9	0.5	1.0	1.0	1.0	1.0	0.9	0.9	0.9	0.9	0.9
Gross Domestic Product	—	7.0	10.4	4.1	7.5	3.0	5.5	5.0	5.9	4.6	5.4	5.9	4.9

[1] July 1 Social Security area population estimates for each year, 1960–98
Note: Numbers and percents may not add to totals because of rounding.

SOURCE: Office of the Actuary, National Health Statistics Group, Health Care Financing Administration, 2000

evaluate the costs or savings of proposed legislative or regulatory changes.

Total Health Care Spending

The HCFA maintains most of the nation's statistics on health care costs. The HCFA reported that the United States spent $1.149 trillion for health care in 1998, up 5.6 percent from the previous year. This rate hovered near the lowest rate of increase since the late 1960s. As a proportion of GDP, health care spending showed little change from 1992 to 1998, averaging around 13.6 percent. (See Table 2.1.)

About 54.5 percent of 1998 health care expenditures, or $626.4 billion, came from private funds, while the remaining 45.5 percent ($522.7 billion) was paid with public money. (See Table 2.4.) This means that 54.5 cents of every dollar spent on health care came from private funds, including out-of-pocket expenses (17.4 cents), private health insurance (32.6 cents), and other private sources (4.5 cents). The remainder (45.5 cents) came from federal (32.8 cents) or state and local governments (12.7 cents). (See Figure 2.2.) The 1998 per capita cost for health care (the average per individual if spending were divided equally among all persons in the country) was $4,094. (See Table 2.1.)

Of the $1.149 trillion spent on health care in 1998, $1.019 trillion (88.7 percent) was spent on personal health services. The remainder went for program administration, government public health programs, research, and construction. (See Tables 2.4 and 2.5.)

In 1998 the nation spent $382.8 billion (33.3 percent of all health expenditures) on hospital costs, by far the largest chunk of health care spending. This expense was followed by $229.5 billion (20 percent) for physicians' services, $121.9 billion (10.6 percent) for drugs and other medical needs, and $87.8 billion (7.6 percent) for nursing home care. (See Table 2.4.) Table 2.5 shows the trends and annual percent changes in personal health care expenditures by category.

TABLE 2.2

Consumer price index and average annual percent change for all items, selected items, and medical care components: selected years 1960–99

Items and medical care components	1960	1970	1980	1990	1995	1996	1997	1998	1999
	Consumer Price Index (CPI)								
All items	29.6	38.8	82.4	130.7	152.4	156.9	160.5	163.0	166.6
All items excluding medical care	30.2	39.2	82.8	128.8	148.6	152.8	156.3	158.6	162.0
All services	24.1	35.0	77.9	139.2	168.7	174.1	179.4	184.2	188.8
Food	30.0	39.2	86.8	132.4	148.4	153.3	157.3	160.7	164.1
Apparel	45.7	59.2	90.9	124.1	132.0	131.7	132.9	133.0	131.3
Housing	—	36.4	81.1	128.5	148.5	152.8	156.8	160.4	163.9
Energy	22.4	25.5	86.0	102.1	105.2	110.1	111.5	102.9	106.6
Medical care	22.3	34.0	74.9	162.8	220.5	228.2	234.6	242.1	250.6
Components of medical care									
Medical care services	19.5	32.3	74.8	162.7	224.2	232.4	239.1	246.8	255.1
Professional services	—	37.0	77.9	156.1	201.0	208.3	215.4	222.2	229.2
Physicians' services	21.9	34.5	76.5	160.8	208.8	216.4	222.9	229.5	236.0
Dental services	27.0	39.2	78.9	155.8	206.8	216.5	226.6	236.2	247.2
Eye glasses and eye care[1]	—	—	—	117.3	137.0	139.3	141.5	144.1	145.5
Services by other medical professionals[1]	—	—	—	120.2	143.9	146.6	151.8	155.4	158.7
Hospital and related services	—	—	69.2	178.0	257.8	269.5	278.4	287.5	299.5
Hospital services[2]	—	—	—	—	—	—	101.7	105.0	109.3
Inpatient hospital services[2]	—	—	—	—	—	—	101.3	104.0	107.9
Outpatient hospital services[1]	—	—	—	138.7	204.6	215.1	224.9	233.2	246.0
Hospital rooms	9.3	23.6	68.0	175.4	251.2	261.0	—	—	—
Other inpatient services[1]	—	—	—	142.7	206.8	216.9	—	—	—
Nursing homes and adult day care	—	—	—	—	—	—	102.3	107.1	111.6
Medical care commodities	46.9	46.5	75.4	163.4	204.5	210.4	215.3	221.8	230.7
Prescription drugs and medical supplies	54.0	47.4	72.5	181.7	235.0	242.9	249.3	258.6	273.4
Nonprescription drugs and medical supplies[1]	—	—	—	120.6	140.5	143.1	145.4	147.7	148.5
Internal and respiratory over-the-counter drugs	—	42.3	74.9	145.9	167.0	170.2	173.1	175.4	175.9
Nonprescription medical equipment and supplies	—	—	79.2	138.0	166.3	169.1	171.5	174.9	176.7
	Average annual percent change from previous year shown								
All items	...	4.3	8.9	4.7	3.1	3.0	2.3	1.6	2.2
All items excluding medical care	...	4.1	8.8	4.5	2.9	2.8	2.3	1.5	2.1
All services	...	5.6	10.2	6.0	3.9	3.2	3.0	2.7	2.5
Food	...	4.0	7.7	4.3	2.3	3.3	2.6	2.2	2.1
Apparel	...	4.4	4.6	3.2	1.2	−0.2	0.9	0.1	−1.3
Housing	...	—	9.9	4.7	2.9	2.9	2.6	2.3	2.2
Energy	...	2.2	15.4	1.7	0.6	4.7	1.3	−7.7	3.6
Medical care	...	6.2	9.5	8.1	6.3	3.5	2.8	3.2	3.5
Components of medical care									
Medical care services	...	7.3	9.9	8.1	6.6	3.7	2.9	3.2	3.4
Professional services	...	—	8.9	7.2	5.2	3.6	3.4	3.2	3.2
Physicians' services	...	6.6	9.7	7.7	5.4	3.6	3.0	3.0	2.8
Dental services	...	5.3	8.2	7.0	5.8	4.7	4.7	4.2	4.7
Eye glasses and eye care[1]	...	—	—	—	3.2	1.7	1.6	1.8	1.0
Services by other medical professionals[1]	...	—	—	—	3.7	1.9	3.5	2.4	2.1
Hospital and related services	...	—	—	9.9	7.7	4.5	3.3	3.3	4.2
Hospital services[2]	...	—	—	—	—	—	—	3.2	4.1
Inpatient hospital services[2]	...	—	—	—	—	—	—	2.7	3.8
Outpatient hospital services[1]	...	—	—	—	8.1	5.1	4.6	3.7	5.5
Hospital rooms	...	13.9	12.2	9.9	7.4	3.9	—	—	—
Other inpatient services[1]	...	—	—	—	7.7	4.9	—	—	—
Nursing homes and adult day care	...	—	—	—	—	—	—	4.7	4.2
Medical care commodities	...	0.7	7.2	8.0	4.6	2.9	2.3	3.0	4.0
Prescription drugs and medical supplies	...	−0.2	7.2	9.6	5.3	3.4	2.6	3.7	5.7
Nonprescription drugs and medical supplies[1]	...	—	—	—	3.1	1.9	1.6	1.6	0.5
Internal and respiratory over-the-counter drugs	...	1.6	7.7	6.9	2.7	1.9	1.7	1.3	0.3
Nonprescription medical equipment and supplies	...	—	—	5.7	3.8	1.7	1.4	2.0	1.0

— Data not available.
... Category not applicable.
[1]Dec. 1986 = 100
[2]Dec. 1996 = 100.
Notes: 1982–84 = 100, except where noted.

SOURCE: *Health, United States, 2000*, National Center for Health Statistics, Hyattsville, MD, 2000

TABLE 2.3

National health expenditure amounts, percent distribution, and average annual percent growth, by source of funds: selected years 1980–2005

Source of funds	Historical							Projected	
	1980	1990	1991	1992	1993	1994	1995	2000	2005
Aggregate amount in billions									
All sources	$251.1	$696.6	$755.6	$820.3	$884.2	$938.3	$1,007.6	$1,481.7	$2,173.7
Private	145.8	410.0	432.9	462.9	496.4	518.1	552.7	807.9	1,171.3
Public	105.3	286.5	322.6	357.5	387.8	420.2	454.9	673.7	1,002.4
By program									
Medicare	37.5	112.1	123.3	136.3	154.2	171.4	190.0	293.5	450.9
Medicaid	26.1	75.4	93.9	108.0	117.9	128.5	138.4	214.5	333.4
Other	41.6	99.0	105.5	111.2	115.7	120.3	126.5	165.7	218.1
By government level									
Federal	72.0	195.8	224.7	254.3	260.6	306.7	334.1	502.5	756.7
State and local	33.3	90.7	98.0	103.2	107.3	113.5	120.8	171.2	245.7
Percent Distribution									
All sources	100.0	100.0	100.0	100.0	100.0	100.0	100.0	100.0	100.0
Private	58.1	58.9	57.3	56.4	56.1	55.2	54.9	54.5	53.9
Public	41.9	41.1	42.7	43.6	43.9	44.8	45.1	45.5	46.1
By program									
Medicare	14.9	16.1	16.3	16.9	17.4	18.3	18.9	19.8	20.7
Medicaid	10.4	10.8	12.4	13.2	13.3	13.7	13.7	14.5	15.3
Other	16.6	14.2	14.0	13.6	13.1	12.8	12.6	11.2	10.0
By government level									
Federal	28.7	28.1	29.7	31.0	31.7	32.7	33.2	33.9	34.8
State and local	13.3	13.0	13.0	12.6	12.1	12.1	12.0	11.6	11.3
Average annual percent change from previous year									
All sources	—	10.7	8.5	8.6	7.8	6.1	7.4	8.0	8.0
Private	—	10.9	5.6	6.9	7.2	4.4	6.7	7.9	7.7
Public	—	10.5	12.6	10.8	8.5	8.3	8.3	8.2	8.3
By program									
Medicare	—	11.6	10.0	12.2	11.5	11.1	10.9	9.1	9.0
Medicaid	—	11.2	24.5	15.0	9.2	9.0	7.7	9.2	9.2
Other	—	9.1	56.	5.5	4.1	4.0	5.2	5.5	5.6
By government level									
Federal	—	10.5	14.8	13.2	10.3	9.3	8.9	8.5	8.5
State and local	—	10.5	8.0	5.3	3.9	5.8	6.4	7.2	7.5
Gross domestic product (billions)	$2,708	$5,546.1	$5,724.8	$6,020.3	$6,343.3	$6,735.0	$7,116.5	$9,310.1	$12,155.5
U.S. population[1]	235.1	259.4	262.8	265.8	268.4	271.0	273.5	285.0	295.7
National health expenditures per capita	$1,068	$2,686	$2,875	$3,086	$3,294	$3,463	$3,685	$5,198	$7,352
National health expenditures as a percent of gross domestic product	9.3	12.6	13.2	13.6	13.9	13.9	14.2	15.9	17.9

[1] July 1 Social Security area population estimates.

Note: Numbers and percents may not add to totals because of rounding.

SOURCE: Katherine R. Levit et al., "National Health Expenditures, 1994," *Health Care Financing Review*, vol. 17, no. 3, Spring 1997

TABLE 2.4

National health expenditures, by source of funds and type of expenditure: selected calendar years 1993–98

Year and Type of Expenditure	Total	All Private Funds	Private Consumer Total	Out of Pocket Payments	Private Health Insurance	Other	Government Total	Federal	State and Local
1993					Amount in Billions				
National Health Expenditures	$898.5	$513.2	$473.9	$167.1	$306.8	$39.3	$385.3	$275.4	$110.0
Health Services and Supplies	869.5	501.3	473.9	167.1	306.8	27.4	368.2	263.3	104.9
Personal Health Care	790.5	459.1	432.3	167.1	265.2	26.8	331.4	252.3	79.1
Hospital Care	323.0	136.7	124.0	14.1	109.9	12.7	186.3	148.8	37.5
Physician Services	185.9	130.4	127.1	33.0	94.1	3.3	55.5	43.4	12.1
Dental Services	39.5	37.6	37.5	18.8	18.7	0.2	1.9	1.1	0.8
Other Professional Services	46.1	36.2	32.8	17.0	15.8	3.4	9.9	7.1	2.8
Home Health Care	23.0	11.9	8.7	5.6	3.1	3.2	11.1	9.5	1.5
Drugs and Other Medical Non-Durables	76.2	66.9	66.9	46.8	20.1	—	9.3	4.9	4.4
Vision Products and Other Medical Durables	12.3	8.0	8.0	7.3	0.7	—	4.3	4.2	0.1
Nursing Home Care	66.4	28.6	27.3	24.5	2.8	1.2	37.9	24.0	13.9
Other Personal Health Care	18.0	2.8	—	—	—	2.8	15.1	9.2	5.9
Program Administration and Net Cost of Private Health Insurance	53.7	42.1	41.6	—	41.6	0.6	11.5	7.7	3.8
Government Public Health Activities	25.3	—	—	—	—	—	25.3	3.3	22.0
Research and Construction	29.0	11.9	—	—	—	11.9	17.1	12.1	5.0
Research	14.5	1.2	—	—	—	1.2	13.3	11.1	2.1
Construction	14.5	10.7	—	—	—	10.7	3.8	0.9	2.9
1994									
National Health Expenditures	$947.7	$524.7	$483.5	$168.2	$315.3	$41.2	$423.0	$301.2	$121.8
Health Services and Supplies	917.3	513.0	483.5	168.2	315.3	29.5	404.3	288.0	116.3
Personal Health Care	834.0	471.8	442.9	168.2	274.7	28.8	362.2	275.7	86.5
Hospital Care	335.7	134.8	121.2	12.6	108.6	13.6	201.0	159.8	41.1
Physician Services	193.0	133.8	130.2	31.3	98.9	3.6	59.2	46.8	12.4
Dental Services	42.4	40.4	40.2	20.0	20.2	0.2	2.0	1.1	0.9
Other Professional Services	49.6	38.5	34.7	18.3	16.4	3.7	11.2	8.3	2.8
Home Health Care	26.2	12.5	9.2	5.8	3.4	3.4	13.7	11.9	1.8
Drugs and Other Medical Non-Durables	81.5	71.2	71.2	47.7	23.4	—	10.4	5.5	4.9
Vision Products and Other Medical Durables	12.6	7.9	7.9	7.2	0.7	—	4.6	4.5	0.1
Nursing Home Care	71.1	29.7	28.3	25.3	3.0	1.3	41.4	26.5	14.9
Other Personal Health Care	21.9	3.1	—	—	—	3.1	18.8	11.3	7.5
Program Administration and Net Cost of Private Health Insurance	55.2	41.2	40.6	—	40.6	0.6	14.0	8.5	5.5
Government Public Health Activities	28.2	—	—	—	—	—	28.2	3.8	24.4
Research and Construction	30.4	11.8	—	—	—	11.8	18.7	13.2	5.5
Research	15.9	1.3	—	—	—	1.3	14.6	12.3	2.3
Construction	14.6	10.5	—	—	—	10.5	4.1	0.9	3.2
1995									
National Health Expenditures	$993.3	$537.3	$494.6	$170.5	$324.0	$42.7	$456.0	$326.1	$129.8
Health Services and Supplies	962.5	526.3	494.6	170.5	324.0	31.8	436.2	312.1	124.0
Personal Health Care	879.1	487.9	456.8	170.5	286.3	31.1	391.2	299.0	92.2
Hospital Care	347.0	132.9	118.2	11.4	106.8	14.7	214.0	170.4	43.6
Physician Services	201.9	138.3	134.5	30.3	104.2	3.8	63.6	50.9	12.6
Dental Services	45.0	43.0	42.8	21.1	21.7	0.2	2.0	1.1	0.9
Other Professional Services	53.6	41.1	37.0	19.8	17.2	4.1	12.5	9.6	2.9
Home Health Care	29.1	13.2	9.6	5.9	3.7	3.5	15.9	14.0	1.9
Drugs and Other Medical Non-Durables	88.6	76.9	76.9	48.3	28.6	—	11.7	6.3	5.5
Vision Products and Other Medical Durables	13.3	7.9	7.9	7.2	0.7	—	5.4	5.3	0.1
Nursing Home Care	75.5	31.4	29.9	26.5	3.4	1.4	44.1	28.5	15.6
Other Personal Health Care	25.1	3.3	—	—	—	3.3	21.9	12.9	9.0
Program Administration and Net Cost of Private Health Insurance	53.6	38.4	37.8	—	37.8	0.7	15.2	9.3	5.9
Government Public Health Activities	29.8	—	—	—	—	—	29.8	3.8	26.0
Research and Construction	30.8	11.0	—	—	—	11.0	19.8	14.0	5.8
Research	16.7	1.3	—	—	—	1.3	15.4	12.9	2.5
Construction	14.0	9.6	—	—	—	9.6	4.4	1.1	3.3

WHO PAYS THE BILL?

Total Expenditures

In general, the government is the fastest-growing payer of health care. From 1990 to 1998, total public share of the nation's total health care bill rose from 40.5 percent to 45.5 percent. This represented the largest increase in the government's contribution to health care since Medicare began covering the disabled population in the early 1970s. (See Table 2.1.)

In 1998 private health insurance, the major non-government payer of health care costs, paid approximate-

TABLE 2.4

National health expenditures, by source of funds and type of expenditure: selected calendar years 1993–98 [CONTINUED]

		Private					Government		
			Consumer						
Year and Type of Expenditure	Total	All Private Funds	Total	Out of Pocket Payments	Private Health Insurance	Other	Total	Federal	State and Local
1996				Amount in Billions					
National Health Expenditures	$1,039.4	$559.0	$513.0	$178.1	$334.9	$46.1	$480.4	$347.3	$133.1
Health Services and Supplies	1007.5	547.5	513.0	178.1	334.9	34.5	460.0	332.9	127.0
Personal Health Care	924.0	510.0	476.2	178.1	298.1	33.8	414.0	319.1	94.9
Hospital Care	359.4	136.0	119.6	11.7	107.9	16.4	223.4	179.3	44.1
Physician Services	208.5	142.0	137.8	31.1	106.7	4.3	66.5	53.7	12.7
Dental Services	47.5	45.4	45.2	22.0	23.2	0.2	2.1	1.2	0.9
Other Professional Services	57.4	44.1	39.8	21.8	18.0	4.2	13.4	10.3	3.0
Home Health Care	31.2	14.1	10.3	6.1	4.2	3.8	17.1	15.1	2.0
Drugs and Other Medical Non-Durables	98.0	84.5	84.5	50.9	33.6	—	13.5	7.6	6.0
Vision Products and Other Medical Durables	14.1	8.3	8.3	7.6	0.8	—	5.8	5.7	0.1
Nursing Home Care	80.2	32.2	30.7	26.9	3.7	1.5	48.1	31.8	16.3
Other Personal Health Care	27.6	3.4	—	—	—	3.4	24.2	14.4	9.8
Program Administration and Net Cost of Private Health Insurance	52.1	37.5	36.8	—	36.8	0.7	14.6	9.9	4.7
Government Public Health Activities	31.3	—	—	—	—	—	31.3	3.9	27.4
Research and Construction	32.0	11.5	—	—	—	11.5	20.4	14.4	6.1
Research	17.2	1.4	—	—	—	1.4	15.7	13.2	2.5
Construction	14.8	10.1	—	—	—	10.1	4.7	1.2	3.5
1997									
National Health Expenditures	$1,088.2	$586.0	$535.7	$189.1	$346.7	$50.3	$502.2	$363.0	$139.2
Health Services and Supplies	1053.5	572.7	535.7	189.1	346.7	37.0	480.7	348.0	132.7
Personal Health Care	968.6	537.7	501.4	189.1	312.4	36.3	430.9	333.4	97.5
Hospital Care	370.2	141.3	123.2	12.2	111.0	18.1	228.9	185.0	43.9
Physician Services	217.8	147.6	143.1	33.8	109.4	4.5	70.1	57.4	12.8
Dental Services	51.1	48.9	48.7	24.3	24.4	0.2	2.2	1.3	1.0
Other Professional Services	61.5	47.6	43.0	24.2	18.8	4.6	13.8	10.8	3.1
Home Health Care	30.5	13.8	10.1	6.1	4.0	3.7	16.7	14.5	2.2
Drugs and Other Medical Non-Durables	108.6	92.8	92.8	52.9	39.9	—	15.8	9.0	6.8
Vision Products and Other Medical Durables	15.1	8.7	8.7	7.9	0.8	—	6.4	6.3	0.1
Nursing Home Care	84.7	33.4	31.9	27.8	4.1	1.6	51.3	34.0	17.2
Other Personal Health Care	29.2	3.6	—	—	—	3.6	25.6	15.2	10.4
Program Administration and Net Cost of Private Health Insurance	50.3	35.0	34.3	—	34.3	0.8	15.2	10.5	4.8
Government Public Health Activities	34.6	—	—	—	—	—	34.6	4.1	30.5
Research and Construction	34.8	13.2	—	—	—	13.2	21.5	15.0	6.5
Research	17.9	1.5	—	—	—	1.5	16.4	13.7	2.6
Construction	16.9	11.8	—	—	—	11.8	5.2	1.3	3.9
1998									
National Health Expenditures	$1,149.1	$626.4	$574.6	$199.5	$375.0	$51.8	$522.7	$376.9	$145.8
Health Services and Supplies	1113.7	613.4	574.6	199.5	375.0	38.8	500.4	360.4	140.0
Personal Health Care	1019.3	574.5	536.5	199.5	337.0	37.9	444.9	343.6	101.3
Hospital Care	382.8	149.9	130.9	12.8	118.0	19.1	232.9	187.4	45.5
Physician Services	229.5	156.2	151.7	35.7	116.0	4.5	73.3	60.8	12.4
Dental Services	53.8	51.5	51.3	25.8	25.5	0.2	2.3	1.3	1.0
Other Professional Services	66.6	52.4	47.4	27.2	20.2	5.0	14.2	11.2	3.0
Home Health Care	29.3	13.7	10.0	6.0	4.0	3.7	15.5	13.1	2.4
Drugs and Other Medical Non-Durables	121.9	103.1	103.1	55.4	47.8	—	18.8	10.7	8.1
Vision Products and Other Medical Durables	15.5	9.0	9.0	8.2	0.8	—	6.5	6.4	0.1
Nursing Home Care	87.8	34.8	33.2	28.5	4.7	1.6	53.0	35.4	17.7
Other Personal Health Care	32.1	3.8	—	—	—	3.8	28.3	17.1	11.2
Program Administration and Net Cost of Private Health Insurance	57.7	38.9	38.0	—	38.0	0.9	18.8	12.6	6.2
Government Public Health Activities	36.6	—	—	—	—	—	36.6	4.2	32.4
Research and Construction	35.3	13.0	—	—	—	13.0	22.3	16.5	5.8
Research	19.9	1.6	—	—	—	1.6	18.3	15.5	2.8
Construction	15.5	11.5	—	—	—	11.5	4.0	1.0	3.0

Note: Research and development expenditures of drug companies and other manufacturers and providers of medical equipment and supplies are excluded from research expenditures, but are included in the expenditure class in which the product falls. Numbers may not add to totals because of rounding.

SOURCE: Office of the Actuary, National Health Statistics Group, Health Care Financing Administration, 2000

FIGURE 2.2

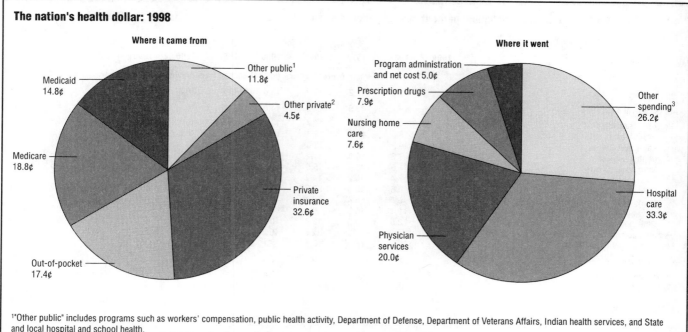

The nation's health dollar: 1998

Where it came from

Other public[1] 11.8¢

Medicaid 14.8¢

Other private[2] 4.5¢

Medicare 18.8¢

Private insurance 32.6¢

Out-of-pocket 17.4¢

Where it went

Program administration and net cost 5.0¢

Prescription drugs 7.9¢

Nursing home care 7.6¢

Other spending[3] 26.2¢

Hospital care 33.3¢

Physician services 20.0¢

[1]"Other public" includes programs such as workers' compensation, public health activity, Department of Defense, Department of Veterans Affairs, Indian health services, and State and local hospital and school health.
[2]"Other private" includes industrial inplant, privately funded construction, and non-patient revenues including philanthropy.
[3]"Other spending" includes dentist services, other professional services, home health, durable medical products, over-the-counter medicines and sundries, public health, research and construction.
Note: Numbers shown may not add to 100.0 because of rounding.

SOURCE: Health Care Financing Administration. Available at: http://www.hcfa.gov/stats/nhe-oact/tables/chart.htm

ly one-third (32.6 percent) of all health expenditures, a proportion that has not changed since 1990. The share, however, of health care spending from private, out-of-pocket (paid by the patient) funds declined, falling from 20.6 percent of total health care spending in 1990 to 17.4 percent in 1998. (See Tables 2.4 and 2.5.)

Different sectors paid more for different types of health services. The public sector paid for more than half (60.8 percent) of all hospital costs, with the federal government providing 49 percent of the nation's hospital bill. The public sector also paid 60.4 percent of all nursing home care and 52.9 percent of all home health care. Private health insurance paid for 50.5 percent of all physicians' services and 47.4 percent of dental bills. Patients paid 48 percent of their dental bills and 45.4 percent of their drug and prescription bills. (See Table 2.4.)

The Personal Health Care Bill

Much of the increase in government spending has occurred in the area of personal health care. In 1980 government sources paid 40.1 percent of personal health care expenditures; by 1998 they covered 43.6 percent ($444.9 billion) of the $1,019.3 billion spent on personal health care services. Of that contribution, 33.7 percent came from the federal government and 9.9 percent from state and local governments. A large proportion of the federal

increase was attributed to Medicare spending, which grew from 11.4 percent of all personal health care expenditures in 1970 to 20.6 percent in 1998. Together, Medicare and Medicaid made up 36.3 percent of all personal health care expenditures. (See Tables 2.4 and 2.6.)

Of the 56.4 percent of personal health costs paid privately, 33.1 percent came from health insurance companies. The patient paid for 19.6 percent out of pocket, and 3.7 percent came from other sources, mainly charities. (See Table 2.6.)

WHY DID HEALTH CARE COSTS INCREASE?

The increase in the cost of medical care is difficult to analyze because the methods and quality of health care change constantly. A hospital stay in 1960 did not include the same services offered in 1999. Furthermore, the care received in today's doctor's office is in no way comparable to that received a generation ago. Part of the rising cost is the increase in medical technology, much of which is now available outside of a hospital.

Many other factors also contribute to the increase in health care costs, however. These include population growth, high salaries for doctors and some other health care workers, and the expense of malpractice insurance. Other factors include advanced medical procedures

TABLE 2.5

National health expenditures, average annual percent change, according to type of expenditure: selected years 1960–98

Type of expenditure	1960	1965	1970	1975	1980	1985	1990	1995	1996	1997	1998
					Average annual percent change from previous year shown						
All expenditures	...	8.9	12.2	12.3	13.6	11.6	10.3	7.3	4.6	4.7	5.6
Health services and supplies	...	8.4	12.5	12.5	14.0	11.8	10.4	7.4	4.7	4.6	5.7
Personal health care	...	8.3	12.7	12.4	13.6	11.6	10.3	7.4	5.1	4.8	5.2
Hospital care	...	8.6	14.8	13.4	14.3	10.4	8.8	6.2	3.6	3.0	3.4
Physician services	...	9.2	10.6	12.0	13.6	13.1	11.8	6.6	3.3	4.5	5.4
Dentist services	...	7.3	10.8	11.2	10.9	10.2	7.8	7.3	5.6	7.6	5.3
Nursing home care	...	11.6	23.4	15.5	15.3	11.7	10.7	8.2	6.3	5.5	3.7
Other professional services	...	7.4	10.2	14.2	18.4	21.2	15.8	9.1	7.1	7.0	8.3
Home health care	...	9.6	19.7	23.2	30.7	18.9	18.4	17.3	7.1	-2.2	-4.0
Drugs and other medical nondurables	...	6.8	8.4	8.1	10.7	11.4	10.1	8.1	10.6	10.8	12.3
Vision products and other medical durables	...	9.1	10.2	9.5	8.1	12.4	9.2	5.0	6.0	6.7	2.7
Other personal health care	...	3.5	9.5	13.8	10.2	8.8	12.9	17.5	9.8	5.9	9.8
Program administration and net cost of health insurance	...	10.6	7.1	12.5	19.3	15.4	10.8	5.7	-2.8	-3.5	14.9
Government public health activities	...	10.8	17.0	16.8	18.1	11.5	11.0	8.7	5.2	10.2	6.0
Research and construction	...	15.1	9.2	9.4	6.8	7.1	8.4	4.6	3.9	8.8	1.6
Noncommercial research	...	17.1	5.1	11.2	10.4	7.5	9.3	6.5	2.6	4.2	11.1
Construction	...	13.7	12.1	8.3	4.1	6.7	7.6	2.7	5.4	14.2	-8.4

... Category not applicable.

SOURCE: *Health, United States, 2000,* National Center for Health Statistics, Hyattsville, MD, 2000

requiring high-technology expertise and equipment; redundant technology in hospitals; cumbersome medical insurance programs; patient demand for the latest and most complete testing and treatment; and the growing number of elderly.

CONTROLLING HEALTH CARE SPENDING

In 1996 national health expenditures topped $1 trillion for the first time, and by 1998 that figure was at $1.149 trillion. Despite the continuing growth in health care spending from year to year—4.6 percent in 1996, 5.6 percent in 1998—these figures represent a steady decline from the skyrocketing costs in the beginning of the 1990s. In 1990, for instance, health costs grew at a staggering 11 percent from the previous year. (See Tables 2.1 and 2.7.)

In order to achieve these results, the nation's health care system underwent some basic changes. Beginning in the late 1980s, employers began looking for new ways to hold down health benefit costs for their workers. Many enrolled their employees in managed care programs, devised by insurance companies as alternatives to traditional, fee-for-service insurance. Managed care programs offered lower premiums by keeping a tighter control on costs and utilization, and by emphasizing the importance of preventive care. This allowed insurers to negotiate discounts with providers in exchange for guaranteed access to employer-insured groups.

New interest has also developed in treatments and technologies designed to reduce the health system's dependence on expensive, inpatient hospital care. Hospital care expenditures were still the single-largest spending component of total health care expenses, at 33.3 percent ($382.8 billion in 1998). The annual hospital cost growth rate, however, dropped from 7.5 percent per year in the early 1990s to around 3.3 percent between 1995 and 1998. (See Tables 2.4 and 2.5.)

Physician services accounted for 20 percent ($229.5 billion) of 1998 national health spending. (See Table 2.4.) Physician spending, however, increased only 5.4 percent from 1997 to 1998, down from 11.8 percent in 1990. (See Table 2.5.) The growing role of managed care has played a large role in this slowdown in growth.

In 1998 spending for freestanding nursing home care (not including hospital-based nursing home care) totaled $87.8 billion, and spending for home health care reached $29.3 billion. (See Table 2.4.) Nursing home expenses increased only 3.7 percent from 1997 to 1998, compared with 9.5 percent annual growth from 1990 to 1995. Home health care expenses also slowed, from 17.3 percent annual growth from 1990 to 1995 to 4 percent between 1997 and 1998. (See Table 2.5.)

On the other hand, one of the fastest-growing elements of health care was the market for drugs and other medical nondurables. In 1998 Americans spent $121.9 billion (Table 2.4) on prescription and nonprescription drugs—a 12.3 percent increase from 1997. (See Table 2.5.) A large part of the increase was driven by private insurers, which paid 39.2 percent of drug costs in 1998, up from 26.4 percent in 1993. In addition, drugs are being substituted more often for other types of health care. For example, antidepressant drugs are being substituted for more expensive psychotherapy and inpatient mental hospital stays, and narcotic analgesics are used in combina-

TABLE 2.6

Personal health care expenditures, aggregate and per capita amounts, and percent distribution, by source of funds: selected calendar years 1960–98

Year	Total	Out-of-Pocket Payments	Third-Party Payments							Medicare[1]	Medicaid[2]
			Total	Private Health Insurance	Other Private Funds	Government				
						Total	Federal	State and Local		
					Amount in Billions						
1960	$23.6	$13.1	$10.6	$5.0	$0.4	$5.1	$2.1	$3.0	—	—
1970	63.8	24.9	38.9	14.8	1.6	22.5	14.7	7.8	7.3	5.1
1980	217.0	60.3	156.8	62.0	7.8	87.0	63.4	23.6	36.4	24.8
1990	614.7	145.0	469.6	207.7	20.8	241.1	177.0	64.2	108.6	71.4
1991	679.6	153.3	526.2	229.8	23.1	273.4	203.2	70.2	117.8	89.6
1992	740.7	161.8	578.9	250.6	24.7	303.6	230.5	73.0	132.7	101.5
1993	790.5	167.1	623.5	265.2	26.8	331.4	252.3	79.1	144.7	115.8
1994	834.0	168.2	665.8	274.7	28.8	362.2	275.7	86.5	162.6	126.9
1995	879.1	170.5	708.6	286.3	31.1	391.2	299.0	92.2	180.8	137.2
1996	924.0	178.1	745.9	298.1	33.8	414.0	319.1	94.9	194.2	146.3
1997	968.6	189.1	779.6	312.4	36.3	430.9	333.4	97.5	205.6	152.2
1998	1,019.3	199.5	819.8	337.0	37.9	444.9	343.6	101.3	210.5	159.6
					Per Capita Amount						
1960	$124.3	$68.7	$55.5	$26.4	$2.2	$26.9	$11.2	$15.7	—	—
1970	297.2	115.9	181.2	68.8	7.6	104.8	68.5	36.4	(3)	(3)
1980	923.0	256.2	666.7	263.7	33.1	369.9	269.6	100.3	(3)	(3)
1990	2,363.0	557.5	1,805.4	798.6	79.8	927.0	680.2	246.8	(3)	(3)
1991	2,585.9	583.5	2,002.4	874.5	87.7	1,040.2	773.1	267.1	(3)	(3)
1992	2,789.6	609.2	2,180.4	944.0	93.1	1,143.3	868.2	275.1	(3)	(3)
1993	2,947.8	622.9	2,324.9	989.1	100.1	1,235.7	940.8	294.9	(3)	(3)
1994	3,080.8	621.5	2,459.4	1,014.8	106.6	1,338.0	1,018.6	319.4	(3)	(3)
1995	3,218.6	624.4	2,594.2	1,048.1	113.8	1,432.3	1,094.8	337.4	(3)	(3)
1996	3,352.8	646.1	2,706.7	1,081.7	122.7	1,502.2	1,157.9	344.4	(3)	(3)
1997	3,482.3	679.7	2,802.6	1,123.1	130.4	1,549.2	1,198.8	350.4	(3)	(3)
1998	3,631.8	710.9	2,920.9	1,200.7	135.1	1,585.1	1,224.1	361.0	(3)	(3)
					Percent Distribution						
1960	100.0	55.3	44.7	21.2	1.8	21.7	9.0	12.6	—	—
1970	100.0	39.0	61.0	23.2	2.6	35.3	23.0	12.2	11.4	7.9
1980	100.0	27.8	72.2	28.6	3.6	40.1	29.2	10.9	16.8	11.4
1990	100.0	23.6	76.4	33.8	3.4	39.2	28.8	10.4	17.7	11.6
1991	100.0	22.6	77.4	33.8	3.4	40.2	29.9	10.3	17.3	13.2
1992	100.0	21.8	78.2	33.8	3.3	41.0	31.1	9.9	17.9	13.7
1993	100.0	21.1	78.9	33.6	3.4	41.9	31.9	10.0	18.3	14.6
1994	100.0	20.2	79.8	32.9	3.5	43.4	33.1	10.4	19.5	15.2
1995	100.0	19.4	80.6	32.6	3.5	44.5	34.0	10.5	20.6	15.6
1996	100.0	19.3	80.7	32.3	3.7	44.8	34.5	10.3	21.0	15.8
1997	100.0	19.5	80.5	32.3	3.7	44.5	34.4	10.1	21.2	15.7
1998	100.0	19.6	80.4	33.1	3.7	43.6	33.7	9.9	20.6	15.7

[1] Subset of Federal funds.
[2] Subset of Federal and State and local funds.
[3] Calculation of per capita estimates is inappropriate.
Notes: Per capita amounts based on July 1 Social Security area population estimates for each year, 1960–98. Numbers and percents may not add to totals because of rounding.
SOURCE: Office of the Actuary, National Health Statistics Group, Health Care Financing Administration, 2000

tion with surgery, making it possible for patients to avoid or shorten inpatient hospital stays.

RATIONING CARE

Many people believe that rationing health care—putting limits on the amount and kind of care Americans can receive—is the only way to help control skyrocketing costs. Others disagree.

Opponents of Rationing

Those who argue against rationing fear that the elderly, poor, and chronically ill would suffer tremendously from cutbacks in care. They believe that improving the efficiency of the U.S. health care system would save enough money to make health care available to all.

Opponents of rationing point out that expenditures for the same procedures vary greatly in different areas of the country. They argue that standardizing fees and costs could realize great savings. Rationing opponents also believe that money could be saved if more emphasis were placed on preventive care and on developing strategies to prevent destructive behavior such as smoking, alcohol abuse, and irresponsible sex. In addition, they insist that the high cost of administering the American health system

TABLE 2.7

National health expenditures, average annual growth from prior year shown: selected years 1960–96

Spending category	1960	1970	1980	1990	1993	1994	1995	1996
National health expenditures	–[a]	10.6%	12.9%	11.0%	8.6%	5.6%	4.8%	4.4%
Health services and supplies	–[a]	10.4	13.3	11.1	8.7	5.7	5.0	4.5
Personal health care	–[a]	10.5	13.0	11.0	8.6	5.3	4.9	4.4
Hospital care	–[a]	11.7	13.9	9.6	8.0	3.9	3.3	3.4
Physician services	–[a]	9.9	12.8	12.5	7.8	3.7	3.1	2.9
Dental services	–[a]	9.1	11.1	9.0	7.4	6.6	7.3	6.4
Other professional services	–[a]	8.8	16.3	18.5	10.1	8.8	7.9	6.8
Home health care[b]	–[a]	14.5	26.9	18.6	20.3	12.2	10.9	6.2
Drugs and other medical nondurables	–[a]	7.6	9.4	10.7	8.0	5.2	6.8	7.7
Prescription drugs	–[a]	7.5	8.2	12.1	9.9	6.2	7.4	9.2
Vision products and other medical durables	–[a]	9.6	8.8	10.7	5.6	1.5	4.9	1.4
Nursing home care[b]	–[a]	17.4	15.4	11.2	9.2	6.8	6.2	4.3
Other personal health care	–[a]	6.5	12.0	10.8	17.0	21.8	15.4	9.4
Program administration and net cost of private health insurance	–[a]	8.9	15.9	13.1	9.8	8.2	3.3	1.2
Government public health activities	–[a]	13.9	17.5	11.3	8.9	12.5	10.7	12.5
Research and construction	–[a]	12.2	8.1	7.7	5.8	5.1	0.8	2.6
Research[c]	–[a]	10.9	10.8	8.4	5.9	9.6	5.0	1.9
Construction	–[a]	12.9	6.2	7.1	5.7	0.5	-3.8	3.4
National health expenditures per capita	–[a]	9.2	11.9	9.8	7.5	4.7	3.9	3.5
Gross domestic product	–[a]	7.0	10.4	7.5	4.5	5.9	4.6	5.1

Note: Numbers may not add to totals because of rounding.

[a] Not available.

[b] Freestanding facilities only. Additional services of this type are provided in hospital-based facilities and are counted as hospital care.

[c] Research and development expenditures of drug companies and other manufacturers and providers of medical equipment and supplies are excluded from "research expenditures" but are included in the expenditure class in which the product falls.

SOURCE: Katherine R. Levit et al., "National Health Spending Trends in 1996," *Health Affairs,* vol. 17, no. 1, January/February 1998

could be streamlined by using a single payer of health care—as in the Canadian system.

Supporters of Rationing

Those who believe that rationing is inevitable argue that the spiraling cost of health care stems from more than simple inefficiency. They note that the population is aging, technological innovation continues to raise the price of care, and the price of labor and supplies is increasing. Rationing supporters believe that the nation's health care system costs too much for what it delivers, and that it fails altogether to deliver to millions of uninsured; in fact, they point out that the United States already rations health care by not covering the uninsured.

These health care rationing advocates argue that the problem is one of basic cultural assumptions, not the economics of the health care industry. Americans value human life, believe in the promise of health for all, and insist that any disease can be cured. The United States spends too much on health in comparison to other needs; too much on the old in comparison to the young; too much on curing and not enough on caring; too much on extending the length of life and not enough on enhancing the quality of life. Supporters of rationing argue instead for a system that guarantees a minimally

decent level of health care for all, while reining in the expensive excesses of the current system, which prolongs life at any cost.

THE OREGON PLAN. In 1987 the state of Oregon began developing a new, universal health care plan that would increase coverage and contain costs by limiting services. Unlike other states, which trimmed budgets by eliminating people from Medicaid eligibility, Oregon wanted to eliminate low-priority services. Their plan, approved in August 1993, aimed to provide Medicaid to 120,000 additional residents living below the poverty level. A 10-cent increase in the state cigarette tax (providing approximately $45 million) helped fund the additional estimated $400 million needed over the next several years.

Oregon worked out a table of health care services and ranked them according to costs and benefits obtained. (See Table 2.8.) Oregon Medicaid would cover the top 565 services on a list of 696 medical procedures. Services that fell below the cutoff point included liver transplants for patients with liver cancer; nutritional counseling for obese people; fertility services; and treatment for the common cold, chronic back pain, and viral hepatitis.

In setting the priorities, prevention and quality of life were the factors that most influenced the ranking of the treatments. Quality of life (quality of well-being, or QWB, in the Oregon plan) drew fire from those who felt such judgments could not be subjectively decided. Active medical or surgical treatment of terminally ill patients also ranked low on the QWB scale, while comfort and hospice care ranked high. The Oregon Health Services Commission emphasized that their QWB judgments were not based on a person's quality of life at a given time; such judgments were ethically inappropriate. Instead they focused on the potential change in a person's life. After treatment, how much better or worse off would the patient be?

Opponents objected that the plan obtained its funding by reducing services that were currently offered to Medicaid recipients (often poor women and children) rather than by emphasizing cost control. Others objected to the ranking and the ethical questions raised by choosing to support some treatments over others.

By 1998 the Oregon Health Plan had developed major problems. The state was no longer promising universal care; doctors were finding ways to get around the rationing; and friction with federal Medicaid regulators was blocking Oregon's efforts to deny more treatments. A plan to have employers insure all their workers or contribute to a fund to cover them failed. Spending for the plan climbed to $2.1 billion in the 1997–99 state budget period, up from $1.7 billion in the 1995–97 period. Higher cigarette taxes did not offset the increase, requiring more money from the state's general fund.

By 1998, five years after the Oregon plan was initiated with the goal of having no uninsured people in the state, coverage was far from universal. Despite the Oregon plan's best efforts, there were still approximately 350,000 people in Oregon who had no insurance.

Rationing by HMOs

More and more Americans receive their health care from health maintenance organizations (HMOs) or other managed care systems. In 1999 national enrollment in HMOs topped 81 million, nearly four times as many as were enrolled just a decade earlier (21 million).

Managed care programs have sought to control costs by limiting their coverage for expensive experimental treatments. Before doctors can perform experimental surgery or prescribe a new treatment plan for a serious illness, they must first get approval from the patient's health care system in order for the expenses to be covered.

Increasingly, patients and doctors are battling HMOs for approval to use new technology and experimental care. Judges and juries, moved by the desperate situations of patients, have generally decided cases against HMOs,

TABLE 2.8

Health care service categories and rankings

Rank	Category ID No.
"Essential" Services	
1. Acute fatal, prevents death, full recovery	15
Examples: Repair of deep, open wound of neck. Appendectomy for appendicitis. Medical therapy for myocarditis.	
2. Maternity care (including care for newborn in first 28 days of life)	12
Examples: Obstetrical care for pregnancy, Medical therapy for drug reactions and intoxications specific to newborn. Medical therapy for low birthweight babies.	
3. Acute fatal, prevents death, w/o full recovery	16
Examples: Surgical treatment for head injury with prolonged loss of consciousness. Medical therapy for acute bacterial meningitis. Reduction of an open fracture of a joint.	
4. Preventive care for children	01
Examples: Immunizations. Medical therapy for streptococcal sore throat and scarlet fever (reduces disability, prevents spread). Screening for specific problems such as vision or hearing problems, or anemia.	
5. Chronic fatal, improves life span and QWB (Quality of Well-Being)	20
Examples: Medical therapy for Type I Diabetes Mellitus. Medical and surgical treatment for treatable cancer of the uterus. Medical therapy for asthma.	
6. Reproductive services (excluding maternity and infertility)	13
Examples: Contraceptive management, vasectomy, tubal ligation.	
7. Comfort care	26
Example: Palliative therapy for conditions in which death is imminent.	
8. Preventive dental (children and adults)	03/07
Example: Cleaning and flouride.	
9. Preventive care for adults (A-B-C)	04
Examples: Mammograms, blood pressure screening, medical therapy and chemoprophylaxis for primary tuberculosis.	
"Very Important" Services	
10. Acute nonfatal, return to previous health	17
Examples: Medical therapy for acute thyroiditis. Medical therapy for vaginitis. Restorative dental service for dental caries.	
11. Chronic nonfatal, one time treatment improves QWB	23
Examples: Hip replacement. Laser surgery for diabetic retinopathy. Medical therapy for rheumatic fever.	
12. Acute nonfatal, w/o return to previous health	18
Examples: Relocation of dislocation of elbow. Arthroscopic repair of internal derangement of knee. Repair of corneal laceration.	
13. Chronic nonfatal, repetitive treatment improves QWB	24
Examples: Medical therapy for chronic sinusitis. Medical therapy for migraine. Medical therapy for psoriasis.	
Services "Valuable to Certain Individuals"	
14. Acute nonfatal, expedites recovery	19
Examples: Medical therapy for diaper rash. Medical therapy for acute conjunctivitis. Medical therapy for acute pharyngitis.	
15. Infertility services	14
Examples: Medical therapy for anovulation. Microsurgery for tubal disease. In-vitro fertilization.	
16. Preventive care for adults (D-E)	05
Examples: Dipstick urinalysis for hematuria in adults less than 60 years of age. Sigmoidoscopy for persons less than 40 years of age. Screening of nonpregnant adults for Type I Diabetes Mellitus.	
17. Fatal or nonfatal, minimal or no improvement in QWB (non-self-limited)	25
Examples: Repair fingertip avulsion that does not include fingernail. Medical therapy for gallstones without cholecystitis. Medical therapy for viral warts.	

SOURCE: Oregon Basic Health Services Program, February 22, 1991

regardless of whether the new treatment had been shown to be effective. (For more information about HMOs, see Chapter 6.)

"SILENT RATIONING." Physicians are concerned that limiting coverage for new, high-cost technology will discourage research and development for new treatments before they have even been developed. This has been

TABLE 2.9

Medicare hospital insurance and/or supplemental medical insurance enrollment demographics, 1997

	Total	Male	Female
	Number in thousands		
All persons	38,455	16,497	21,958
Aged persons	33,608	13,694	19,914
65-74	17,916	8,035	9,881
75-84	11,619	4,521	7,098
85 and over	4,073	1,138	2,935
Disabled Persons	4,846	2,803	2,043
Under 45	1,610	967	643
45-54	1,388	804	584
55-64	1,848	1,032	816
White	32,709	14,005	18,704
Black	3,486	1,475	2,011
All Other	2,065	942	1,123
Native American	58	29	29
Asian/Pacific	412	184	228
Hispanic	866	415	451
Other	728	314	414
Unknown race	195	75	120

Note: Data as of December 1997. Totals do not necessarily equal the sum of the rounded components.

SOURCE: *1998 Data Compendium,* Health Care Financing Administration, Baltimore, MD, 1998

called "silent rationing," because patients will never know what they have missed.

While new technology is thought to contribute heavily to the growth of the nation's health care bill, exactly how much is unknown. Some estimates have put the share at 30–50 percent. On the other hand, new technologies often save money through more effective medical care, although they frequently increase the volume of services, thereby hiking total spending.

In an effort to control costs, some HMOs have discouraged doctors from telling patients about certain treatment options—those that are very expensive or not covered by the HMO. This has proved to be a highly controversial issue, both politically and ethically. In December 1996 HHS ruled that HMOs and other health plans cannot prevent doctors from telling Medicare patients about all available treatment options.

HEALTH CARE FOR THE ELDERLY, THE DISABLED, AND THE POOR

The United States is one of the few industrialized nations that does not have national health care programs. In most other developed countries, government programs cover almost all health-related costs, from maternity care to long-term care.

In the United States, the major government health care programs are Medicare and Medicaid. They provide financial assistance for the elderly, the poor, and the disabled. Before the existence of these programs, a large number of older Americans could not afford adequate medical care. Medicare mainly reimburses for hospital and physician care, while Medicaid provides much of the cost of nursing home care.

Medicare

The Medicare program, enacted under Title XVIII ("Health Insurance for the Aged") of the Social Security Act (PL 89-97), went into effect on July 1, 1966. The program is composed of two parts:

- Part A provides hospital insurance. Coverage includes doctors' fees, nursing services, meals, semiprivate rooms, special-care units, operating room costs, laboratory tests, and some drugs and supplies. Part A also covers rehabilitation services, limited posthospital care in a skilled nursing facility, home health care, and hospice care for the terminally ill.

- Part B (Supplemental Medical Insurance, or SMI) is elective medical insurance; that is, enrollees must pay premiums to get coverage. SMI covers private physicians' services, diagnostic tests, outpatient hospital services, outpatient physical therapy, speech pathology services, home health services, and medical equipment and supplies.

In 1997 more than 38 million persons were enrolled in Medicare: 16.5 million males and 22 million females. Most (87.4 percent, or 33.6 million) were 65 and older. The majority (53.3 percent) of elderly persons were between the ages of 65 and 74; a third (34.6 percent) were between the ages of 75 and 84; and 12.1 percent were 85 and older. (See Table 2.9.) The relative proportion of those between the ages of 65 and 69 has steadily declined, while the proportion of those 85 and older has steadily increased. The HCFA estimated that by 2050, 69 million people aged 65 and older would be eligible for Medicare; of those, 15 million would be 85 or older.

In general, Medicare reimburses doctors on a fee-for-service basis, which presents a number of problems. Because of paperwork, reduced compensation, and delays in reimbursements, some doctors will not provide services under the Medicare program.

Because of these problems, the Tax Equity and Fiscal Responsibility Act of 1982 (PL 97-248) authorized a "risk managed care" option for Medicare, based on agreed-upon prepayments. Beginning in 1985, the HCFA could contract to pay health care providers, such as HMOs or health care prepayment plans, to serve Medicare and Medicaid patients. These groups are paid a predetermined cost per patient for their services. Continued cuts in payments, however, have made what once was a profitable enterprise for managed care companies a riskier venture. In fact, many managed care companies are no longer offering their services to the elderly and are withdrawing existing policies.

TABLE 2.10

Medicaid recipients and medical vendor payments, according to type of service: selected fiscal years 1972–98

Type of service	1972	1975	1980	1985	1990	1995	1996	1997	1998[1]
Recipients					**Number in millions**				
All recipients	17.6	22.0	21.6	21.8	25.3	36.3	36.1	34.9	40.6
					Percent of recipients				
Inpatient general hospitals	16.1	15.6	17.0	15.7	18.2	15.3	14.8	13.6	10.5
Inpatient mental hospitals	0.2	0.3	0.3	0.3	0.4	0.2	0.3	0.3	0.3
Mentally retarded intermediate care facilities	—	0.3	0.6	0.7	0.6	0.4	0.4	0.4	0.3
Nursing facilities	—	—	—	—	—	4.6	4.4	4.6	4.0
Skilled	3.1	2.9	2.8	2.5	2.4	—	—	—	—
Intermediate care	—	3.1	3.7	3.8	3.4	—	—	—	—
Physician	69.8	69.1	63.7	66.0	67.6	65.6	63.3	60.7	45.6
Dental	13.6	17.9	21.5	21.4	18.0	17.6	17.2	17.0	12.2
Other practitioner	9.1	12.1	15.0	15.4	15.3	15.2	14.8	14.7	10.7
Outpatient hospital	29.6	33.8	44.9	46.2	49.0	46.1	44.0	39.1	29.9
Clinic	2.8	4.9	7.1	9.7	11.1	14.7	14.0	13.5	13.0
Laboratory and radiological	20.0	21.5	14.9	29.1	35.5	36.0	34.9	31.8	23.1
Home health	0.6	1.6	1.8	2.5	2.8	4.5	4.8	5.3	3.0
Prescribed drugs	63.3	64.3	63.4	63.8	68.5	65.4	62.5	60.1	47.6
Family planning	...	5.5	5.2	7.5	6.9	6.9	6.6	6.0	4.9
Early and periodic screening	...	...	...	8.7	11.7	18.2	18.2	18.5	15.2
Rural health clinic	...	...	...	0.4	0.9	3.4	3.9	4.1	—
Prepaid health care	—	—	—	—	—	—	—	—	49.7
Other care	14.4	13.2	11.9	15.5	20.3	31.5	36.3	35.5	36.0
Vendor payments[2]					**Amount in billions**				
All payments	$6.3	$12.2	$23.3	$37.5	$64.9	$120.1	$121.7	$124.4	$142.3
					Percent distribution				
Total	100.0	100.0	100.0	100.0	100.0	100.0	100.0	100.0	100.0
Inpatient general hospitals	40.6	27.6	27.5	25.2	25.7	21.9	20.7	18.6	15.1
Inpatient mental hospitals	1.8	3.3	3.3	3.2	2.6	2.1	1.7	1.6	2.0
Mentally retarded intermediate care facilities	—	3.1	8.5	12.6	11.3	8.6	7.9	7.9	6.7
Nursing facilities	—	—	—	—	—	24.2	24.3	24.5	22.4
Skilled	23.3	19.9	15.8	13.5	12.4	—	—	—	—
Intermediate care	—	15.4	18.0	17.4	14.9	—	—	—	—
Physician	12.6	10.0	8.0	6.3	6.2	6.1	5.9	5.7	4.3
Dental	2.7	2.8	2.0	1.2	0.9	0.8	0.8	0.8	0.6
Other practitioner	0.9	1.0	0.8	0.7	0.6	0.8	0.9	0.8	0.4
Outpatient hospital	5.8	3.0	4.7	4.8	5.1	5.5	5.3	5.0	4.0
Clinic	0.7	3.2	1.4	1.9	2.6	3.6	3.5	3.4	2.8
Laboratory and radiological	1.3	1.0	0.5	0.9	1.1	1.0	1.0	0.8	0.7
Home health	0.4	0.6	1.4	3.0	5.2	7.8	8.9	9.8	1.9
Prescribed drugs	8.1	6.7	5.7	6.2	6.8	8.1	8.8	9.6	9.5
Family planning	...	0.5	0.3	0.5	0.4	0.4	0.4	0.3	0.3
Early and periodic screening	...	...	...	0.2	0.3	1.0	1.1	1.3	0.9
Rural health clinic	...	...	...	0.0	0.1	0.2	0.2	0.2	—
Prepaid health care	—	—	—	—	—	—	—	—	13.6
Other care	1.8	1.9	1.9	2.5	3.7	7.7	8.4	8.9	13.6

Medicaid

Medicaid was enacted by Congress in 1965 under "Grants to States for Medical Assistance Programs," Title XIX of the Social Security Act. It is a joint federal/state program that provides medical assistance to certain categories of low-income Americans: the aged, the blind, the disabled, or families with dependent children. Medicaid covers hospitalization, doctors' fees, laboratory fees, X rays, and long-term care in nursing homes.

In 1998, 40.6 million people received Medicaid services—an 88 percent increase over 1980. Of Medicaid dollars spent in 1998, 22.4 percent went to nursing facilities, while 15.1 percent was spent in inpatient general hospitals. (See Table 2.10.)

The Personal Responsibility and Work Opportunity Reconciliation Act (PL 104-193)—federal welfare reform— was signed into law in August 1996, replacing the American Families with Dependent Children program (AFDC) with Temporary Assistance for Needy Families (TANF). Under TANF, Medicaid coverage was no longer guaranteed, as it was for recipients of AFDC. The new law, however, required states to continue benefits to those who would have been eligible under the AFDC requirements that each state had in place on July 16, 1996.

Medicaid is the largest third-party payer of long-term care in the United States, financing 47.8 percent of nursing home care in 1996. Under current law, an elderly person must have less than $2,500 in savings or assets (with some exceptions) to qualify for nursing home care paid for by Medicaid. Although home health services currently account for a small share of Medicaid expenditures for the aged, they are the fastest-growing expense.

TABLE 2.10

Medicaid recipients and medical vendor payments, according to type of service: selected fiscal years 1972–98 [CONTINUED]

Type of service	1972	1975	1980	1985	1990	1995	1996	1997	1998[1]
Vendor payments per recipient[2]					Amount				
Total payment per recipient	$ 358	$ 556	$ 1,079	$ 1,719	$ 2,568	$ 3,311	$ 3,369	$ 3,568	$ 3,501
Inpatient general hospitals	903	983	1,742	2,753	3,630	4,735	4,696	4,877	5,031
Inpatient mental hospitals	2,825	6,045	11,742	19,867	18,548	29,847	21,873	22,990	20,701
Mentally retarded intermediate care facilities	—	5,507	16,438	32,102	50,048	68,613	68,232	72,033	74,960
Nursing facilities	—					17,424	18,589	19,029	19,379
Skilled	2,665	3,864	6,081	9,274	13,356	—	—	—	—
Intermediate care	—	2,764	5,326	7,882	11,236	—	—	—	—
Physician	65	81	136	163	235	309	317	333	327
Dental	71	86	99	98	130	160	166	175	182
Other practitioner	37	48	61	75	96	178	205	190	135
Outpatient hospital	70	50	113	178	269	397	409	453	474
Clinic	82	358	209	337	602	804	833	902	742
Laboratory and radiological	23	27	38	53	80	90	96	93	100
Home health	229	204	847	2,094	4,733	5,740	6,293	6,575	2,206
Prescribed drugs	46	58	96	166	256	413	474	571	699
Family planning	...	55	72	119	151	206	200	200	223
Early and periodic screening	...	...	...	45	67	177	212	251	216
Rural health clinic	...	...	...	81	154	174	215	213	—
Prepaid health care	—	—	—	—	—	—	—	—	955
Other care	44	80	172	274	465	807	782	891	1,331

— Data not available.
... Category not applicable.
[1]Prior to 1998 recipient counts exclude those individuals who only received coverage under prepaid health care and for whom no direct vendor payments were made during the year. Prior to 1998 vendor payments exclude payments to health maintenance organizations and other prepaid health plans ($19.3 billion in 1998 and $18 billion in 1997). The total number of persons who were Medicaid eligible and enrolled was 41.4 million in 1998, 41.6 million in 1997, and 41.2 million in 1996 (HCFA Medicaid Statistics, Program and Financial Statistics FY1996, FY1997, and FY1998. unpublished).
[2]Payments exclude disproportionate share hospital payments ($16 billion in 1997 and $15 billion in 1998).
Notes: 1972 and 1975 data are for fiscal year ending June 30. All other years are for fiscal year ending September 30.
SOURCE: *Health, United States, 2000*, National Center for Health Statistics, Hyattsville, MD, 2000

LONG-TERM HEALTH CARE

One of the most pressing and difficult health care problems facing America today is long-term care. Long-term care refers to services needed by individuals with chronic illnesses or mental or physical conditions so severe that they cannot care for themselves on a daily basis. Longer life spans and improved life-sustaining technologies are increasing the possibility that an individual may eventually require costly, long-term care.

Limited and Expensive Options

Caring for chronically ill or elderly patients presents difficult and expensive choices for Americans: either provide long-term care at home or rely on a nursing home. Home health care was the fastest-growing segment of the health care industry in the first half of the 1990s. Although the rate of growth dropped in 1997 and 1998, the home health care sector was expected to more than double, from $29.3 billion to $68 billion, by 2005.

The situation of the disabled elderly who remain at home can be grim. Nine out of 10 disabled elderly persons rely on their families for some degree of care, and 80 percent rely totally on their families, often creating a tremendous financial and emotional drain. Women are usually the caregivers, whether the elderly person is her own parent or her husband's, and sometimes she must give up her job and income to care for elderly dependents. Hiring an unskilled worker to care for the sick or elderly in the home can cost over $25,000 a year; skilled care costs much more.

Nursing homes are an even more costly option. In the late 1990s, one year's stay in a freestanding nursing home averaged $40,000, with actual costs ranging from $20,000 to $80,000, depending on the amount of care required. Lifetime savings are often consumed before the need for care ends, and Medicaid often must pay for the remainder.

In 1998 Americans spent $87.8 billion on nursing homes (both freestanding and hospital-based). About 40 percent of payments came from personal funds and private insurance, and 60 percent from government sources. The HCFA estimated that nursing home expenditures would reach $179.6 billion by 2005 (Sally T. Burner and Daniel R. Waldo, "National Health Expenditure Projections, 1994–2005," *Health Care Financing Review*, Vol. 16, No. 4, Summer 1995).

Of the nearly 1.6 million residents in nursing homes in 1995, approximately 90 percent (1.4 million) were 65 years or older, and 37 percent (557,100) were 85 years or older. According to the U.S. Bureau of the Census projections, the number of nursing home residents aged 85 or over might be two or three times as high by 2040 (Achinta N. Dey, "Characteristics of Elderly Nursing Home Residents: Data from the 1995 National Nursing Home Survey," *Advance Data,* no. 289, July 2, 1997).

The increasing cost of long-term care frightens health care reform advocates. Daniel Callahan, of the Hastings Center, and former Colorado governor Dick Lamm have both argued that, after a natural life span (somewhere in the seventies or eighties), health care should be limited to relieving suffering. Opponents of such reforms believe that the new proposals for rationing will cut off support to the elderly. They fear that rationing for the elderly will happen by age, not by possible benefit to the patient. This, they claim, would be a form of age discrimination that most people would find unacceptable.

AIDS

Although deaths due to the HIV/AIDS epidemic have slowed in the United States since new drugs became available in the late 1990s, the cost of care for patients continues to be expensive. In 1996 the National Institute for Allergy and Infectious Diseases budgeted $1.4 billion for AIDS research. A full-scale clinical trial for an AIDS drug cost between $9 million and $18 million. The cost of AIDS drugs per patient fell between $12,000 and $70,000 a year, depending on the severity of the patient's condition.

In 1988 the average lifetime cost (the treatment cost over the life of the patient) of treating an AIDS patient was $57,000; in 1991 it was $85,333; and because of new, expensive drug therapies, it shot up to $102,000 in 1992, the last year for which this data are available. The yearly cost of treating an HIV-infected patient who has not yet developed AIDS nearly doubled from $5,100 in 1991 to $10,000 in 1992, and ranged from $12,000 to $20,000 in 1998. In comparison, AIDS treatments cost approximately $22,300 per year in Europe, $2,000 in Latin America, and $393 in Africa, although treatment in Latin America and Africa was usually minimal.

The Centers for Disease Control and Prevention no longer tracks annual or lifetime costs of treatments for AIDS patients because treatment costs and patients' life spans now vary widely. The retroviral drugs that bring hope to many AIDS patients are expensive, and not every AIDS patient is able to get them. Furthermore, individual states now have programs in place to help AIDS patients obtain treatment, but the benefits offered vary from state to state.

Federal government spending on HIV-related care and activities has increased steadily since 1985. The Public Health Service reported that federal spending for HIV-related expenses in 1997 exceeded $8.4 billion, $4.8 billion of which was spent on medical care. Other costs financed by taxpayers included research ($1.7 billion), education and prevention ($678 million), and cash assistance ($1.3 billion), which is provided through the Social Security Administration and the U.S. Department of Housing and Urban Development.

Cancer

Cancer, in all its forms, is extremely expensive to treat. Americans often resort to many different methods of treatment in search of a cure. In addition, it can be costly to treat the adverse side effects of radiation, chemotherapy, and other therapies. Pain management is also expensive for cancer patients. The National Cancer Institute estimated the overall annual cost for cancer at $107 billion, of which $37 billion goes for direct costs.

Generally, the younger a patient, the higher the cost, since younger patients can often fight the disease longer than older patients can. Most expenses for cancer treatment occur at the end of life: hospitalization for the initial phase of treatment costs only 38 percent as much as terminal care.

THE HARDSHIP OF HIGH HEALTH CARE COSTS ON FAMILIES

Families USA Foundation is a consumer organization based in Washington, D.C., that is concerned with affordable, quality health care and long-term care for American families. The foundation reported, in *Skyrocketing Health Inflation 1980-1993-2000, the Burden on Families and Businesses* (1993), that American families paid about two-thirds of the nation's health care bill, while American businesses paid the other third. These percentages are based on the premise that families and businesses pay for health care in several ways:

- Directly, through out-of-pocket health payments and insurance expenses, such as premiums, deductibles (annual amounts that must be paid by the employee before the insurance plan begins paying), and copayments.

- Indirectly, through Medicare payroll, income, and other federal, state, and local taxes that support public health programs. These include veterans' health benefits, military health benefits, the Medicaid program, and a variety of smaller public health programs.

Therefore, these estimates of per capita health spending differ from other reports, such as those from the HCFA and the Census Bureau, which take into account only direct payments.

Rising Premiums

In the 1990s the cost of premiums paid by employees in employer-sponsored insurance programs accelerated. In 1988 the average employee contribution for family insurance coverage in a conventional insurance plan was $48 per month, or about one-fourth (24 percent) of the total premium (Jon Gabel et al., "Employer-Sponsored

Health Insurance in America," *Health Affairs,* Vol. 8, No. 1, Spring 1989).

By 1993 the average family-paid premium was $149.48 per month, or 37 percent of the average total monthly premium. This change represented a threefold increase in average family-paid monthly premiums in only five years (Joel C. Cantor et al., "Private Employment-Based Health Insurance in Ten States," *Health Affairs,* Vol. 14, No. 2, Summer 1995). It is not unusual today for union-management negotiations to stall over the issue of what percentage employees should pay toward their health insurance.

Families also purchase insurance themselves when they work for employers who do not offer group health insurance, or when insurers refuse to insure certain groups they consider to be high risk (for example, those with certain chronic diseases, such as asthma). Workers who retire before reaching age 65 and are not eligible for Medicare coverage also must purchase insurance on their own. In addition, many Medicare beneficiaries pay insurance premiums for supplemental (Medigap) insurance to cover the difference in charges that Medicare does not pay, as well as uncovered costs, such as prescription drugs.

Private insurance and Medicare premiums were the fastest-growing elements of family payments from 1980 to 1998. Families also paid for much of their health care directly through copayments and deductibles. (See Chapter 4 for more information about health insurance.) In 1998 out-of-pocket payments made up 17.4 percent of all national health expenditures. In 1995 Americans spent nearly 7 percent of disposable personal income for health insurance premiums, according to the *Source Book of Health Insurance Data—1997* (Health Insurance Association of America, Washington, D.C., 1998).

CHAPTER 3
INTERNATIONAL COMPARISONS OF HEALTH CARE

International comparisons are often difficult to make, because cultures and values differ. What is important in one society may be unimportant in another. A political or human right in one nation may not exist in a neighboring state. The question of quality in health care, for example, may be difficult to measure from one culture to another. Thus, a comparison as subjective as health care should be done with great caution.

A COMPARISON OF SIMILAR COUNTRIES

The 30 member nations of the Organisation for Economic Co-operation and Development (OECD) are generally considered the wealthier, more developed nations in the world. The OECD includes the Western European nations, Canada, the United States, Japan, Australia, New Zealand, Mexico, the Czech Republic, South Korea, Poland, Hungary, and the Slovak Republic (the Slovak Republic joined the OECD in 2000).

Percentage of Gross Domestic Product Spent on Health Care

Although health has always been a concern for Americans, the growth in the health care industry since the mid-1970s has made it a major factor in the American economy. For many years, the United States has spent a larger proportion of its gross domestic product (GDP) on health care than have other nations with similar economic development. From 1975 through 1990, total health care expenditures as a percentage of the U.S. GDP rose from 8 to 12.7 percent. From 1990 to 1996, the ratio rose to 14.2 percent, the highest rate in the OECD. Other nations that spent large percentages of GDP on health care in 1995 and 1996 included Germany (10.5 percent), Switzerland (9.8 percent), France (9.6 percent), and Canada (9.2 percent). Ireland (4.9 percent), Mexico (4.5 percent), and Poland (4.4 percent) spent the least in the OECD. (See Table 3.1.)

TABLE 3.1

Spending on health care: 1990 and 1996

Country	Percent of GDP spent on health		Per capita spending[a] (in U.S. dollars)	
	1990	1996	1990	1996
Australia	8.2%	8.4%	$1,316	$1,776
Austria	7.1	7.9	1,180	1,681
Belgium	7.6	7.9	1,247	1,693
Canada	9.2	9.2	1,691	2,002
Czech Republic	5.5	7.9[b]	538	749[b]
Denmark	6.5	6.4	1,069	1,430
Finland	8.0	7.5	1,292	1,389
France	8.9	9.6	1,539	1,978
Germany	8.2	10.5	1,642	2,222
Greece	4.2	5.9	389	748
Hungary	6.6	6.7	—[c]	—[c]
Iceland	8.0	7.9	1,375	1,839
Ireland	6.6	4.9	748	923
Italy	8.1	7.6	1,322	1,520
Japan	6.0	7.2[b]	1,082	1,581[b]
Korea	3.9	5.3[b]	310	666[b]
Luxembourg	6.6	7.0[b]	1,499	2,206[b]
Mexico	—[c]	4.5	—[c]	384
Netherlands	8.3	8.6	1,325	1,756
New Zealand	7.0	7.2	937	1,251
Norway	7.8	7.9	1,365	1,937
Poland	4.4	4.4	—[c]	—[c]
Portugal	6.5	8.2	616	1,077
Spain	6.9	7.6[b]	813	1,131
Sweden	8.8	7.2[b]	1,492	1,405
Switzerland	8.4	9.8[b]	1,782	2,412b
Turkey	2.5	—[c]	119	—[c]
United Kingdom	6.0	6.9	957	1,304
United States	12.7	14.2	2,689	3,708

Note: GDP is gross domestic product.

[a] Per capita spending is adjusted for purchasing power parities. Purchasing power parities express the rate at which one currency should be converted to another for a given expenditure to purchase the same set of goods and services in both countries.
[b] 1995 data.
[c] Not available.

SOURCE: Gerard F. Anderson, "In Search of Value: An International Comparison of Cost, Access, and Outcomes," *Health Affairs,* 16:6, November/December 1997. The People-to-People Health Foundation, Inc.

TABLE 3.2

Distribution of health care spending: 1990 and 1995

Country	Hospitals		Physicians		Drugs	
	1990	1995	1990	1995	1990	1995
Canada	48%	46%	15%	14%	11%	13%
France	44	44	12	12	17	17
Germany	34	36	17	17	14	13
Italy	45	47	20	21	18	17
Japan	33	29[a]	36	35[a]	21	20[a]
United Kingdom	44	40[a]	—[b]	—[b]	14	16[a]
United States	44	43	21	20	9	8

[a] 1994 data.
[b] Not available.

SOURCE: Gerard F. Anderson, "In Search of Value: An International Comparison of Cost, Access, and Outcomes," *Health Affairs*, 16:6, November/December 1997

The exponential growth in health care spending in the United States during the 1990s was not an international trend, although a number of other countries also experienced rapid increases in the percentage of GDP spent on health care from 1990 to 1995–96. These included the Czech Republic (from 5.5 to 7.9 percent), Germany (from 8.2 to 10.5 percent), Greece (from 4.2 to 5.9 percent) Japan (from 6 to 7.2 percent), South Korea (from 3.9 to 5.3 percent), and Portugal (from 6.5 to 8.2 percent). These countries, however, were spending a relatively small percentage of their GDP on health care in 1990. Six countries—Denmark, Finland, Iceland, Ireland, Italy, and Sweden—spent less of their GDP on health care in 1996 than they did in 1990. The majority of other countries experienced small increases. (See Table 3.1.)

Per Capita Spending on Health Care

In 1996 the United States also enjoyed the highest per capita spending for health care services, spending an average of $3,708 per citizen (that number had risen to $4,094 by 1998). No other country came close to spending that amount per capita in 1995 and 1996: Switzerland spent $2,412 per citizen; Germany spent $2,222; Luxembourg spent $2,206; and Canada spent $2,002. In 1995 South Korea spent the least of any OECD nation on health care: 5.3 percent of its GDP and $666 per capita. (See Table 3.1.)

Proportional Spending on Health Care

In 1995, in a ranking of the proportion of health care resources spent on hospitals, the United States, at 43 percent, placed in the middle of the Group of 7 (G7) nations, a group of countries (which originally consisted of Canada, France, Germany, Italy, Japan, the United Kingdom, and the United States, and later included Russia, thereby becoming the G8) whose representatives meet to discuss economic concerns. Canada and France used the largest chunk of their health care dollars on hospitals (46 and 44 percent, respectively), while Japan spent the least (29 percent).

Of all the G7 nations, the United States spent the third-highest proportion on physicians (20 percent), after Japan and Italy. (Japan consistently spent the highest percentage on physicians: 35 percent in 1994.) France spent the least: only 12 percent of its overall health care spending went to its physicians.

Only 8 percent of U.S. health care resources was spent on drugs. This number was considerably lower than any other industrialized country. Japan had the highest distribution of drug spending in 1994, at 20 percent. Germany and Canada also used relatively small proportions of their overall spending on drugs, at 13 percent each. (See Table 3.2.)

Hospitalization Statistics

Of all the G7 countries, Japan had the highest number of inpatient hospital beds in 1990 and 1994 (16 and 16.2 beds per 1,000 population respectively). This is probably because Japan does not distinguish between acute and long-term care beds. Germany had the next-highest number of beds, at 9.7 per 1,000 population in 1995. The United States had the lowest, 4.1 in 1995, and the United Kingdom and Canada followed with 4.7 and 5.1 beds, respectively, per 1,000 population. (See Table 3.3.)

Japan also had the longest average hospital stay, by far, of all the G7 nations: 45.5 days in 1995, down from 50.5 days in 1990. This compares with 14.2 days in Germany and 12.2 days in Canada. The United States permitted its patients to stay in the hospital for the fewest average days of any country: 8 days in 1995. (See Table 3.3.) These figures included stays in community hospitals, federal hospitals, and psychiatric hospitals.

France had the highest hospitalization rate of any of the G7 nations. More than one in five of its citizens—22.7 percent—were admitted to a hospital in 1995. Germany and the United Kingdom also had relatively high hospital-

TABLE 3.3

Inpatient hospital data: A comparison of G7 member nations: 1990 and 1995

Country	Inpatient hospital beds per 1,000 population		Average length-of-stay (days)[a]		Percent of population admitted		Hospital staffing ratios[b]	
	1990	1995	1990	1995	1990	1995	1990	1995
Canada	6.2	5.1	13.0	12.2	13.6%	12.5%[c]	2.8	—[d]
France	9.7	8.9	13.3	11.2	23.2	22.7	1.09	1.05
Germany	10.4	9.7	16.7	14.2	19.0	20.7	—[d]	1.95
Italy	7.2	6.4	11.7	10.5	15.5	16.0[e]	1.5	1.67[e]
Japan	16.0	16.2[e]	50.5	45.5	8.2	8.9[e]	0.88	0.88[e]
United Kingdom	5.9	4.7	15.6	9.9	18.4	20.8	3.1	—[d]
United States	4.7	4.1	9.1	8.0	13.7	12.4	3.435	—[d]

Note: G7 refers to the Group of Seven industrialized nations.
[a] Includes community hospitals, federal hospitals, and psychiatric hospitals.
[b] Acute care hospitals only.
[c] 1993 data.
[d] Not available.
[e] 1994 data.

SOURCE: Gerard F. Anderson, "In Search of Value: An International Comparison of Cost, Access, and Outcomes," *Health Affairs,*16:6, November/December 1997

ization rates: 20.7 and 20.8 percent, respectively. Japan had the lowest rate, at 8.9 percent. Approximately 13.7 percent of the U.S. population was hospitalized in 1995.

OVERVIEWS OF SELECTED HEALTH CARE SYSTEMS

In 1992 a group of academics examined the operation of health systems in the United States and several other developed countries. The authors studied the methods of financing and providing health care in the United States, Germany, Canada, the United Kingdom, France, and Japan, and issued a detailed report on the differences between the systems (George Schieber, Jean-Pierre Poullier, and Leslie Greenwald, "U.S. Health Expenditure Performance: An International Comparison and Data Update," *Health Care Financing Review,* Summer 1992). Although some aspects of those systems have changed since 1992, the essential models remain the same. Summaries from this article follow, with updates since the article was written.

United States

The U.S. health care financing system is based on the consumer sovereignty, or private insurance, model. There are more than 1,000 private insurance companies in the United States. Employer-based health insurance is tax-subsidized: health insurance premiums are a tax-deductible business expense but are not taxed as employee compensation. Individually purchased policies are partially tax-subsidized for self-employed Americans. Benefits, premiums, and provider reimbursement methods differ among private insurance plans, and among public programs as well.

Physicians who provide both office visits and inpatient care are generally reimbursed on a fee-for-service basis, and payment rates vary among insurers. Hospitals are paid on the basis of charges, costs, negotiated rates, or diagnosis-related groups, depending on the patient's insurer. There are no overall global budgets or expenditure limits. Nevertheless, managed care (oversight by some group or authority to verify the medical necessity of treatments and to control the cost of health care) has played an increasing role. Health maintenance organizations and health insurance companies now exert greater control over the practices of individual doctors, in an effort to control costs.

A growing number of doctors are finding their decisions and fees open to question by insurers, and health insurance companies may deny coverage for a procedure selected by the physician. Many doctors are joining group practices or organizations, or are being forced to lower their fees so they can treat patients covered by large insurers.

In 1996 there were 6,201 hospitals in the United States: 290 federal hospitals and 5,911 nonfederal hospitals. About 59 percent of nonfederal community hospitals were nonprofit; 15 percent were proprietary (privately owned); and 26 percent were operated by state and local governments. Increasingly, hospitals are being absorbed into for-profit operations.

Germany

The German health care system is based on the social insurance model. Statutory sickness funds and private insurance cover the entire population. Approximately 1,200 sickness funds cover about 88 percent of the population. Employees and employers finance these sickness funds through payroll contributions. Almost all employers, including small businesses and low-wage industries, must participate.

In the mid-1990s, contributions to sickness funds averaged about 13 percent of a worker's salary. About 9 percent of sickness fund members purchased complementary private insurance. Another 7 percent of the population chose not to participate in the public system and were fully covered by private insurance. Seventy-three percent of all health expenditures were public, and about 11 percent were direct, out-of-pocket payments. Under the sickness funds, losing or changing jobs does not affect health insurance protection.

Ambulatory (outpatient) and inpatient care are completely separate in the German health care system. German hospitals generally do not have outpatient departments. Ambulatory care physicians are paid on the basis of fee schedules negotiated between the organizations of sickness funds and organizations of physicians. A separate fee schedule for private patients uses a similar scale. Hospitals were previously paid on the basis of negotiated per diem (or length of stay) payments, but the 1993 Health Care Reform law (see below) instituted a sliding scale based on specific fees for specific procedures.

Public (federal, state, and local) hospitals account for about 51 percent of hospital beds; private voluntary hospitals, often run by religious organizations, account for 35 percent of beds; and private for-profit hospitals, generally owned by physicians, account for 14 percent. Ambulatory care physicians are generally self-employed professionals, while most hospital-based physicians are salaried employees of the hospital.

On January 1, 1993, Germany's new Health Care Reform law went into effect. Among its many provisions, the new law tied increases in physician, dental, and hospital expenditures to the income growth rate of members of the sickness funds. This limited the licensing of new ambulatory care physicians (based on the number of physicians already in an area) and set a cap for overall pharmaceutical outlays. It also changed the hospital compensation system from per diem payments to specific fees for individual procedures and conditions. The government was also trying to limit what it considered excessive health benefits, such as cutting back on how often a patient might visit a health spa to recuperate.

Canada

The Canadian system has been characterized as a provincial government health insurance model, in which each of the 10 provinces runs its own health system under general federal rules and with a fixed federal contribution. Entitlement to benefits is linked to residency, and the system is financed through general taxation. Private insurance is prohibited from covering the same benefits covered by the public system. More than 60 percent of Canadians, however, are covered by complementary private policies. Seventy-three percent of all health expendi-

tures are public, and consumers pay an estimated 20 percent of health care expenditures out of pocket.

In Canada, all citizens have equal access to medical care, regardless of their ability to pay. Canadian health insurance covers all medically necessary services, including hospital care and physician services. Some provinces also cover preventive services, routine dental care for children, and outpatient drugs for the elderly and the poor. No restrictions are placed on a patient's choice of physicians. For some time, the government reimbursed patients in full for hospital treatment and doctors' services. Now, however, individuals incur additional out-of-pocket expenses for services such as adult dental care, cosmetic surgery, and private or semiprivate hospital rooms. Many Canadians purchase additional health insurance to cover these charges.

Hospitals are funded on the basis of global budgets, and physicians in both inpatient and outpatient settings are paid on a negotiated, fee-for-service basis. (A global budget is one that authorizes a lump sum of money to a large department or area. Then all the groups in that department or area must negotiate to see how much of the total money each group receives.) The systems vary somewhat from province to province, and certain provinces, such as Quebec, have also established global budgets for physician services. The federal government's share of spending has progressively declined, from a historic high of 50 percent to 38 percent in 1990, 30 percent in 1993, and less than 20 percent in 1997. The delivery system is composed largely of nonprofit community hospitals and self-employed physicians. About 95 percent of Canadian hospital beds are public; private hospitals do not participate in the public insurance program.

FINANCIAL PROBLEMS. In the 1990s public revenues did not increase fast enough in Canada to cover rising health care costs. The Canadian government attributed many of the financial problems to lower revenue from taxes, higher prices for medical technology, relatively lengthy hospital stays, and too many doctors paid on a fee-for-service basis. In 1993, for the first time since Canada instituted universal health insurance 27 years earlier, Canadians had to pay for common services such as strep throat tests.

As a result of cutbacks and inadequate equipment, waiting times for nonemergency surgery, such as hip replacement, and high-technology diagnostic tools, such as computerized axial tomography (CAT scans), could amount to months, or even years. Although Canadians generally still support their present system, there has been growing dissatisfaction with the rising costs and long waiting periods among both patients and doctors.

THE SAFETY VALVE TO THE SOUTH. Some Canadians have begun to cross the border to avoid the lines in their hospitals. Canadian doctors sometimes refer their more seriously ill patients who need immediate attention to American hospitals in such cities as nearby Buffalo, New York; Cleveland, Ohio; and Detroit, Michigan. In fact, many American hospitals have begun to market medical services, most notably cardiac care and addiction treatment, to the Canadian public. Overall, however, there has been very little border-jumping. Canadians accounted for less than 1 percent of total admissions in each of the nine border hospitals surveyed by the American Medical Association.

CUTTING COSTS. The general consensus is that no one wants to disassemble what has become Canada's most popular social program, but most agree that change is inevitable. The Ontario Health Insurance Plan insures 10 million people, or almost 40 percent of all Canadians. They have managed to cut costs in several ways:

- Reducing fees to commercial laboratories and allowing them to bill patients directly for tests performed.

- Stopping payment for certain services connected with employment. For example, someone who needs a physical examination to qualify for a job must pay for it.

- Ending coverage of electrolysis (removal of unwanted hair) and reviewing coverage of such items as psychoanalysis, vasectomies, newborn circumcision, in vitro fertilization, and chiropractic, podiatric, and osteopathic services.

- Increasing the amount that patients must pay for prescriptions covered under the Ontario Drug Benefit Plan, which is used mainly by persons over age 65.

Similarly, in an effort to cut hospital costs, British Columbia was moving to shift some services away from hospitals to outpatient clinics, public health programs, and home care. Canadian officials hoped that cutbacks in covered services and caps on doctors' fees and hospital budgets could keep the popular health care system afloat.

United Kingdom

The United Kingdom employs the National Health Service, or Beveridge, model to finance and deliver health care. The entire population is covered under a system that is financed mainly from general taxation. There is minimal cost sharing. About 15 percent of the population also purchases private insurance as a supplement to the public system. Eighty-four percent of all health spending is from public funds, and about 4 percent of all spending represents direct, out-of-pocket payments.

Services are organized and managed by regional and local public authorities. General practitioners serve as primary care physicians and are reimbursed on the basis of a combination of capitation payments (payments for each person served), fees, and other allowances. Hospitals receive overall budget allotments from district health authorities, and hospital-based physicians are salaried.

Private insurance reimburses both physicians and hospitals on a fee-for-service basis.

Self-employed general practitioners are considered independent contractors, and salaried hospital-based physicians are public employees. Of the United Kingdom's hospital beds, 90 percent are public and generally owned by the National Health Service. As of 1991, it became possible for large physician practices to become "budget holders," and receive a larger capitation payment. Similarly, individual hospitals may become "self-governing trust hospitals," whereby they may compete for patients and sell their services. While emergency health service is immediate, persons needing elective surgery, such as hip replacement, may end up on a waiting list for years.

France

The French health care system is based on the social insurance, or Bismarck, model. Virtually the entire population is covered by a legislated, compulsory health insurance plan that is financed through the social security system. Three major programs, and several smaller ones, are quasi-autonomous, nongovernmental bodies. The system is financed through employee and employer payroll tax contributions. More than 80 percent of the population supplements their public benefits by purchasing insurance from private, nonprofit *mutuels,* and about 2 percent of the population has private commercial insurance.

The public share of total health spending is 74 percent, and about 17 percent of expenditures represent direct, out-of-pocket payments. Physicians practicing in municipal health centers and public hospitals are salaried, but physicians in private hospitals and in ambulatory care settings are typically paid on a negotiated, fee-for-service basis. Public hospitals are granted lump-sum budgets, and private hospitals are paid on the basis of negotiated per diem payment rates. About 65 percent of hospital beds are public, while the remaining 35 percent are private (and equally divided between profit and nonprofit).

In April 1996, the French government announced major reforms aimed at containing rising costs in the national health care system. The new system would monitor each patient's total health costs and penalize doctors if they overran their budgets for specific types of care and prescriptions. In addition, French citizens would be required to consult general practitioners before going to specialists. Doctors—specialists, in particular—denounced the reforms and warned that they could lead to rationing and low-quality health care.

Japan

Japan's health care financing is also based on the social insurance model and, in particular, on the German health care system. Three general schemes cover the entire population: Employee Health Insurance, Communi-

TABLE 3.4

Infant mortality and life expectancy, OECD countries: 1990 and 1995

Country	Infant mortality per 1,000 live births		Life expectancy at birth, males (years)		Life expectancy at birth, females (years)	
	1990	1995	1990	1995	1990	1995
Australia	8.2	5.7	73.9	75.0	80.1	80.9
Austria	7.8	5.4	72.3	73.5	78.9	80.1
Belgium	8.0	7.0	72.4	73.3	79.1	80.0
Canada	6.8	6.0	73.8	75.3	80.4	81.3
Czech Republic	10.8	7.7	67.5	70.0	76.0	76.9
Denmark	7.5	5.5	72.0	72.5	77.7	77.8
Finland	5.6	4.0	70.9	72.8	78.9	80.2
France	7.3	5.0	72.7	73.9	80.9	81.9
Germany	7.1	5.3	72.7	73.0	79.1	79.5
Greece	9.7	8.1	74.6	75.1	79.4	80.3
Hungary	15.0	11.0	65.1	65.3	73.7	74.5
Iceland	5.9	6.1	75.7	76.5	80.3	80.6
Ireland	8.2	6.3	72.0	72.9	77.5	78.5
Italy	8.2	6.2	73.5	74.4	80.0	80.8
Japan	4.6	4.3	75.9	76.4	81.9	82.8
Korea	13.0	9.0	67.4	70.0	75.4	76.0
Luxembourg	7.4	5.0	72.3	72.5	78.5	79.5
Mexico	24.0	16.5	67.7	69.5	74.0	76.0
Netherlands	7.1	5.5	73.8	74.6	80.1	80.4
New Zealand	8.4	7.0	72.4	73.8	78.3	79.2
Norway	7.0	4.0	73.4	74.8	79.8	80.8
Poland	19.3	13.6	66.5	67.6	75.5	76.4
Portugal	11.0	7.4	70.9	71.5	77.9	78.6
Spain	7.6	5.5	73.4	73.2	80.5	81.2
Sweden	6.0	4.1	74.8	76.2	80.4	81.5
Switzerland	6.8	5.0	74.0	75.3	80.9	81.7
Turkey	59.3	45.0	64.1	65.4[a]	68.4	70.0[a]
United Kingdom	7.9	6.0	72.9	74.3	78.6	79.7
United States	9.2	8.0	71.8	72.5	78.8	79.2

[a] 1994 data.

SOURCE: Gerard F. Anderson, "In Search of Value: An International Comparison of Cost, Access, and Outcomes," *Health Affairs,* 16:6, November/December 1997

ty Health Insurance, and Health and Medical Services for the Aged. About 62 percent of the population receives coverage through about 1,800 employer-sponsored plans. Small businesses, the self-employed, and farmers are covered through Community Health Insurance, which is administered by a conglomeration of local governmental and private bodies. The elderly are covered by a separate plan that largely pools funds from the other plans. The emphasis is on the government, not business, bearing the major financial burden for the nation's health care.

The system is financed through employer and employee income-related premiums. There are different levels of public subsidization of the three different schemes. Limited private insurance exists for supplemental coverage. Public expenditures account for 72 percent of total health spending, while out-of-pocket expenses account for about 12 percent.

Physicians and hospitals are paid on the basis of national, negotiated fee schedules. Physicians practicing in public hospitals are salaried, while those practicing in physician-owned clinics and private hospitals are reimbursed on a fee-for-service basis. The amount paid for each medical procedure is rigidly controlled. Physicians prescribe and dispense pharmaceuticals. Perhaps because of this, the Japanese take about 50 percent more drugs than Americans do.

A close doctor–patient relationship is unusual in Japan; the typical doctor tries to see as many patients as possible in a day in order to earn a living. A patient going to a clinic for treatment may have to wait many hours in a very crowded facility. As a result, health care is rarely a joint doctor–patient effort. Instead, doctors tend to dictate treatment without fully informing patients of their conditions or of the drugs and therapy that have been prescribed.

About 80 percent of Japan's hospitals are privately operated (and often physician-owned) and the remaining 20 percent are public. For-profit hospitals are prohibited. Hospital stays are typically far longer than in the United States, or any other G7 country, allowing hospitals and doctors to overcome the limitations of the fee schedules.

Despite the limitations of Japan's health care system, Japanese men and women had the longest life expectancy in the world in 1995: 82.8 years for women and 76.4 years for men. The Japanese infant mortality rate in 1995, at 4.3 per 1,000 live births, was the lowest in the world. (See Table 3.4.) These two statistics are usually considered reliable indicators of a successful medical system. It must be noted, though, that Japan does not have a large impoverished class, as does the United States, and its diet is among the healthiest in the world.

CHAPTER 4

INSURANCE—THOSE WITH AND THOSE WITHOUT

In 1798 Congress established the U.S. Marine Hospital Services for seamen. It was the first time an employer offered health insurance in the United States. Payments for hospital services were deducted from the sailors' salaries.

Today, many factors affect the availability of health insurance, including employment, income, and age. As a result, an individual's or family's health insurance status often changes as circumstances change. In 1999, 7 of every 10 Americans (71 percent) were covered during all or some part of the year by private insurance, mostly through their employers (62.8 percent). Medicare, the government's health insurance program for elderly and disabled persons, covered 13.2 percent of Americans, and Medicaid, the government's health insurance program for the poor, covered 10.2 percent. Note that percentages total more than 100 percent because some persons are covered by more than one type of insurance program. (See Figure 4.1.)

In 1998, 15.5 percent of the American population was without health coverage during the entire year, down from 16.3 percent in 1998. This marked the first time since 1987 that the share of the population without health insurance declined. In the 11-year period from 1987 (the first year comparable health statistics were available) to 1998, the uninsured rate either increased or remained unchanged from one year to the next. The number of uninsured children also dropped between 1998 and 1999, from 15.4 percent to 13.9 percent (Robert J. Mills, *Current Population Reports 1999,* U.S. Census Bureau, September 2000).

WHO WAS UNINSURED IN 1999?

The poor were the income group most likely to be without insurance coverage. In 1999, 32.4 percent of the nation's poor went without insurance. Across every demo-

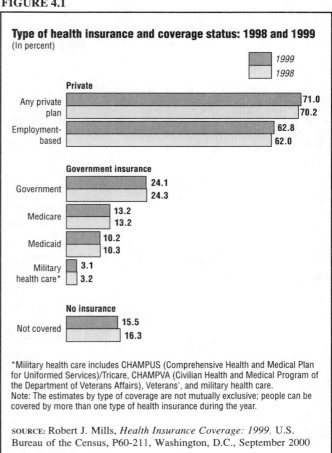

FIGURE 4.1

Type of health insurance and coverage status: 1998 and 1999
(In percent)

1999
1998

Private

Any private plan — 71.0 / 70.2
Employment-based — 62.8 / 62.0

Government insurance

Government — 24.1 / 24.3
Medicare — 13.2 / 13.2
Medicaid — 10.2 / 10.3
Military health care* — 3.1 / 3.2

No insurance

Not covered — 15.5 / 16.3

*Military health care includes CHAMPUS (Comprehensive Health and Medical Plan for Uniformed Services)/Tricare, CHAMPVA (Civilian Health and Medical Program of the Department of Veterans Affairs), Veterans', and military health care.
Note: The estimates by type of coverage are not mutually exclusive; people can be covered by more than one type of health insurance during the year.

SOURCE: Robert J. Mills, *Health Insurance Coverage: 1999,* U.S. Bureau of the Census, P60-211, Washington, D.C., September 2000

graphic category—age, race, citizenship status, education, and work experience—higher proportions of the poor went uninsured in 1999.

Gender, Age, and Race/Ethnicity

More males than females lacked insurance in 1999—16.5 percent of males lacked insurance, compared to 14.6 percent of females. As would be expected,

FIGURE 4.2

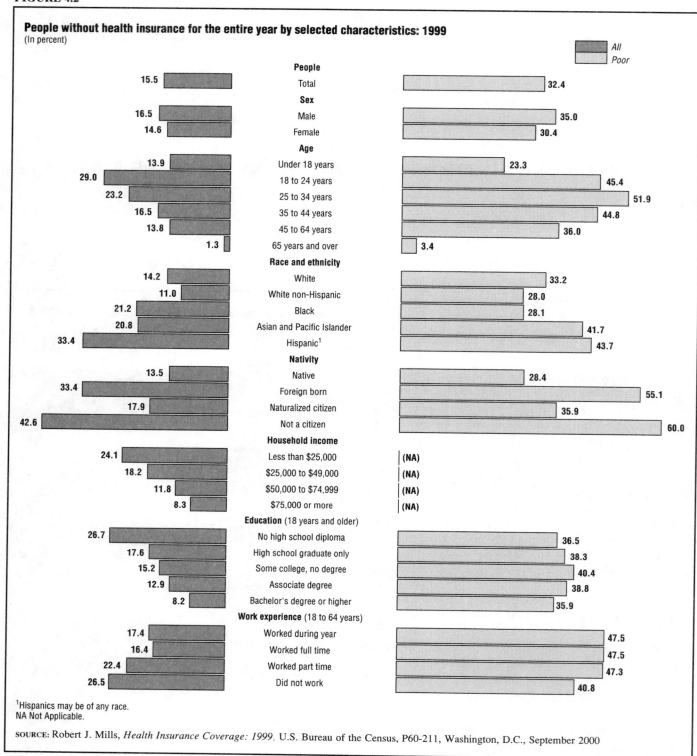

People without health insurance for the entire year by selected characteristics: 1999
(In percent)

Legend: All (dark), Poor (light)

People
- Total: 15.5 | 32.4

Sex
- Male: 16.5 | 35.0
- Female: 14.6 | 30.4

Age
- Under 18 years: 13.9 | 23.3
- 18 to 24 years: 29.0 | 45.4
- 25 to 34 years: 23.2 | 51.9
- 35 to 44 years: 16.5 | 44.8
- 45 to 64 years: 13.8 | 36.0
- 65 years and over: 1.3 | 3.4

Race and ethnicity
- White: 14.2 | 33.2
- White non-Hispanic: 11.0 | 28.0
- Black: 21.2 | 28.1
- Asian and Pacific Islander: 20.8 | 41.7
- Hispanic[1]: 33.4 | 43.7

Nativity
- Native: 13.5 | 28.4
- Foreign born: 33.4 | 55.1
- Naturalized citizen: 17.9 | 35.9
- Not a citizen: 42.6 | 60.0

Household income
- Less than $25,000: 24.1 | (NA)
- $25,000 to $49,000: 18.2 | (NA)
- $50,000 to $74,999: 11.8 | (NA)
- $75,000 or more: 8.3 | (NA)

Education (18 years and older)
- No high school diploma: 26.7 | 36.5
- High school graduate only: 17.6 | 38.3
- Some college, no degree: 15.2 | 40.4
- Associate degree: 12.9 | 38.8
- Bachelor's degree or higher: 8.2 | 35.9

Work experience (18 to 64 years)
- Worked during year: 17.4 | 47.5
- Worked full time: 16.4 | 47.5
- Worked part time: 22.4 | 47.3
- Did not work: 26.5 | 40.8

[1]Hispanics may be of any race.
NA Not Applicable.

SOURCE: Robert J. Mills, *Health Insurance Coverage: 1999*, U.S. Bureau of the Census, P60-211, Washington, D.C., September 2000

those aged 65 and over were most likely to be covered by insurance, since almost all of them qualified for Medicare (and possibly Medicaid also). Only 1.3 percent of the elderly went without health insurance in 1999. Persons 18 to 24 years of age had the least insurance coverage—29 percent of Americans in that age group lacked health insurance in 1999. Hispanics were most likely to be uninsured (33.4 percent), followed by blacks (21.2 percent), and Asians and Pacific Islanders (20.8 percent). Only 11 percent of non-Hispanic whites had no coverage. (See Figure 4.2.)

While only 13.5 percent of native-born Americans went without coverage, 33.4 percent of foreign-born per-

FIGURE 4.3

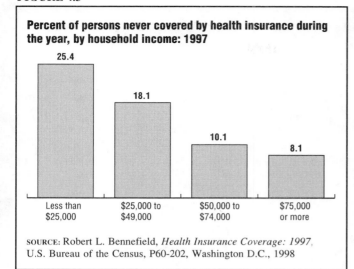

Percent of persons never covered by health insurance during the year, by household income: 1997

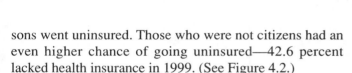

SOURCE: Robert L. Bennefield, *Health Insurance Coverage: 1997*, U.S. Bureau of the Census, P60-202, Washington D.C., 1998

FIGURE 4.4

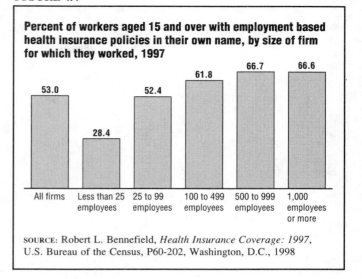

Percent of workers aged 15 and over with employment based health insurance policies in their own name, by size of firm for which they worked, 1997

SOURCE: Robert L. Bennefield, *Health Insurance Coverage: 1997*, U.S. Bureau of the Census, P60-202, Washington, D.C., 1998

sons went uninsured. Those who were not citizens had an even higher chance of going uninsured—42.6 percent lacked health insurance in 1999. (See Figure 4.2.)

Effects of Education Level, Income, and Employment

Education levels and health coverage are closely related. Generally, the better educated a person, the more likely he or she is to have a job with health insurance and other benefits. In 1999 those who had not completed high school were more than three times as likely to be uninsured as those who held bachelor's degrees (26.7 percent versus 8.2 percent). (See Figure 4.2.)

As household income increases, the chances of being uninsured drop dramatically. Figure 4.3 shows the 1997 percentages of uninsured persons according to income level. While only 8.1 percent of individuals with an income of $75,000 or more lacked insurance, one-fourth (25.4 percent) of those with incomes under $25,000 were uninsured. The same was true in 1999—only 8.3 percent of high-income individuals were uninsured, while 24.1 percent of Americans in the lowest income bracket went without insurance.

Not surprisingly, persons who worked full-time were most likely to have health insurance. In 1999 about 16.4 percent of full-time workers were uninsured, compared to 22.4 percent of part-time workers and 26.5 percent of those who did not work. Among the poor population, however, the proportions of uninsured workers were considerably higher. (See Figure 4.2.)

Large companies were more likely to provide health insurance coverage than were smaller firms. (See Figure 4.4.) Many small firms cannot afford health insurance for their employees. Insurers charge higher premiums for small firms because of the higher administrative costs of small groups.

SOURCES OF HEALTH INSURANCE

Persons under Age 65

For persons under age 65, there are two sources of health insurance coverage: private insurance (from employers or private policies) and Medicaid (the government program for low-income or disabled persons). From 1984 to 1997, the proportion of those covered by private insurance declined, while the percentage covered by Medicaid and the proportion of uninsured increased.

In 1997 the National Center for Health Statistics estimated that about 70.9 percent of the under-65 population had private health policies, with 65.1 percent covered through the workplace. These figures were down from 77.1 percent (69.2 through the workplace) 13 years before. In 1997 about 9.6 percent had Medicaid coverage, up from 6.7 percent in 1984. Persons under 65 without health insurance accounted for 17.4 percent of the population in 1997, up from 14.3 percent in 1984. (See Table 4.1.)

There are three major factors contributing to the long-term decline in private health insurance. The first is the rising cost of health care, which frequently leads to greater cost-sharing between employers and employees. Some workers can simply no longer afford the higher premiums and copayments (the share of medical bills the employee pays). A second factor is the shift in American commerce from the goods-producing sector, where health benefits have traditionally been provided, to the service sector, where many employers do not offer health insurance.

A third factor is the changing nature of the relationship between employer and employee. In the past, many companies took a paternalistic (fatherly) approach to employee welfare to promote both a healthy workforce

TABLE 4.1

Health care coverage for persons under 65 years of age, according to type of coverage and selected characteristics: selected years 1984–97

Characteristic	Private insurance						Private insurance obtained through workplace[1]					
	1984	1989	1994[2]	1995	1996	1997[2,3]	1984	1989	1994[2]	1995	1996	1997[2,3]
						Number in millions						
Total[4]	157.5	162.7	160.7	165.0	165.9	165.8	141.8	146.3	146.7	151.4	151.4	152.5
						Percent of population						
Total, age adjusted[4,5]	77.1	76.2	70.7	71.9	71.6	70.9	69.2	68.4	64.5	66.0	65.3	65.1
Total, crude[4]	76.8	75.9	70.3	71.6	71.4	70.7	69.1	68.3	64.2	65.7	65.1	65.0
Age												
Under 18 years	72.6	71.8	63.8	65.7	66.4	66.1	66.5	65.8	59.0	60.9	61.1	61.4
Under 6 years	68.1	67.9	58.3	60.1	61.1	61.3	62.1	62.3	53.9	55.6	56.5	57.3
6–17 years	74.9	74.0	66.8	68.7	69.1	68.5	68.7	67.7	61.8	63.7	63.4	63.4
18–44 years	76.5	75.5	69.8	71.2	70.6	69.4	69.6	68.4	63.9	65.6	64.7	64.4
18–24 years	67.4	64.5	58.3	61.2	60.4	59.3	58.7	55.3	50.7	53.9	52.3	53.8
25–34 years	77.4	75.9	69.4	70.3	69.5	68.1	71.2	69.5	64.1	65.3	64.4	63.6
35–44 years	83.9	82.7	77.1	78.0	77.5	76.4	77.4	76.2	71.6	72.9	72.0	71.2
45–64 years	83.3	82.5	80.3	80.4	79.5	79.0	71.8	71.6	71.8	72.4	71.4	70.8
45–54 years	83.3	83.4	81.3	81.1	80.4	80.4	74.6	74.4	74.6	74.9	74.0	73.6
55–64 years	83.3	81.6	78.8	79.3	78.1	76.9	69.0	68.3	67.9	68.6	67.5	66.6
Sex[5]												
Male	77.7	76.5	71.2	72.3	72.0	71.2	70.1	68.9	65.0	66.5	65.8	65.4
Female	76.5	75.9	70.2	71.6	71.3	70.6	68.4	67.9	64.0	65.4	64.9	64.9
Race[5,6]												
White	80.1	79.3	74.1	74.9	74.6	74.3	72.0	71.2	67.4	68.8	67.9	68.0
Black	59.2	58.7	53.0	55.6	56.2	56.1	53.3	53.6	50.2	51.8	53.0	53.7
Asian or Pacific Islander	70.9	71.6	67.9	68.8	68.3	68.2	64.4	60.2	57.8	60.2	59.4	60.5
Hispanic origin and race[5,6]												
All Hispanic	57.1	53.2	49.4	48.3	48.4	47.9	52.9	48.6	45.1	44.9	44.6	44.5
Mexican	54.9	48.5	46.4	44.7	44.4	43.9	51.7	45.6	44.3	42.7	41.5	41.8
Puerto Rican	51.0	46.8	49.5	49.1	52.5	48.2	48.3	43.4	46.3	45.9	49.9	45.5
Cuban	72.1	70.0	63.7	63.4	65.7	70.7	57.6	56.3	45.7	53.8	54.8	55.9
Other Hispanic	62.0	62.4	53.1	53.1	53.4	51.2	57.7	55.7	47.1	47.9	48.4	47.6
White, non-Hispanic	82.4	82.5	77.7	78.9	78.6	78.0	74.0	74.0	70.7	72.3	71.5	71.4
Black, non-Hispanic	59.4	58.8	53.4	56.1	56.7	56.3	53.4	53.7	50.6	52.3	53.3	53.9
Age and percent of poverty level[7]												
All ages:[5]												
Below 100 percent	33.0	27.5	22.3	22.7	20.7	23.6	23.8	19.7	16.8	17.7	15.8	19.6
100–149 percent	61.8	54.2	46.6	47.7	46.8	42.0	51.1	45.0	40.6	41.7	40.4	36.8
150–199 percent	77.2	70.6	65.2	66.1	67.1	63.6	68.6	61.9	58.3	60.0	60.0	58.1
200 percent or more	91.6	91.0	88.8	89.1	89.3	87.6	85.0	83.9	82.7	83.4	83.0	82.0
Under 18 years:												
Below 100 percent	28.7	22.3	14.9	16.8	16.1	17.5	23.2	17.5	12.4	13.4	13.4	15.4
100–149 percent	66.2	59.6	47.8	48.5	49.5	42.5	58.3	52.5	43.2	43.6	43.7	38.4
150–199 percent	80.9	75.9	69.3	68.5	73.0	66.8	75.8	70.1	64.0	63.0	67.4	63.1
200 percent or more	92.3	92.7	89.7	90.4	90.7	88.9	86.9	86.7	84.5	85.5	84.6	83.7
Geographic region[5]												
Northeast	80.7	82.1	75.3	75.7	75.5	74.3	74.1	75.1	70.0	70.1	69.2	69.7
Midwest	80.9	81.7	77.7	77.8	78.8	77.3	72.1	73.4	71.4	71.6	72.6	71.4
South	74.5	71.7	66.0	67.6	66.7	67.5	66.2	63.8	60.0	62.4	61.0	61.6
West	72.3	71.8	66.0	68.5	67.7	65.8	64.9	64.2	58.8	61.2	60.1	59.4
Location of residence[5]												
Within MSA[8]	77.8	76.8	71.3	72.8	73.0	71.5	71.0	69.8	65.5	67.2	67.0	66.0
Outside MSA[8]	75.5	74.0	68.7	68.3	66.4	68.5	65.3	63.5	60.8	61.0	59.0	61.7

and employee loyalty. Today, many companies feel less responsibility for their workers and consider cutting the cost of health care a good way to cut expenditures ("Sources of Health Insurance and Characteristics of the Uninsured," *EBRI Issue Brief,* no. 170, February 1996).

RACE AND ETHNICITY. In the under-65 age group, more than three-fourths of non-Hispanic whites (78 percent) had private health insurance in 1997, down from 82.4 percent in 1984. A little over half (56.3 percent) of non-Hispanic blacks had private policies in 1997, while 59.4 percent were insured in 1984. In 1997 two-thirds (68.2 percent) of Asians and Pacific Islanders (APIs) had private policies. The pro-

portion of privately insured APIs also declined from 1984, when 70.9 percent held private coverage.

The most dramatic drop in private coverage was among Hispanics. In 1997 less than half (47.9 percent) of Hispanic Americans had private coverage, down from 57.1 percent in 1984. (See Table 4.1.)

INCOME AND LOCATION. Not surprisingly, persons under 65 with higher incomes in 1997 were more likely to have private health insurance. All income levels, however, were less likely to have private insurance than in 1984. In 1984, 33 percent of individuals living at or below the

TABLE 4.1

Health care coverage for persons under 65 years of age, according to type of coverage and selected characteristics: selected years 1984–97 [CONTINUED]

Characteristic	Medicaid[9]						Not covered[10]					
	1984	1989	1994[2]	1995	1996	1997[2,3]	1984	1989	1994[2]	1995	1996	1997[2,3]
	Number in millions											
Total[4]	14.0	15.4	24.1	25.3	25.0	22.9	29.8	33.4	40.4	37.4	38.9	41.0
	Percent of population											
Total, age adjusted[4,5]	6.7	7.1	10.3	10.8	10.5	9.6	14.3	15.3	17.4	16.0	16.6	17.4
Total, crude[4]	6.8	7.2	10.6	11.0	10.8	9.7	14.5	15.6	17.7	16.2	16.7	17.5
Age												
Under 18 years	11.9	12.6	20.0	20.6	20.1	18.4	13.9	14.7	15.3	13.6	13.4	14.0
Under 6 years	15.5	15.7	27.2	28.3	27.4	24.7	14.9	15.1	13.7	11.9	11.9	12.5
6–17 years	10.1	10.9	16.2	16.6	16.4	15.2	13.4	14.5	16.2	14.5	14.1	14.7
18–44 years	5.1	5.2	7.3	7.4	7.3	6.6	17.1	18.4	21.9	20.5	21.2	22.4
18–24 years	6.4	6.8	9.6	9.7	9.2	8.8	25.0	27.1	31.1	28.2	29.6	30.1
25–34 years	5.3	5.2	7.7	7.7	7.5	6.8	16.2	18.3	22.1	21.3	22.5	23.8
35–44 years	3.5	4.0	5.4	5.6	6.0	5.2	11.2	12.3	16.0	15.2	15.2	16.7
45–64 years	3.4	4.3	4.5	5.3	5.2	4.6	9.6	10.5	12.0	11.0	12.1	12.4
45–54 years	3.2	3.8	3.8	4.9	4.8	4.0	10.5	11.0	12.6	11.7	12.5	12.8
55–64 years	3.6	4.9	5.5	6.0	5.7	5.6	8.7	10.0	11.2	10.0	11.6	11.8
Sex[5]												
Male	5.2	5.6	8.3	8.9	8.7	8.1	15.0	16.4	18.6	17.3	17.8	18.5
Female	8.0	8.6	12.2	12.6	12.4	11.0	13.6	14.3	16.3	14.8	15.4	16.2
Race[5,6]												
White	4.6	5.1	7.8	8.4	8.4	7.5	13.4	14.2	16.7	15.4	15.9	16.3
Black	18.9	17.8	24.5	24.6	22.2	20.5	20.0	21.4	20.2	18.6	19.8	20.2
Asian or Pacific Islander	9.1	11.3	9.2	10.1	11.3	9.4	18.0	18.5	20.3	18.3	19.1	19.3
Hispanic origin and race[5,6]												
All Hispanic	12.2	12.7	17.8	19.1	17.9	16.0	29.1	32.4	32.3	31.7	32.7	34.3
Mexican	11.1	11.5	16.5	18.0	16.8	15.3	33.2	38.8	36.7	36.5	38.0	39.2
Puerto Rican	28.6	26.9	33.8	30.5	31.1	28.9	18.1	23.3	16.3	18.5	15.1	19.4
Cuban	4.8	7.8	8.4	13.7	12.6	8.2	21.6	20.9	27.5	22.1	18.9	20.5
Other Hispanic	7.4	10.4	14.6	16.5	14.5	13.9	27.5	25.2	31.0	29.9	30.8	32.9
White, non-Hispanic	3.7	4.2	6.3	6.8	6.8	6.2	11.8	11.9	14.5	13.0	13.3	13.7
Black, non-Hispanic	19.1	17.8	24.5	24.3	21.9	20.3	19.7	21.3	19.8	18.5	19.7	20.1
Age and percent of poverty level[7]												
All ages:[5]												
Below 100 percent	30.5	35.3	42.3	44.1	43.9	38.8	34.7	35.8	34.0	32.4	34.4	34.4
100–149 percent	7.5	11.0	15.0	17.2	16.1	17.5	27.0	31.3	35.0	32.1	34.0	36.1
150–199 percent	3.1	5.0	5.5	7.1	7.2	7.4	17.4	21.8	25.8	23.6	23.5	25.9
200 percent or more	0.6	1.1	1.3	1.5	1.5	1.7	5.8	6.8	8.7	8.1	7.8	8.8
Under 18 years:												
Below 100 percent	43.1	47.8	63.6	65.6	65.9	59.7	28.9	31.6	23.3	20.6	21.3	22.4
100–149 percent	9.0	12.3	22.9	26.3	24.8	30.2	22.8	26.1	27.7	25.5	25.2	26.1
150–199 percent	4.4	6.1	8.6	11.7	10.8	12.2	12.7	15.8	19.0	17.7	16.1	19.7
200 percent or more	0.8	1.6	2.2	2.7	2.6	2.9	4.2	4.4	6.8	6.0	5.3	6.1
Geographic regions[5]												
Northeast	8.5	6.8	10.8	11.3	11.2	11.2	10.1	10.7	13.7	13.1	13.6	13.4
Midwest	7.2	7.5	9.4	9.8	8.4	8.2	11.1	10.5	12.3	12.2	12.3	13.1
South	5.0	6.4	10.0	10.3	10.7	8.6	17.4	19.4	21.2	19.4	20.1	20.7
West	6.9	8.2	11.4	11.9	12.1	11.4	17.8	18.4	20.6	17.8	18.7	20.4
Location of residence[5]												
Within MSA[8]	7.1	7.0	10.4	10.6	10.0	9.5	13.3	14.9	17.0	15.3	15.8	16.7
Outside MSA[8]	5.9	7.8	10.0	11.6	12.5	9.9	16.4	16.9	19.2	18.8	19.7	19.9

[1] Private insurance originally obtained through a present or former employer or union.
[2] The questionnaire changed compared with previous years.
[3] Preliminary data.
[4] Includes all other races not shown separately and unknown poverty level.
[5] Estimates are age adjusted to the year 2000 standard using three age groups: Under 18 years, 18–44 years, and 45–64 years.
[6] The race groups white, black, and Asian or Pacific Islander include persons of Hispanic and non-Hispanic origin; persons of Hispanic origin may be of any race.
[7] Poverty level is based on family income and family size using Bureau of the Census poverty thresholds.
[8] Metropolitan statistical area.
[9] Includes other public assistance through 1996. In 1997 includes state-sponsored health plans. In 1997 the age-adjusted percent of the population under 65 years of age covered by Medicaid was 9.5 percent, and 1.2 percent were covered by state-sponsored health plans.
[10] Includes persons not covered by private insurance, Medicaid, public assistance (through 1996), state-sponsored or other government-sponsored health plans (1997), Medicare, or military plans.
Note: Percents do not add to 100 because the percent with other types of health insurance (for example, Medicare, military) is not shown, and because persons with both private insurance and Medicaid appear in both columns.

SOURCE: *Health, United States, 2000*, National Center for Health Statistics, Hyattsville, MD, 2000

TABLE 4.2

Health care coverage for persons 65 years of age and over, according to type of coverage and selected characteristics: selected years 1984–97

Characteristic	Private insurance[1]						Private insurance obtained through workplace[1, 2]					
	1984	1989	1994[3]	1995	1996	1997[3,4]	1984	1989	1994[3]	1995	1996	1997[3,4]
						Number in millions						
Total[5]	19.4	22.4	24.0	23.5	22.9	22.3	10.2	11.2	12.5	12.5	12.1	12.0
						Percent of population						
Total, age adjusted[5,6]	72.5	76.1	77.2	74.8	71.9	69.5	37.2	37.3	39.6	39.0	37.6	37.0
Total, crude[5]	73.3	76.5	77.3	74.8	72.0	69.5	38.8	38.4	40.4	39.6	38.1	37.5
Age												
65–74 years	76.5	78.2	78.4	75.3	72.4	69.9	45.1	43.7	45.6	43.3	41.5	42.0
75 years and over	68.1	73.9	75.8	74.2	71.3	69.1	28.6	30.2	33.0	34.3	33.3	31.6
75–84 years	70.8	75.9	77.9	76.0	73.3	70.2	30.8	32.0	35.0	36.1	35.5	33.2
85 years and over	56.8	65.5	67.9	67.8	63.9	64.7	18.9	22.8	25.1	27.5	25.3	25.6
Sex[6]												
Male	73.4	77.4	78.9	76.6	73.8	72.1	42.5	42.1	43.9	43.3	42.0	42.0
Female	71.9	75.4	76.1	73.6	70.7	67.7	33.7	34.0	36.6	36.0	34.5	33.5
Race[6,7]												
White	75.7	79.8	80.9	78.4	75.2	72.7	38.8	38.7	41.2	40.5	38.8	37.9
Black	41.3	42.3	43.6	40.8	42.9	42.5	22.9	23.7	25.3	24.9	28.6	30.8
Hispanic origin and race[6,7]												
All Hispanic	38.2	42.3	50.0	39.9	37.7	30.6	23.1	22.2	20.5	18.4	18.0	17.7
Mexican	39.1	33.5	42.5	31.9	34.4	31.8	23.9	20.2	20.8	15.9	17.3	17.7
White, non-Hispanic	76.9	81.0	82.3	80.5	77.0	74.9	39.4	39.3	42.2	41.7	39.9	39.0
Black, non-Hispanic	41.0	42.4	44.2	40.6	43.5	42.6	22.6	23.7	25.7	24.7	29.2	30.7
Percent of poverty level[6,8]												
Below 100 percent	43.4	46.1	41.6	38.3	34.3	31.9	12.9	11.6	10.7	11.5	10.6	7.2
100–149 percent	67.1	67.7	69.1	68.6	59.0	54.5	27.2	22.2	25.1	25.3	22.2	17.4
150–199 percent	77.9	81.1	81.4	77.8	75.6	69.8	39.7	39.0	37.3	39.5	37.2	33.3
200 percent or more	85.0	85.5	88.5	86.2	84.1	81.8	50.9	49.4	52.4	50.5	48.9	48.5
Geographic region[6]												
Northeast	76.1	76.1	78.0	76.3	72.8	72.7	41.8	42.2	43.9	44.6	41.6	42.3
Midwest	79.0	81.9	84.4	82.4	80.5	78.5	38.9	40.0	42.2	44.8	41.7	40.7
South	66.8	73.0	70.7	71.1	67.3	66.0	33.4	32.0	35.5	33.9	33.6	32.9
West	69.3	74.7	77.9	69.1	68.7	59.9	36.0	37.1	38.0	33.7	35.0	33.6
Location of residence[6]												
Within MSA[9]	73.6	76.6	77.7	75.0	72.1	68.4	40.3	39.9	41.2	41.1	39.6	38.6
Outside MSA[9]	70.7	74.8	75.7	74.0	71.2	73.2	32.0	30.2	35.1	32.2	31.1	31.8

poverty level had private insurance; by 1997 the proportion sank to 23.6 percent. For people earning 200 percent or more above the poverty line, 91.6 percent were covered by private insurance in 1984, compared to 87.6 percent in 1997. (See Table 4.1.)

Accompanying the declines in private health insurance for those under 65 from 1984 to 1997 was the significant increase in the proportion of individuals receiving Medicaid health benefits at all income levels. Most surprising was the sharp increase in Medicaid participation by people living above the poverty level—who qualify for the federal program due to disabilities of some sort. Until a slight dip in 1996, the proportion of uninsured persons increased at all income levels, except those living below the poverty level. (See Table 4.1.)

From 1984 to 1997, all geographic regions showed decreases in the percentage of persons under 65 covered by private health insurance (except for persons covered through the workplace in the Midwest) and increases in the percentages of uninsured and Medicaid recipients. In 1997 persons in the South and West were least likely to have private insurance and the most likely to be unin-

sured. In 1984 and in 1997, more people living within metropolitan statistical areas (large cities and their surrounding suburbs) had private insurance than did those living in more rural areas. (See Table 4.1.)

Persons Aged 65 and Over

There are three sources of health insurance for elderly persons age 65 and over: private insurance, Medicare, and Medicaid. Medicare is the government's primary health program for those 65 years old and older. Medicaid is the government's program for the poor and the disabled. In 1999 only 1.3 percent of elderly persons went without health insurance.

Elderly persons may be covered by a combination of private health insurance and Medicare, or Medicare and Medicaid, depending on their incomes and levels of disability. In 1997, 69.5 percent of all the elderly had a combination of private insurance and Medicare, 7.9 percent had a combination of Medicare and Medicaid, and 20.1 percent had Medicare only.

Whites were far more likely to have both Medicare and private insurance (74.9 percent) than any other ethnic

TABLE 4.2

Health care coverage for persons 65 years of age and over, according to type of coverage and selected characteristics: selected years 1984–97 [CONTINUED]

Characteristic	Medicaid[1,10]						Medicare only[11]					
	1984	1989	1994[3]	1995	1996	1997[3,4]	1984	1989	1994[3]	1995	1996	1997[3,4]
	Number in millions											
Total[5]	1.8	2.0	2.5	2.9	2.7	2.5	4.7	4.5	4.1	4.6	5.7	6.7
	Percent of population											
Total, age adjusted[5,6]	7.2	7.2	8.1	9.3	8.6	7.9	18.6	15.7	13.4	14.8	18.1	20.8
Total, crude[5]	7.0	7.0	7.9	9.2	8.5	7.9	17.9	15.4	13.2	14.8	18.1	20.8
Age												
65–74 years	6.0	6.3	6.8	8.3	7.5	7.5	15.2	13.8	12.3	14.4	18.0	20.3
75 years and over	8.5	8.2	9.6	10.4	9.9	8.4	22.3	17.8	14.5	15.2	18.2	21.5
75–84 years	7.7	7.9	8.4	9.5	9.0	7.9	20.6	16.2	13.3	14.1	16.8	20.5
85 years and over	11.7	9.7	14.2	13.7	13.0	10.2	29.8	24.9	19.0	19.3	23.4	25.2
Sex[6]												
Male	4.6	5.2	4.9	5.7	5.6	5.1	18.4	14.9	13.0	14.3	16.9	19.6
Female	8.9	8.6	10.4	11.8	10.7	9.9	18.8	16.2	13.6	15.1	18.8	21.7
Race[6,7]												
White	5.3	5.6	6.3	7.1	6.9	6.5	17.3	13.9	11.9	13.5	16.9	19.3
Black	25.9	21.2	23.0	27.4	22.4	19.7	31.2	34.9	29.2	29.4	30.6	34.8
Hispanic origin and race[6,7]												
All Hispanic	26.6	26.4	27.9	32.5	29.7	29.0	29.1	22.7	18.5	23.8	28.8	35.1
White, non-Hispanic	4.6	4.9	5.3	5.8	5.7	5.4	17.0	13.6	11.5	12.9	16.4	18.4
Black, non-Hispanic	26.2	21.1	22.3	27.5	22.5	19.5	31.3	34.9	29.4	29.5	29.7	34.8
Percent of poverty level[6,8]												
Below 100 percent	27.6	28.2	37.0	39.9	38.7	40.0	27.9	26.4	22.6	21.8	25.4	27.0
100–149 percent	7.1	9.0	10.6	13.0	12.7	13.9	22.8	20.7	18.5	17.7	26.5	28.3
150–199 percent	3.4	4.7	3.8	5.4	5.1	5.1	16.9	13.6	12.9	15.9	18.9	22.7
200 percent or more	1.9	2.4	2.0	1.9	2.0	2.7	11.6	11.0	8.1	10.1	12.4	14.6
Geographic region[6]												
Northeast	5.4	5.4	7.5	8.9	7.7	6.5	17.8	17.4	14.4	15.3	20.2	19.8
Midwest	4.4	3.7	3.8	5.7	5.0	5.0	15.8	13.8	10.9	11.1	13.3	15.4
South	9.9	9.7	10.9	11.4	10.3	10.0	20.7	16.6	16.2	15.9	19.4	21.6
West	8.3	9.4	9.7	11.1	11.0	9.9	19.5	14.4	10.5	17.3	18.8	28.3
Location of residence[6]												
Within MSA[9]	6.4	6.5	7.5	8.6	7.9	7.5	18.4	15.9	13.2	15.0	18.8	22.3
Outside MSA[9]	8.5	8.8	9.7	11.6	10.9	9.4	18.9	15.5	14.0	14.2	15.7	15.9

[1]Almost all persons 65 years of age and over are covered by Medicare also. In 1997, 92 percent of older persons with private insurance also had Medicare.
[2]Private insurance originally obtained through a present or former employer or union.
[3]The questionnaire changed compared with previous years.
[4]Preliminary data.
[5]Includes all other races not shown separately and unknown poverty level.
[6]Estimates are age adjusted to the year 2000 standard using two age groups: 65–74 years and 75 years and over.
[7]The race groups white and black include persons of Hispanic and non-Hispanic origin; persons of Hispanic origin may be of any race.
[8]Poverty level is based on family income and family size using Bureau of the Census poverty thresholds.
[9]Metropolitan statistical area.
[10]Includes public assistance through 1996. In 1997 includes state-sponsored health plans. In 1997 the age-adjusted percent of the population 65 years of age and over covered by Medicaid was 7.4 percent, and 0.4 percent were covered by state-sponsored health plans.
[11]Persons covered by Medicare but not covered by private health insurance, Medicaid, public assistance (through 1996), state-sponsored or other government-sponsored health plans (1997), or military plans.
Note: Percents do not add to 100 because persons with both private health insurance and Medicaid appear in more than one column, and because the percent of persons without health insurance (1.1 percent in 1997) is not shown.

SOURCE: *Health, United States, 2000*, National Center for Health Statistics, Hyattsville, MD, 2000

or racial group. Only 3 of 10 Hispanics (30.6 percent), and 4 in 10 blacks (42.6 percent) had both Medicare and private coverage. (See Table 4.2.)

SPELLS OF BEING UNINSURED

Through its longitudinal (long term) *Survey of Income and Program Participation (SIPP)*, the U.S. Bureau of the Census has surveyed the changes in health insurance coverage over time and estimated the number of persons who experience a lapse in health coverage. The most recent *SIPP* covered the 36-month period between February 1993 and January 1996.

Who Lost Coverage?

The survey found that 29 percent of the population was without health insurance for at least one month during the survey period. Males (31 percent) were somewhat more likely than females (27 percent) to have a lapse in coverage. (Females were more likely to participate in a government assistance program such as Medicaid.) Persons who lacked high school diplomas (36 percent) and those with high school diplomas only (30 percent) were more likely to be without coverage for at least one month than were those who completed one or more years of college (22 percent). (See Figure 4.5.)

FIGURE 4.5

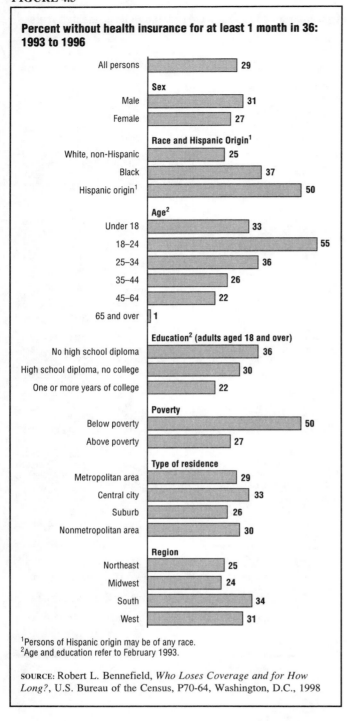

Percent without health insurance for at least 1 month in 36: 1993 to 1996

All persons	29
Sex	
Male	31
Female	27
Race and Hispanic Origin[1]	
White, non-Hispanic	25
Black	37
Hispanic origin[1]	50
Age[2]	
Under 18	33
18–24	55
25–34	36
35–44	26
45–64	22
65 and over	1
Education[2] (adults aged 18 and over)	
No high school diploma	36
High school diploma, no college	30
One or more years of college	22
Poverty	
Below poverty	50
Above poverty	27
Type of residence	
Metropolitan area	29
Central city	33
Suburb	26
Nonmetropolitan area	30
Region	
Northeast	25
Midwest	24
South	34
West	31

[1]Persons of Hispanic origin may be of any race.
[2]Age and education refer to February 1993.

SOURCE: Robert L. Bennefield, *Who Loses Coverage and for How Long?*, U.S. Bureau of the Census, P70-64, Washington, D.C., 1998

FIGURE 4.6

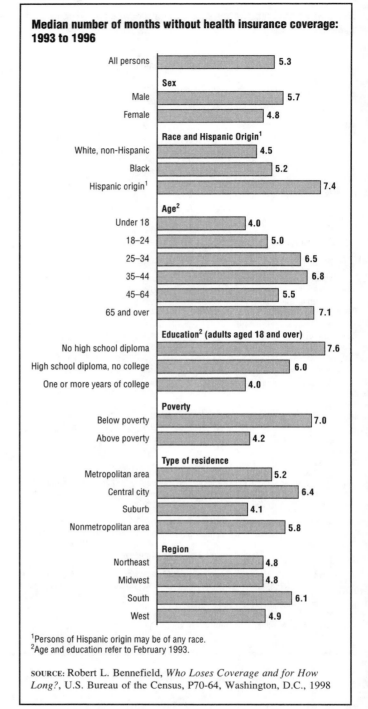

Median number of months without health insurance coverage: 1993 to 1996

All persons	5.3
Sex	
Male	5.7
Female	4.8
Race and Hispanic Origin[1]	
White, non-Hispanic	4.5
Black	5.2
Hispanic origin[1]	7.4
Age[2]	
Under 18	4.0
18–24	5.0
25–34	6.5
35–44	6.8
45–64	5.5
65 and over	7.1
Education[2] (adults aged 18 and over)	
No high school diploma	7.6
High school diploma, no college	6.0
One or more years of college	4.0
Poverty	
Below poverty	7.0
Above poverty	4.2
Type of residence	
Metropolitan area	5.2
Central city	6.4
Suburb	4.1
Nonmetropolitan area	5.8
Region	
Northeast	4.8
Midwest	4.8
South	6.1
West	4.9

[1]Persons of Hispanic origin may be of any race.
[2]Age and education refer to February 1993.

SOURCE: Robert L. Bennefield, *Who Loses Coverage and for How Long?*, U.S. Bureau of the Census, P70-64, Washington, D.C., 1998

Three of every 10 children under the age of 18 lacked continuous health insurance between 1993 and 1996. More than half (55 percent) of young adults between the ages of 18 and 24 had at least one month's lapse in coverage. Coverage improved with age. Less than one-fourth (22 percent) of those 45 to 64 had interrupted coverage during the survey period. (See Figure 4.5.)

Whites were least likely to lose health insurance coverage, although one-fourth (25 percent) lacked insurance for at least one month during the survey period. Half of all Hispanics (50 percent) and over one-third (37 percent) of blacks were without coverage at some time during this period. (See Figure 4.5.)

Durations of Spells without Insurance

The *SIPP* found that the median number of months a person was without health insurance was 5.3 months—5.7 months for males and 4.8 months for females. Persons of Hispanic origin averaged longer spells without coverage (7.4 months) than blacks (5.2 months) or whites (4.5

FIGURE 4.7

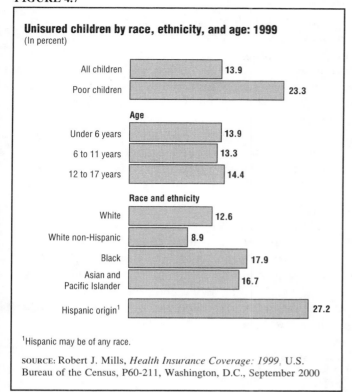

Unisured children by race, ethnicity, and age: 1999
(In percent)

All children — 13.9
Poor children — 23.3

Age

Under 6 years — 13.9
6 to 11 years — 13.3
12 to 17 years — 14.4

Race and ethnicity

White — 12.6
White non-Hispanic — 8.9
Black — 17.9
Asian and Pacific Islander — 16.7
Hispanic origin[1] — 27.2

[1]Hispanic may be of any race.

SOURCE: Robert J. Mills, *Health Insurance Coverage: 1999*, U.S. Bureau of the Census, P60-211, Washington, D.C., September 2000

FIGURE 4.8

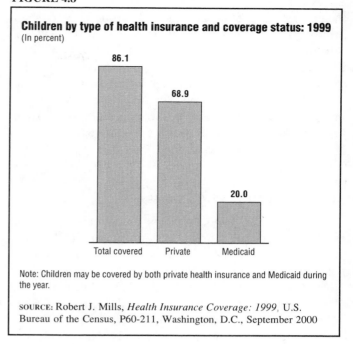

Children by type of health insurance and coverage status: 1999
(In percent)

Total covered — 86.1
Private — 68.9
Medicaid — 20.0

Note: Children may be covered by both private health insurance and Medicaid during the year.

SOURCE: Robert J. Mills, *Health Insurance Coverage: 1999*, U.S. Bureau of the Census, P60-211, Washington, D.C., September 2000

FIGURE 4.9

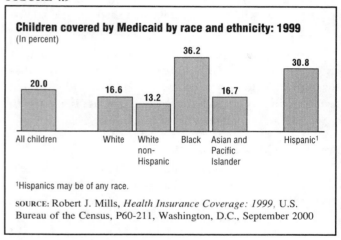

Children covered by Medicaid by race and ethnicity: 1999
(In percent)

All children — 20.0
White — 16.6
White non-Hispanic — 13.2
Black — 36.2
Asian and Pacific Islander — 16.7
Hispanic[1] — 30.8

[1]Hispanics may be of any race.

SOURCE: Robert J. Mills, *Health Insurance Coverage: 1999*, U.S. Bureau of the Census, P60-211, Washington, D.C., September 2000

months). Those living in rural areas (5.8 months) and central cities (6.4 months) were without insurance longer than those living in metropolitan areas or suburbs (5.2 and 4.1 months, respectively). (See Figure 4.6.)

Adults between the ages of 25 and 34 (6.5 months), 35 to 44 years of age (6.8 months), and age 65 and older (7.1 months) were likely to suffer longer spells without coverage than other age groups. High school dropouts (7.6 months) and those with a high school diploma only (6 months) averaged longer lapses in coverage than persons with one year or more of college (4 months). (See Figure 4.6.)

CHILDREN

In 1999, 13.9 million children under the age of 18 were uninsured. Among poor children under the age of 18, 23.3 percent had no health insurance. Hispanic children were the most likely to be uninsured—27.2 percent in 1999. Almost one-fifth (17.9 percent) of black children were without insurance, as were 16.7 percent of APIs and 8.9 percent of non-Hispanic whites. Older children, aged 12 through 17, were more likely to be uninsured (14.4 percent) than children under 6 (13.9 percent) and aged 6 to 11 (13.3 percent). (See Figure 4.7.)

In 1999, 68.9 percent of American children were insured under private health insurance plans, either privately purchased or obtained through the parents' workplace, and one-fifth (20 percent) were covered by Medicaid. (See Figure 4.8.) Medicaid covered a higher

percentage of black children (36.2 percent) and Hispanic children (30.8 percent) than API (16.7 percent) or non-Hispanic white children (13.2 percent). (See Figure 4.9.)

Some observers believed that the 1996 welfare reform law, the Personal Responsibility and Work Opportunity Reconciliation Act (PL 104-193), would lead to lower enrollment in Medicaid. Under the 1996 law, federal money once dispensed through the American Families with Dependent Children (AFDC) program was now given as a block grant (a lump sum of money) to states. In addition, the law no longer required that children who received cash assistance automatically be enrolled in the Medicaid program. The law gave states greater leeway in defining their requirements for AFDC eligibility, and in some states, some families were no longer eligible for Medicaid.

After three previous years of fairly steady enrollment, the percentage of children under 18 enrolled in Medicaid dropped from 20.1 percent in 1996, when the welfare reform legislation was enacted, to 18.4 percent in 1997. Medicaid enrollment dropped from 10.5 percent to 9.6 percent among the general population. The economic boom of the late 1990s, however, may have played a role in the decline of Medicaid enrollments, and it is too soon to tell whether figures from more recent years will bear out the drop in enrollment.

HEALTH INSURANCE PORTABILITY AND ACCOUNTABILITY ACT OF 1996

On August 21, 1996, President Bill Clinton signed the Health Insurance Portability and Accountability Act (PL 104-191). The new law stipulated that American workers who had previous insurance coverage were immediately eligible for new coverage. The law prohibited group health plans from denying new coverage based on past or present poor health and guaranteed that employees could keep existing coverage even after they left their jobs. New employers could still require a routine waiting period (usually no more than three months) before paying health benefits, but the new employee who applied for insurance coverage could be continuously covered during the waiting period.

What follows is a description of some of the major provisions of the act. In addition to the provisions discussed below, the act clarified current law and stiffened penalties for fraud and abuse. The law applies to both group and individual health insurance policies.

Preexisting Medical Conditions

In the past, insurers could refuse to cover a medical condition that had been treated or diagnosed before a person enrolled in the insurance program. Under the new law, if the condition was treated or diagnosed within six months of the patient's enrollment in the insurance program, the insurance company could withhold coverage for that condition no longer than 12 months. If the preexisting condition was not treated or diagnosed within six months of changing insurance, there was no waiting period beyond the short time an employer may require before providing benefits to a new employee.

This provision, along with the portability provision, means that insured employees are no longer "locked" into their present employment by fear of losing their health insurance if they lose or leave their present jobs. In the past, many workers stayed in unsatisfactory jobs because they were ill or had dependents with existing medical conditions. They were afraid to change jobs for fear of losing coverage or having to wait a long time before obtaining coverage.

Pregnancies are exempt from the 12-month waiting period and are covered within 30 days. Newborns and adopted children are also covered within 30 days.

Medical Savings Accounts

The new law also authorized a pilot program designed to test the concept of medical savings accounts. Beginning January 1, 1997, about 750,000 people with high-deductible health plans could make tax-deductible contributions into savings accounts designed to pay medical expenses. They could also deduct any employer contributions into the accounts as tax-deductible income. If a person does not spend all the money in the account during the year, he or she may keep the money as savings. Supporters of the medical savings account believe that people will be less likely to seek medical care if they know they can keep the money left in the account for themselves at the end of the year.

The pilot program lasted for four years and included people from companies with 50 or fewer employees, as well as self-employed persons and uninsured persons. Congress planned to review the program in its 2001–2 session, determine whether it was successful, and decide whether to make it available to everyone.

Tax Benefits of the New Law

The act also changed several tax provisions involving health expenses:

- Health premium tax deductions for the self-employed increased. Formerly, self-employed persons could deduct only 30 percent of their premiums from their taxes. The new law set up a graduated increasing scale of deductions—45 percent in 1998, 60 percent in 1999–2001, 70 percent in 2002, and 100 percent thereafter.

- Long-term care plan contributions. If an employer contributes to a long-term health care plan for a worker, a spouse, and dependents, those contributions will not be counted as taxable employee income. Long-term care includes rehabilitative care and personal care, such as feeding, bathing, and dressing, for a chronically ill person, defined as a person who has been unable for 12 months to perform activities of daily living, such as eating and bathing.

- Individual retirement account (IRA) withdrawals. Ordinarily, withdrawals from an IRA before age 59 carry a 10 percent penalty. If medical expenses, however, exceed 7.5 percent of a person's annual income, he or she may withdraw from an IRA without penalty. This provision also would allow persons who have collected federal or state unemployment benefits for at least 12 weeks to withdraw money from their IRAs without penalty.

MEDICARE C

Medicare C, or Medicare+Choice, became available to Medicare recipients on January 1, 1999. Medicare C came about as a result of the Balanced Budget Act of 1997 and was designed to supplement Medicare Parts A and B. Medicare C offers Medicare beneficiaries up to six different coverage options, including traditional Medicare and Medicare health maintenance organizations (HMOs). Traditional Medicare (fee-for-service) is the only option that would be available to everyone on Medicare.

Medicare provider sponsored organizations are like HMOs, except that doctors and hospitals run them. Medicare preferred provider organizations (PPOs) are similar to HMOs but permit patients to see providers outside the network and do not require that patients choose a primary care physician. Patients in PPOs may go to any doctor associated with the plan. Medicare private fee-for-service plans are more like traditional Medicare, except patients may pay more out-of-pocket expenses. Medical savings accounts (MSAs) have two parts—an insurance policy and a savings account. Medicare will pay the insurance premium and deposit a set amount in an MSA each year to pay for an individual's health care.

THE FUTURE: FURTHER HEALTH CARE REFORM

In 2001 members of Congress vowed to implement further health care reforms. Proposed "Patients' Bill of Rights" legislation would give consumers the right to challenge an HMO's decision not to cover procedures it considers unnecessary or expensive. Critics of the proposed legislation believed that permitting patients to challenge HMOs in court would subject insurers to astronomical legal expenses and increase the costs of health care for all Americans.

In addition, members of Congress and President George W. Bush vowed to reform the Medicare system to keep it solvent as the population of baby boomers hits retirement age. They also planned to pass legislation making prescription drugs more affordable for senior citizens enrolled in the Medicare program.

CHAPTER 5

DOCTORS, NURSES, DENTISTS, AND OTHER HEALTH CARE PROFESSIONALS

PHYSICIANS

Physicians routinely perform medical examinations, diagnose illness, treat patients suffering from injury or disease, and advise people on good health practices. There are two types of physicians: the MD (Doctor of Medicine) and the DO (Doctor of Osteopathy). While MDs and DOs may use all accepted methods of treatment, including drugs and surgery, DOs place special emphasis on the body's muscles and bones. DOs believe that good health requires the proper alignment of bones, muscles, ligaments, and nerves.

Modern medicine requires a great deal of skill and training. Recent advances in medical technologies have created new medical procedures, such as multiple organ transplants and laser surgery, and sophisticated diagnostic equipment, such as magnetic resonance imaging, ultrasound, and positron-emission tomography (PET scans).

Medical School Training and Qualifications

The road to becoming a physician is long and difficult. Applicants to medical school should have good college grades and achieve high scores on the entrance exams to be admitted to medical school. Once admitted to a medical school program, students spend the first two years primarily in laboratories and classrooms taking basic medical courses. They also learn how to take case histories, perform routine examinations, and recognize symptoms of diseases. During their last two years, the medical students work under supervision at hospitals and clinics to learn acute, chronic, preventive, and rehabilitative care. By spending time in different specialties—internal medicine, obstetrics and gynecology, pediatrics, psychology, and surgery—they acquire the necessary experience to diagnose and treat a wide variety of illnesses.

Following medical school, new physicians must complete a year of internship emphasizing one of the specialties and providing clinical experience in various hospital services—wards, clinics, emergency rooms, and operating rooms.

In the past, many doctors began practice after this first year of postgraduate training. In the present era of specialization, doctors continue in residence training, which lasts an additional three to six years, depending on the specialty. Those who choose a subspecialty must spend another one or two years in residency. Immediately after residency, they must take a final exam to be certified.

The training is difficult and involves long hours. Residents typically work 24- to 36-hour shifts and more than 80 hours a week. Lack of sleep and low wages are a way of life for most medical students, although the 36-hour shift has come under criticism as an unnecessary, and possibly dangerous, practice. In 1995 New York State limited most residents to 24-hour shifts and 80-hour weeks. The regulations were the first of their kind in the country. New York has almost 150 teaching hospitals and trains 16 percent of the nation's doctors.

In the 1999 school year, median annual medical school costs ranged from $11,375 for in-state residents at a public school, to $25,195 for nonresidents. Students at private institutions paid even more—$26,991 for residents and $28,733 for nonresidents. In 2000 the Association of American Medical Colleges reported that, by graduation, the average medical school student had incurred an average debt of $95,000. Medical school debt has increased a staggering 58.3 percent since 1993, when students owed an average of $60,000 at graduation. Their potential earnings, however, usually make this debt a wise investment.

Applying to Medical School

The average premedical student applies to 12 medical schools. There is an average of 2.6 applicants for every available opening. The ratio, however, jumps as high as 70 to 1 for small, selective schools such as the Mayo Medical School in Rochester, Minnesota. The Association of

TABLE 5.1

Active health personnel according to occupation: 1980–97

Occupation	1980	1985[1]	1990	1995	1997[2]
	Number of active health personnel				
Chiropractors	25,600	—	41,500	47,200	—
Dentists[3]	121,240	135,500	146,600	—	159,500
Nutritionists/Dieticians	32,000	—	67,000	—	69,000
Nurses, registered	1,272,900	1,531,200	1,789,600	2,115,800	2,161,700
Associate and diploma	908,300	1,016,700	1,107,300	1,235,000	1,252,600
Baccalaureate	297,300	419,200	549,000	673,200	693,200
Masters and doctorate	67,300	95,300	133,300	207,500	215,900
Occupational therapists	25,000	—	34,000	—	45,000
Optometrists	22,330	23,900	26,000	28,900	29,500
Pharmacists	142,780	159,200	161,900	182,300	185,000
Physical therapists	50,000	—	92,000	—	107,000
Physicians	427,122	542,653	567,611	672,859	723,507
Federal	17,642	23,305	20,784	21,153	20,619
Doctors of medicine[4]	16,585	21,938	19,166	19,830	19,353
Doctors of osteopathy	1,057	1,367	1,618	1,323	1,266
Non-Federal	409,480	519,348	546,826	651,706	702,888
Doctors of medicine[4]	393,407	497,473	520,450	617,362	665,252
Doctors of osteopathy	16,073	21,875	26,376	34,344	37,636
Podiatrists[5]	7,000	9,700	10,600	10,300	—
Speech therapists	50,000	—	65,000	—	97,000
	Number per 100,000 population				
Chiropractors	11.2	—	16.5	17.8	—
Dentists[3]	53.5	56.9	58.8	—	58.2
Nutritionists/Dieticians	14.0	—	26.7	—	25.9
Nurses, registered	560.0	641.4	713.7	797.6	814.9
Associate and diploma	399.9	425.8	441.6	465.5	472.2
Baccalaureate	130.9	175.6	218.9	253.8	261.3
Masters and doctorate	29.6	39.9	53.2	78.2	81.4
Occupational therapists	10.9	—	13.5	—	16.9
Optometrists	9.8	9.9	10.4	10.9	11.1
Pharmacists	62.5	66.3	64.4	68.9	69.4
Physical therapists	21.8	—	36.6	—	40.1
Physicians	189.8	221.3	230.2	255.9	265.9
Federal	7.8	9.5	8.4	8.0	7.6
Doctors of medicine[4]	7.4	8.9	7.7	7.5	7.1
Doctors of osteopathy	0.5	0.6	0.7	0.5	0.5
Non-Federal	182.0	211.8	221.8	247.9	258.3
Doctors of medicine[4]	174.9	202.9	211.1	234.8	244.5
Doctors of osteopathy	7.1	8.9	10.7	13.1	13.8
Podiatrists[5]	3.0	4.2	4.2	3.9	—
Speech therapists	21.8	—	25.9	—	36.4

— Data not available.
[1] Osteopath data are for 1986 and podiatric data are for 1984.
[2] All physician data are for 1997, other occupations are for 1996.
[3] Excludes dentists in military service, U.S. Public Health Service, and Department of Veterans Affairs.
[4] Excludes physicians with unknown addresses and those who do not practice or practice less than 20 hours per week.
[5] Podiatrists in patient care.
Notes: Ratios for physicians and dentists are based on civilian population; ratios for all other health occupations are based on resident population. From 1989 to 1994 data for doctors of medicine are as of January 1; in other years these data are as of December 31.

SOURCE: *Health, United States, 2000*, National Center for Health Statistics, Hyattsville, MD, 2000

American Medical Colleges reported 37,092 medical school applications for the 2000–2001 school year, down from an all-time high of 45,365 in 1995. These applicants were vying for 16,500 available places. After a drop in the 1980s, medical school applications increased steadily throughout the 1990s.

The decline in medical school applications may have a number of explanations. With the exponential growth in the cost of medical school, some prospective students may no longer be willing to incur such significant debt. Another factor may be concerns voiced by doctors about the growing bureaucracy and unavoidable paperwork, including requirements to seek approval from health insurers for many diagnostic tests, surgical procedures, and admissions of patients to hospitals.

Still, despite mounting costs for medical education and growing constraints on practices, a medical degree still offers economic security and a way to help people. Many potential doctors consider medicine a relatively "recession-proof" way of earning a living.

APPLICANTS OLDER AND MORE DIVERSE. Classes in American medical schools more closely resemble the American population in sex and ethnic background than in previous years. In 1996, 43 percent of students were women, 17 percent Asians, 8 percent blacks, and 6.5 percent Hispanics. Medical students are also older than they used to be. In the past, almost all students went to medical school straight from undergraduate college. While the majority of students in the mid-1990s were still straight from college, 20 percent were now between the ages of 24 and 27 upon application to medical school, and nearly 10 percent were between the ages of 28 and 31. Some medical school officials believe older students present difficulties because they are more willing to challenge their professors. At the same time, medical schools have come to value maturity and experience among their older students.

Number of Physicians Increasing

In 1997 an estimated 723,507 physicians practiced medicine in the United States, up 27.4 percent from 1990, when 567,611 were in practice. (See Table 5.1.) The overwhelming majority (94.7 percent) were MDs; the remainder were DOs. The proportion of doctors also increased dramatically—from 189.8 per 100,000 population in 1980, to 265.9 in 1997.

In 1996 New England and the Middle Atlantic states had the highest ratio (294 and 284 per 100,000, respectively) of physicians to population. The East South Central states—Kentucky, Tennessee, Alabama, and Mississippi—had the fewest physicians (184 per 100,000).

Many Specialists

Most doctors are specialists. Of those professionally active doctors not employed by the federal government, only 9.5 percent are in general and family practice, 12 percent are in internal medicine, and 5.5 percent are in pediatrics. These physicians are considered primary care physicians and together account for 27 percent of nonfederal doctors. The rest are specialists. The most common specialists are surgeons (8.7 percent), obstetricians and gynecologists (4.6 percent), anesthesiologists (3.8 percent), and psychiatrists (3.7 percent). About 69 percent

(445,765) of all nonfederal doctors are office-based rather than hospital-based.

Working Conditions

Most doctors work long, irregular hours. The American Medical Association (AMA) reported that the average physician worked 59 hours a week on patient care and office management. Physicians in salaried positions, such as those employed by health maintenance organizations, usually have shorter and more regular hours and enjoy more flexible work schedules than those in private practice. A growing number of doctors are partners in group practices. Medical doctors working in groups can pool their money for more expensive medical equipment and also are able to adapt more easily to changes in the health care environment.

In the 1990s the typical doctor spent 49 hours per week on patient care. Most (54 percent) of it was spent in the office, while about 18 percent was spent making hospital rounds, and 13 percent was in surgery. Naturally, the hours differed somewhat depending on the specialty. General and family practitioners and pediatricians spent far more time with office visits, while surgeons, obstetricians, and gynecologists spent more time at the hospital. According to the AMA, the average doctor saw a total (hospital and office visits) of 118.4 patients per week. General and family practitioners examined 144.4 patients; pediatricians, 133.5; obstetricians and gynecologists, 112.2; internists, 110.7; and surgeons, 106.9.

The average physician had 79.2 office visits per week. These ranged from 111.6 office visits for general and family practitioners, 104.4 for pediatricians, 86.6 for obstetricians and gynecologists, 75.4 for surgeons, and 64.3 for doctors in internal medicine.

Physicians' Earnings

According to the AMA, the average annual income for physicians in 1998 was $200,000. The range of salaries varies widely and is often based on a doctor's specialty, the number of years in practice, hours worked, and geographic location. Cardiovascular surgeons earned the most, with an average income of $363,300 in 1997. Neurosurgeons were next, with an average income of $317,700, while pediatricians earned the least, $137,100 a year. Other specialties included gastroenterology (the digestive system; $198,700), dermatology ($166,500), internal medicine ($143,900), and family practice physicians ($138,300).

Visiting the Doctor

In 1995 the typical American consulted a doctor 5.8 times per year. Women (6.5 times) saw the doctor more often than men (4.9 times). As would be expected, persons over 65 years of age saw doctors more frequently than younger persons. Families with less than $15,000 annual income contacted doctors more often than families with higher incomes. (See Table 5.2.)

Most often the patient saw the physician at the doctor's office (56.6 percent), but he or she sometimes saw the doctor in a hospital outpatient department (12.6 percent) or talked on the telephone (13.5 percent). About 14.1 percent saw a physician in another setting, usually a clinic. The home visit (3.2 percent) has almost disappeared in the United States, though some doctors make house calls to older Americans, a practice that has actually increased since 1990. (See Table 5.3.)

The higher the family income, the more likely patients were to consult with doctors in their offices or over the telephone. The lower the income, the more likely the patients were to see physicians in the hospital outpatient department or in another setting.

Whites were more likely than blacks to visit doctors in their offices (58 percent versus 48.3 percent) or to speak over the telephone (14 percent versus 10.1 percent). On the other hand, blacks were more likely than whites to see a physician in the hospital outpatient department (19.5 percent versus 11.5 percent) or in an "other" setting (18.8 percent versus 13.2 percent). Not surprisingly, older Americans were more likely to receive home visits than were younger ones—in fact, home visits accounted for 22.4 percent of all physician contacts with patients 75 years old and over. (See Table 5.3.)

Interval since Last Visit

In 1998 more than four of every five Americans (83.1 percent) had visited a doctor within the past year. Only 5.8 percent had gone without seeing a physician for at least three years. Males (76.5 percent) were somewhat less likely than females (89.5 percent) to have seen a doctor in the past year and three times as likely to have gone three years without seeing a doctor (8.8 percent versus 2.9 percent). While there was little difference in the interval between doctor visits for blacks and whites, American Indians and Asian/Pacific Islanders went longer between appointments. Those patients with higher incomes went to the doctor more frequently than the poor and near-poor. (See Table 5.4.)

NURSE PRACTITIONERS AND PHYSICIAN ASSISTANTS

Many of the decisions usually made by a physician can also be made by individuals with less training. Nurse practitioners and physician assistants usually work under the direction of a physician and treat minor ailments and injuries, make diagnoses and write prescriptions for patients. These professionals are trained to recognize symptoms that indicate more serious problems, even though they cannot treat them, and to refer those patients

TABLE 5.2

Physician contacts, according to selected patient characteristics: 1987–95

[Data are based on household interviews of a sample of the civilian noninstitutionalized population]

Characteristic	1987	1988	1989	1990	1991	1992	1993	1994	1995
	\multicolumn{9}{c}{Physician contacts per person}								
Total[1,2]	5.4	5.3	5.3	5.5	5.6	5.9	6.0	6.0	5.8
Age									
Under 15 years	4.5	4.6	4.6	4.5	4.7	4.6	4.9	4.6	4.5
Under 5 years	6.7	7.0	6.7	6.9	7.1	6.9	7.2	6.8	6.5
5-14 years	3.3	3.3	3.5	3.2	3.4	3.4	3.6	3.4	3.4
15-44 years	4.6	4.7	4.6	4.8	4.7	5.0	5.0	5.0	4.8
45-64 years	6.4	6.1	6.1	6.4	6.6	7.2	7.1	7.3	7.1
65 years and over	8.9	8.7	8.9	9.2	10.4	10.6	10.9	11.3	11.1
65-74 years	8.4	8.4	8.2	8.5	9.2	9.7	9.9	10.3	9.8
75 years and over	9.7	9.2	9.9	10.1	12.3	12.1	12.3	12.7	12.9
Sex and age									
Male[1]	4.6	4.6	4.8	4.7	4.9	5.1	5.2	5.2	4.9
Under 5 years	6.7	7.3	7.5	7.2	7.6	7.1	7.5	7.0	6.8
5-14 years	3.4	3.4	3.7	3.3	3.5	3.5	3.8	3.5	3.6
15-44 years	3.3	3.3	3.4	3.4	3.4	3.7	3.6	3.7	3.3
45-64 years	5.5	5.2	5.2	5.6	5.8	6.1	6.1	6.3	6.0
65-74 years	8.1	7.9	8.5	8.0	8.6	9.2	9.3	10.1	9.5
75 years and over	9.2	9.6	9.9	10.0	11.6	12.2	11.7	11.6	11.9
Female[1]	6.0	6.0	5.9	6.1	6.3	6.6	6.7	6.7	6.5
Under 5 years	6.7	6.8	5.9	6.5	6.6	6.7	6.9	6.5	6.3
5-14 years	3.1	3.3	3.3	3.2	3.2	3.3	3.4	3.3	3.1
15-44 years	5.8	6.0	5.9	6.0	5.9	6.2	6.4	6.2	6.2
45-64 years	7.2	6.9	7.0	7.1	7.4	8.2	8.1	8.3	8.1
65-74 years	8.6	8.8	7.9	9.0	9.7	10.1	10.4	10.5	10.1
75 years and over	10.0	9.0	9.9	10.2	12.7	12.1	12.8	13.4	13.5
Race and age									
White[1]	5.5	5.5	5.5	5.6	5.8	6.0	6.0	6.1	5.9
Under 5 years	7.1	7.6	7.1	7.1	7.4	7.3	7.5	7.1	6.7
5-14 years	3.5	3.6	3.8	3.5	3.7	3.7	3.9	3.7	3.6
15-44 years	4.7	4.8	4.8	4.9	4.9	5.0	5.1	5.1	4.9
45-64 years	6.4	6.1	6.2	6.4	6.6	7.2	7.0	7.4	7.0
65-74 years	8.4	8.3	8.0	8.5	9.4	9.6	9.7	10.5	9.9
75 years and over	9.7	9.3	9.7	10.1	12.1	12.0	12.2	12.4	13.1
Black[1]	5.1	4.8	4.9	5.1	5.2	5.9	6.0	5.7	5.5
Under 5 years	5.1	4.6	5.3	5.6	6.0	5.6	6.2	5.2	5.8
5-14 years	2.3	2.2	2.3	2.2	2.1	2.3	2.4	2.5	2.5
15-44 years	4.2	4.2	3.9	4.2	4.0	5.3	4.7	4.8	4.3
45-64 years	7.3	6.6	6.3	7.1	7.5	7.8	8.7	7.7	8.0
65-74 years	8.6	9.1	10.0	9.2	7.3	10.9	11.5	9.3	9.9
75 years and over	10.8	8.7	12.7	10.4	15.7	13.7	13.1	16.3	11.5
Family income[1,3]									
Less than $15,000	6.8	6.2	6.3	6.3	6.8	7.3	7.3	7.6	7.4
$15,000-$24,999	5.6	5.3	5.2	5.6	5.6	6.0	5.7	5.9	6.1
$25,000-$34,999	5.2	5.0	5.5	5.2	5.5	5.7	6.0	5.8	5.3
$35,000-$49,999	5.2	5.5	5.2	5.7	5.8	5.9	6.0	6.2	5.7
$50,000 or more	5.4	5.5	6.0	5.6	5.8	5.8	5.8	6.0	5.6
Geographic region[1]									
Northeast	5.2	5.0	5.3	5.2	5.4	5.9	5.9	5.9	5.6
Midwest	5.6	5.4	5.4	5.3	5.8	5.9	6.2	6.0	5.8
South	5.1	5.2	5.3	5.6	5.5	5.8	5.7	5.6	5.8
West	5.5	5.9	5.5	5.6	5.9	6.1	6.0	6.4	5.8
Location of residence[1]									
Within MSA[4]	5.5	5.5	5.4	5.6	5.8	6.0	6.1	6.0	5.9
Outside MSA[4]	4.8	4.9	5.2	4.9	5.1	5.6	5.6	5.7	5.3

[1] Age adjusted.

[2] Includes all other races not shown separately and unknown family income.

[3] Family income categories for 1995. In 1989-94 the two lowest income categories are less than $14,000 and $14,000-$24,999; the three higher income categories are as shown. Income categories for 1988 are less than $13,000; $13,000-$18,999; $19,000-$24,999; $25,000-$44,999; and $45,000 or more. Income categories for 1987 are less than $10,000; $10,000-$14,999; $15,000-$19,999; $20,000-$34,999 and $35,000 or more.

[4] Metropolitan statistical area.

SOURCE: *Health, United States, 1998,* National Center for Health Statistics, Hyattsville, MD, 1998

to the doctor. According to the American Academy of Physician Assistants, there were 31,084 physician assistants in the United States in 1998, 11.9 per every 100,000 population. The numbers of physician assistants and nurse practitioners have increased dramatically since the beginning of the 1990s.

TABLE 5.3

Physician contacts, according to place of contact and selected patient characteristics: 1990 and 1995
[Data are based on household interviews of a sample of the civilian noninstitutionalized population]

| | | Place of contact | | | | | | | | | | |
| | | Doctor's office | | Hospital outpatient department[1] | | Telephone | | Home | | Other[2] | |
Characteristic	Total	1990	1995	1990	1995	1990	1995	1990	1995	1990	1995
					Percent distribution						
Total[3,4]	100.0	59.9	56.6	13.7	12.6	12.7	13.5	2.1	3.2	11.6	14.1
Age											
Under 15 years	100.0	60.7	59.3	13.6	12.4	14.9	14.6	0.9	*0.7	9.9	13.0
Under 5 years	100.0	59.1	58.9	14.0	12.5	15.9	15.0	*1.1	*1.2	9.8	12.4
5-14 years	100.0	62.6	59.6	13.1	12.2	13.7	14.2	*0.6	*0.3	10.0	13.6
15-44 years	100.0	59.4	55.7	14.3	13.1	12.0	14.0	0.6	1.8	13.7	15.5
45-64 years	100.0	60.4	55.4	14.1	13.0	12.2	12.7	2.0	4.4	11.4	14.5
65 years and over	100.0	58.7	54.4	11.1	10.4	9.9	10.3	11.8	14.1	8.4	10.8
65-74 years	100.0	60.2	57.7	13.7	12.5	9.7	10.8	7.0	6.5	9.4	12.5
75 years and over	100.0	56.8	50.7	7.8	8.2	10.2	9.7	18.1	22.4	7.0	9.0
Sex[3]											
Male	100.0	57.6	55.7	16.1	13.9	11.3	12.2	2.1	2.7	12.9	15.4
Female	100.0	61.6	57.0	12.2	11.8	13.4	14.2	2.0	3.5	10.9	13.5
Race[3]											
White	100.0	61.7	58.0	12.3	11.5	13.1	14.0	1.9	3.2	11.0	13.2
Black	100.0	48.2	48.3	24.3	19.5	9.1	10.1	2.8	3.3	15.6	18.8
Family income[3,5]											
Less than $15,000	100.0	48.9	46.4	19.9	15.7	11.5	11.0	3.2	5.0	16.4	21.9
$15,000-$24,999	100.0	56.9	54.3	16.0	15.0	11.8	11.4	1.7	3.6	13.5	15.7
$25,00-$34,999	100.0	60.9	56.7	13.8	13.0	13.2	13.9	1.6	2.5	10.4	14.1
$35,000-$49,999	100.0	62.0	58.7	11.5	10.6	14.6	16.2	1.1	3.0	10.9	11.5
$50,000 or more	100.0	66.1	62.1	8.9	10.0	14.1	16.1	1.5	2.0	9.5	9.7
Geographic region[3]											
Northeast	100.0	62.6	60.9	13.0	12.2	11.7	14.5	1.9	2.3	10.8	10.1
Midwest	100.0	55.8	52.9	14.7	13.8	15.4	15.8	1.9	1.8	12.3	15.7
South	100.0	61.1	57.3	13.6	12.4	11.3	12.7	2.6	4.5	11.3	13.1
West	100.0	60.4	55.8	13.6	12.0	12.8	11.3	1.4	3.4	12.0	17.4
Location of residence[3]											
Within MSA[6]	100.0	59.6	56.7	13.7	12.7	13.1	13.9	1.9	3.1	11.7	13.7
Outside MSA[6]	100.0	61.4	56.3	14.1	12.1	10.7	12.0	2.6	3.6	11.2	16.1

* Relative standard error greater than 30 percent.
[1] Includes hospital outpatient clinic, emergency room, and other hospital contacts.
[2] Includes clinics or other places outside a hospital.
[3] Age adjusted.
[4] Includes all other races not shown separately and unknown family income.
[5] Family income categories for 1995. In 1990 the two lowest income categories are less than $14,000 and $14,000-$24,999; the three higher income categories are as shown.
[6] Metropolitan statistical area.

SOURCE: *Health, United States, 1998*, National Center for Health Statistics, Hyattsville, MD, 1998

DENTISTS

Dentists diagnose and treat problems of the teeth and tissues of the mouth, take X rays, place protective plastic sealant on children's teeth, fill cavities, straighten teeth, and treat gum disease. In 1995 there were approximately 150,000 practicing dentists in the United States (excluding military personnel).

Fluoridation of community water supplies and improved dental hygiene have dramatically improved the dental health of the American population. Dental caries (cavities) among all age groups have declined significantly. As a result, many dental services are shifting focus from young people to adults. Many adults today are choosing to have orthodontic services, such as straightening their teeth.

In addition, the older population generally requires more complex dental procedures, such as endodontic (root canal) services, bridges, and dentures.

Most Dentists Have Their Own Practices

The overwhelming majority of dentists own solo dental practices, where only one dentist operates in each office. According to the American Dental Association (ADA), more than three-fourths (79 percent) of the nation's private dentists were working alone in the mid-1990s, while 13 percent were practicing with one other dentist. About 91 percent of all private-practice dentists owned their own operations. Most dentists (89 percent) started their careers owning their own dental practice. In the 1990s, however, this became more difficult, and an

TABLE 5.4

Interval since last health care contact among adults 18 years of age and over, according to selected characteristics: 1997 and 1998

Characteristic	Total	1 year or less		More than 1 year to 3 years		More than 3 years	
		1997	1998	1997	1998	1997	1998
		Percent distribution[1]					
All adults 18 years of age and over[2,3]	100.0	82.4	83.1	12.0	11.1	5.6	5.8
Age							
18–44 years	100.0	78.8	79.0	14.6	14.1	6.6	6.9
18–24 years	100.0	78.2	78.9	16.1	14.4	5.7	6.8
25–44 years	100.0	78.9	79.1	14.2	14.0	6.9	6.9
45–64 years	100.0	83.6	84.6	11.0	9.6	5.4	5.7
45–54 years	100.0	82.8	83.8	11.7	10.4	5.5	5.9
55–64 years	100.0	84.9	86.0	9.8	8.5	5.3	5.5
65 years and over	100.0	91.6	93.3	5.4	4.2	3.0	2.5
65–74 years	100.0	90.4	92.2	6.1	4.8	3.5	3.0
75 years and over	100.0	93.1	94.7	4.5	3.5	2.3	1.8
Sex[3]							
Male	100.0	75.3	76.5	16.3	14.7	8.4	8.8
Female	100.0	89.3	89.5	7.8	7.6	2.9	2.9
Race[3,4]							
White	100.0	82.8	83.3	11.8	11.0	5.4	5.7
Black	100.0	83.3	84.7	11.2	10.3	5.4	5.0
American Indian or Alaska Native	100.0	80.4	77.2	11.4	13.0	*8.1	9.8
Asian or Pacific Islander	100.0	76.8	78.0	15.9	13.6	7.3	8.4
Race and Hispanic origin[3]							
White, non-Hispanic	100.0	83.9	84.3	11.5	10.8	4.6	5.0
Black, non-Hispanic	100.0	83.2	84.6	11.4	10.4	5.4	4.9
Hispanic[4]	100.0	74.3	76.1	14.2	12.9	11.5	11.0
Mexican[4]	100.0	69.7	70.8	15.3	14.5	15.0	14.7
Poverty status[3,5]							
Poor	100.0	79.4	78.4	12.0	12.6	8.6	9.0
Near poor	100.0	79.0	79.0	12.8	12.7	8.2	8.3
Nonpoor	100.0	84.5	85.3	11.3	10.3	4.2	4.4
Race and Hispanic origin and poverty status[3,5]							
White, non-Hispanic							
Poor	100.0	83.3	81.1	10.8	12.3	5.8	6.6
Near poor	100.0	81.4	81.4	12.0	11.7	6.7	7.0
Nonpoor	100.0	85.1	85.8	10.9	10.1	4.0	4.2
Black, non-Hispanic:							
Poor	100.0	83.7	84.2	10.2	10.2	6.1	5.6
Near poor	100.0	81.7	80.3	11.8	13.6	6.4	*6.1
Nonpoor	100.0	84.5	86.1	11.2	9.8	4.3	4.1
Hispanic:[4]							
Poor	100.0	67.4	68.4	15.7	15.2	16.9	16.4
Near poor	100.0	69.6	73.1	15.5	14.5	14.9	12.4
Nonpoor	100.0	79.8	82.0	13.7	11.6	6.5	6.4
Health insurance status[6,7]							
18–64 years of age:							
Insured	100.0	84.2	—	11.7	—	4.1	—
Private	100.0	83.5	—	12.3	—	4.2	—
Medicaid	100.0	91.5	—	5.2	—	3.3	—
Uninsured	100.0	63.5	—	20.8	—	15.8	—
65 years of age and over:							
Private	100.0	93.3	—	4.6	—	2.2	—
Medicaid	100.0	91.2	—	5.6	—	*3.1	—
Medicare only	100.0	86.9	—	7.8	—	5.3	—

TABLE 5.4

Interval since last health care contact among adults 18 years of age and over, according to selected characteristics: 1997 and 1998 [CONTINUED]

Characteristic	Total	1 year or less		More than 1 year to 3 years		More than 3 years	
		1997	1998	1997	1998	1997	1998
Poverty status and health insurance status[5,6]							
18–64 years of age:							
Poor:							
Insured	100.0	86.5	—	9.3	—	4.1	—
Uninsured	100.0	62.4	—	19.2	—	18.4	—
Near poor:							
Insured	100.0	83.8	—	10.6	—	5.6	—
Uninsured	100.0	61.4	—	21.9	—	16.6	—
Nonpoor:							
Insured	100.0	84.5	—	11.8	—	3.7	—
Uninsured	100.0	66.8	—	20.0	—	13.3	—
Geographic region[3]							
Northeast	100.0	85.6	86.0	10.1	9.3	4.4	4.6
Midwest	100.0	82.8	83.2	12.3	11.4	4.8	5.4
South	100.0	81.9	82.7	12.3	11.3	5.9	6.0
West	100.0	79.7	81.0	12.8	12.0	7.5	7.0
Location of residence[3]							
Within MSA[8]	100.0	82.7	83.4	11.7	10.9	5.6	5.7
Outside MSA[8]	100.0	81.4	82.4	12.9	11.7	5.7	5.9

* Data preceded by an asterisk have a relative standard error of 20–30 percent.
— Data not available as of publication date.

[1] Respondents were asked "About how long has it been since you last saw or talked to a doctor or other health care professional about your own health? Include doctors seen while a patient in a hospital."

[2] Includes all other races not shown separately, unknown poverty status, and unknown health insurance status.

[3] Estimates are for persons 18 years of age and over and are age adjusted to the year 2000 standard using five age groups: 18–44 years, 45–54 years, 55–64 years, 65–74 years, and 75 years and over.

[4] The race groups white, black, American Indian or Alaska Native, and Asian or Pacific Islander include persons of Hispanic and non-Hispanic origin; persons of Hispanic origin may be of any race.

[5] Poverty status is based on family income, family size, number of children in the family, and for families with two or fewer adults the age of the adults in the family using Bureau of the Census poverty thresholds. Poor persons are defined as below the poverty threshold. Near poor persons have incomes of 100 percent to less than 200 percent of poverty threshold. Nonpoor persons have incomes of 200 percent or greater than the poverty threshold. Poverty status was unknown for 22 percent of adults in the sample in 1997 and 27 percent in 1998.

[6] Estimates for persons 18–64 years of age are age adjusted to the year 2000 standard using three age groups: 18–44 years, 45–54 years, and 55–64 years of age. Estimates for persons 65 years of age and over are age adjusted to the year 2000 standard using two age groups: 65–74 years and 75 years and over

[7] Health insurance categories are mutually exclusive. Persons who reported both Medicaid and private coverage are classified as having Medicaid coverage.

[8] MSA is metropolitan statistical area.

SOURCE: *Health, United States, 2000,* National Center for Health Statistics, Hyattsville, MD, 2000

geons, operate on the mouth and jaws. The rest of the specialists concentrate in pediatric dentistry (dentistry for children), periodontics (treating the gums), prosthodontics (making dentures and artificial teeth), endodontics (root canals), public health dentistry (community dental health), and oral pathology (diseases of the mouth). Cosmetic dentistry is also one of the newest and fastest-growing specialties.

Training to Become a Dentist

Entry into dental schools requires two to four years of college-level predental education—most dental students

increasing number of dentists are beginning their careers working in a clinic or in another dentist's private practice.

Dental Specialists

In 1995 about 20 percent of all dentists practiced in one of the eight specialty areas recognized by the ADA. Orthodontists, who straighten teeth, make up the largest group of specialists. The next largest group, oral and maxillofacial sur-

have at least a bachelor's degree when they enter dental school. Dental school usually lasts four academic years. A student begins by studying the basic sciences, including anatomy, microbiology, biochemistry, and physiology. During the last two years, students receive practical experience by treating patients, usually in dental clinics supervised by licensed dentists.

In 1996, 3,768 students were graduated from the nation's 53 dental schools. Men outnumbered women graduates by about two to one. Of the graduates, 68 percent were white and only 5.8 percent were black. Other minorities made up about 26 percent.

Earnings of Dentists

Just as among medical doctors, dental specialists earn more than do those offering primary care. According to the ADA, the net median (half earned more, and half earned less) annual income of dentists in private practice was $100,000 in 1994. The net median income for general practitioners was $97,450, while the net median income for specialists was $132,500.

Visiting the Dentist

In 1998, 66.2 percent of Americans had visited their dentists at least once in the past year. Children aged 2 to 17 (73.5 percent) were more likely to have visited the dentist than any other age group, and women (68.8 percent) were somewhat more likely to see the dentist than men (63.6 percent). The proportion of non-Hispanic whites visiting dentists (69.5 percent) was considerably higher than the proportions of blacks (58 percent) and Hispanics (54.1 percent). The higher the income level, the more likely the person was to visit the dentist annually. (See Table 5.5.)

REGISTERED NURSES

Registered nurses (RNs) are licensed by the state to care for the sick and to promote health. RNs supervise hospital care, give drugs and treatment as prescribed by doctors, monitor the progress of patients, and provide health education. Nurses work in a variety of health settings, including hospitals, nursing homes, physicians' offices, clinics, and schools.

Education for Nurses

There are three types of education for registered nurses. These include associate degrees (two-year community college programs), baccalaureate programs (four years of college), and postgraduate (master's degree and doctorate) programs. The baccalaureate degree provides more knowledge of community health services, as well as the psychological and social aspects of caring for patients, than does the associate degree. Those who complete the four-year baccalaureate degree and the other advanced degrees are better prepared to eventually attain manage-

TABLE 5.5

Dental visits in the past year according to selected patient characteristics: 1997 and 1998

Characteristic	2 years of age and over[1]		2–17 years of age		18–64 years of age		65 years of age and over[2]	
	1997	1998	1997	1998	1997	1998	1997	1998
	Percent of persons with a dental visit in the past year[3]							
Total[4]	64.9	66.2	72.7	73.5	64.1	65.6	54.8	56.4
Sex								
Male	62.6	63.6	72.3	72.0	60.4	61.7	55.4	57.8
Female	67.2	68.8	73.0	75.1	67.7	69.2	54.4	55.4
Race[5]								
White	66.5	67.8	74.0	74.9	65.7	67.2	56.8	58.2
Black	56.5	58.0	68.8	69.8	57.0	58.3	35.4	36.9
American Indian or Alaska Native	51.5	56.1	66.8	72.6	49.9	53.7	*	*41.1
Asian or Pacific Islander	61.8	65.5	69.9	67.8	60.3	63.4	53.9	67.4
Race and Hispanic origin								
White, non-Hispanic	68.2	69.5	76.4	77.1	67.5	68.9	57.2	58.7
Black, non-Hispanic	56.5	58.0	68.8	69.8	56.9	58.1	35.3	37.3
Hispanic[5]	52.9	54.1	61.0	62.4	50.8	52.2	47.8	46.8
Poverty status[6]								
Poor	47.2	48.3	62.0	63.5	46.4	47.1	30.3	32.6
Near poor	48.9	50.5	61.6	61.2	46.4	49.0	39.6	41.8
Nonpoor	72.3	73.2	79.7	80.4	71.1	72.0	66.3	66.8
Race and Hispanic origin and poverty status[6]								
White, non-Hispanic:								
Poor	49.9	51.8	63.3	64.1	50.3	51.8	31.1	34.0
Near poor	51.0	52.6	64.8	63.5	48.2	51.4	41.2	43.0
Nonpoor	73.6	74.4	80.7	81.5	72.5	73.3	67.6	67.7
Black, non-Hispanic:								
Poor	46.7	47.1	66.7	67.7	44.5	46.6	26.2	22.5
Near poor	44.9	47.8	60.1	61.3	44.7	46.4	23.6	33.9
Nonpoor	65.4	65.4	75.5	76.1	66.2	65.5	48.9	48.4
Hispanic:[5]								
Poor	41.9	41.7	56.8	58.7	39.0	37.4	33.0	36.3
Near poor	46.2	45.3	54.1	53.1	42.6	43.7	49.2	40.3
Nonpoor	65.1	67.2	74.8	75.5	62.5	65.4	56.5	59.4
Geographic region								
Northeast	69.6	70.4	77.5	80.5	69.6	69.6	55.5	56.3
Midwest	68.3	69.4	76.4	76.9	67.4	69.2	57.6	56.2
South	60.0	62.2	68.0	69.1	59.4	61.2	49.0	53.9
West	64.9	65.6	71.5	70.1	62.9	64.7	61.9	61.2
Location of residence								
Within MSA[7]	66.5	67.9	73.6	74.6	65.7	67.2	57.6	59.1
Outside MSA[7]	59.1	60.3	69.3	69.6	58.0	59.5	46.1	47.6

* Data preceded by an asterisk have a relative standard error of 20–30 percent. Data not shown have a relative standard error greater than 30 percent.
[1] Estimates are age adjusted to the year 2000 standard using six age groups: 2–17 years, 18–44 years, 45–54 years, 55–64 years, 65–74 years, and 75 years and over.
[2] Estimates for the elderly present the percent of persons 65 years of age and over with a dental visit in the past year. Data from the 1997 and 1998 National Health Interview Survey estimate that 29–30 percent of persons 65 years of age and over were edentulous (having lost all their natural teeth). In 1997 and 1998, 70–71 percent of elderly dentate persons compared with 18 percent of elderly edentate persons had a dental visit in the past year.
[3] Respondents were asked "About how long has it been since you last saw or talked to a dentist? Include all types of dentists, such as orthodontists, oral surgeons, and all other dental specialists as well as dental hygienists." This question was not asked for children under two years of age. This table presents the percent of persons with a visit in the past one year or less.
[4] Includes all other races not shown separately and unknown poverty status.
[5] The race groups white, black, American Indian or Alaska Native, and Asian or Pacific Islander include persons of Hispanic and non-Hispanic origin; persons of Hispanic origin may be of any race.
[6] Poverty status is based on family income, family size, number of children in the family, and for families with two or fewer adults the age of the adults in the family, using Bureau of the Census poverty thresholds. Poor persons are defined as below the poverty threshold. Near poor persons have incomes of 100 percent to less than 200 percent of poverty threshold. Nonpoor persons have incomes of 200 percent or greater than the poverty threshold. Poverty status was unknown for 20 percent of persons in 1997 and 25 percent in 1998 in the sample.
[7] MSA is metropolitan statistical area.
SOURCE: *Health, United States, 2000*, National Center for Health Statistics, Hyattsville, MD, 2000

TABLE 5.6

Allied health care providers

Dental hygienists provide services for maintaining oral health. Their primary duty is to clean teeth.

Emergency Medical Technicians (EMTs) provide immediate care to critically ill or injured people in emergency situations.

Home health aides provide nursing, household, and personal care services to patients who are homebound or disabled.

Licensed practical nurses (LPNs) are trained and licensed to provide basic nursing care under the supervision of registered nurses and doctors.

Medical records personnel analyze patient records and keep them up-to-date, complete, accurate, and confidential.

Medical technologists perform laboratory tests to help diagnose diseases and to aid in identifying their causes and extent.

Nurses' Aides, Orderlies, and Attendants help nurses in hospitals, nursing homes and other facilities.

Occupational therapists help disabled persons adapt to their disabilities. This may include helping a patient relearn basic living skills or modifying the environment.

Optometrists measure vision for corrective lenses and prescribe glasses.

Pharmacists are trained and licensed to make up and dispense drugs in accordance with a physician's prescription.

Physician assistants (PAs) work under a doctor's supervision. Their duties include performing routine physical exams, prescribing certain drugs, and providing medical counseling.

Physical therapists work with disabled patients to help restore function, strength and mobility. PTs use exercise, heat, cold, water, and electricity to relieve pain and restore function.

Podiatrists diagnose and treat diseases, injuries, and abnormalities of the feet. They may use drugs and surgery to treat foot problems.

Psychologists are trained in human behavior and provide counseling and testing services related to mental health.

Radiation technicians take and develop x-ray photographs for medical purposes.

Registered dietitians (RDs) are licensed to use dietary principles to maintain health and treat disease.

Respiratory therapists treat breathing problems under a doctor's supervision and help in respiratory rehabilitation.

Social workers help patients to handle social problems such as finances, housing, and social and family problems that arise out of illness or disability.

Speech pathologists diagnose and treat disorders of speech and communication.

SOURCE: U.S. Department of Commerce

ment roles and to make more comprehensive decisions about patient care.

Between 1980 and 1997, the number of registered nurses increased by 69.2 percent, from 1.3 to 2.2 million. Over the same period, the proportion of nurses per 100,000 population rose from 560 per 100,000 to 815 per 100,000. The largest percentage increases occurred among those holding baccalaureate, master's, and doctorate degrees. (See Table 5.1.)

Although the number of registered nurses holding baccalaureate degrees increased sharply in the 1990s, there is still a shortage of nurses. Some experts believe that the shortage is because more lucrative fields are now open to women, the traditional nursing population. Others feel the shortage results from the increased demand due to the spread of drug abuse, the AIDS epidemic, an aging population, and cost-control measures. In addition, the rapid development of new technology and medical techniques enables many people to live longer than they would have only a few years earlier, but they may require more hospital time for treatment, thus increasing the need for nurses.

ALLIED HEALTH CARE PROVIDERS

The total health care team includes other professionals who work with physicians, nurses, and dentists to provide medical care. These allied health workers include nurses' aides, home health aides, pharmacists, dental hygienists, and many others. (See Table 5.6.)

INCREASE IN HEALTH CARE EMPLOYMENT

In 1999, 11.6 million persons worked in health care services, a 46.8 percent increase since 1985, when 7.9 million worked in the health field. Workers in health care professions accounted for 8.7 percent of all employed Americans (excluding military personnel). In 1970 only 5.5 percent of employed civilians worked in health care services. (See Table 5.7.)

Since 1970 the proportion of health care workers employed in hospitals has dropped dramatically. More than 6 in 10 (63.4 percent) of health services personnel worked in hospitals in 1970. By 1990 that number had dropped to 49.6 percent employed in hospitals, and by 1999 that number fell again, to 43.9 percent. While hospitals still employ a larger proportion of health workers than any other service locations, more patients are now able to receive treatment in doctors' offices, clinics, and other outpatient settings. In addition, insurers are probably less willing to pay for lengthy hospitalizations than they were in the past.

Why Is Health Care Booming?

Three major factors appear to have influenced the escalation in health care employment: advances in technology, the increasing amounts of money spent on health care, and the aging of the nation's population. In other sectors of the economy, technology often replaces humans in the labor force. But health care technology has increased the demand for highly trained specialists to operate the sophisticated equipment. Because of technological advances, patients are likely to undergo more tests and diagnostic procedures, take more drugs, see more specialists, and be subjected to more aggressive treatments than ever before.

The second factor in the increase in health care employment involves the amount of money the nation

TABLE 5.7

Persons employed in health service sites: selected years 1970–99

Site	1970	1975	1980	1985	1990	1993	1994	1995	1996	1997	1998	1999
					Number of persons in thousands							
All employed civilians	76,805	85,846	99,303	107,150	117,914	119,306	123,060	124,900	126,708	129,558	131,463	133,488
All health service sites	4,246	5,945	7,339	7,910	9,447	10,553	10,587	10,928	11,199	11,525	11,504	11,646
Offices and clinics of physicians	477	618	777	894	1,098	1,450	1,404	1,512	1,501	1,559	1,581	1,624
Offices and clinics of dentists	222	331	415	480	580	567	596	644	614	662	666	694
Offices and clinics of chiropractors	19	30	40	59	90	116	105	99	99	118	127	142
Hospitals	2,690	3,441	4,036	4,269	4,690	5,032	5,009	4,961	5,041	5,130	5,116	5,117
Nursing and personal care facilities	509	891	1,199	1,309	1,543	1,752	1,692	1,718	1,765	1,755	1,801	1,786
Other health service sites	330	634	872	899	1,446	1,635	1,781	1,995	2,178	2,301	2,213	2,283
					Percent of employed civilians							
All health service sites	5.5	6.9	7.4	7.4	8.0	8.8	8.6	8.7	8.8	8.9	8.8	8.7
					Percent distribution							
All health service sites	100.0	100.0	100.0	100.0	100.0	100.0	100.0	100.0	100.0	100.0	100.0	100.0
Offices and clinics of physicians	11.2	10.4	10.6	11.3	11.6	13.7	13.3	13.8	13.4	13.5	13.7	13.9
Offices and clinics of dentists	5.2	5.6	5.7	6.1	6.1	5.4	5.6	5.9	5.5	5.7	5.8	6.0
Offices and clinics of chiropractors	0.4	0.5	0.5	0.7	1.0	1.1	1.0	0.9	0.9	1.0	1.1	1.2
Hospitals	63.4	57.9	55.0	54.0	49.6	47.7	47.3	45.4	45.0	44.5	44.5	43.9
Nursing and personal care facilities	12.0	15.0	16.3	16.5	16.3	16.6	16.0	15.7	15.8	15.2	15.7	15.3
Other health service sites	7.8	10.7	11.9	11.4	15.3	15.5	16.8	18.3	19.4	20.0	19.2	19.6

Notes: Employment is full- or part-time work. Totals exclude persons in health-related occupations who are working in nonhealth industries, as classified by the U.S. Bureau of the Census, such as pharmacists employed in drugstores, school nurses, and nurses working in private households. Totals include federal, state, and county health workers. In 1970–82, employed persons were classified according to the industry groups used in the 1970 Census of Population. In 1983–91, persons were classified according to the system used in the 1980 Census of Population. Beginning in 1992 persons were classified according to the system used in the 1990 Census of Population.

SOURCE: *Health, United States, 2000*, National Center for Health Statistics, Hyattsville, MD, 2000

spends on keeping its citizens in good health. Americans spent $1.149 trillion on health care in 1998, and each year that the amount of money spent on health care continues to grow, employment in the field grows as well. Some believe that financing for the health care industry, unlike other fields, is virtually unlimited.

The third factor contributing to the rise in the number of health care workers is the aging of the nation's population. There are greater numbers of elderly people in the United States than ever before, and they are living longer. According to the U.S. Bureau of the Census, in 1997 there were 3.9 million people aged 85 and older. Experts estimated that by 2005 there would be 4.9 million Americans aged 85 or older; and by 2030 there would be 18.2 million people over the age of 85.

The increase in the number of older people is expected to raise the demand for health care services in the home and in nursing homes. Many nursing homes now offer special care to stroke victims and those who need the help of a respirator to breathe. To care for such patients, nursing homes need more physical therapists and respiratory therapists—two of the fastest-growing occupations. The U.S. Bureau of Labor Statistics estimated that by 2006 the number of physical therapists would increase 70.8 percent, to 196,000, and the number of respiratory therapists would grow 45.8 percent, to 119,000.

ALTERNATIVE OR COMPLEMENTARY HEALTH CARE

More and more Americans are turning to alternative forms of health care that emphasize wellness and rely on the body's own ability to heal itself. In 1997 some 83 million Americans used some form of alternative medicine. According to the *Journal of the American Medical Association,* that figure represented a 30 percent increase over 1990. Although these alternatives to traditional medicine are gaining in popularity throughout the United States, many medical doctors still regard them with skepticism because they have not been thoroughly tested.

Acupuncture

Chinese medicine believes that a cycle of energy called Qi (pronounced chee) is essential to good health. This cycle of energy is thought to flow through the human body in meridians, or channels. The Chinese believe that pain and disease develop when there is any sort of disturbance in the natural flow. After a diagnosis of an imbalance in the flow of energy, the acupuncturist inserts long, thin needles at specific points along the 12 to 14 meridians. Each point controls a different part of the body. Once the needles are in place, they are rotated gently or are charged with a small electric current for a short time. Because acupuncture can control pain, it is also used as a type of anesthesia. Some Western doctors think that inserting the needles may alter the balance between the different parts of the nervous system.

In 1997 an independent panel of experts concluded that acupuncture was an effective remedial treatment for certain ailments, especially those that include nausea and pain, and should be used in standard medical treatment for these problems. The 12-member panel was convened by various agencies of the National Institutes of Health, including its newly minted Office of Alternative Medicine (now known as the National Center for Complementary and Alternative Medicine [NCCAM]).

Chiropractic

Chiropractors treat patients whose health problems are associated mainly with the body's structural and neurological systems, especially the spine. These practitioners believe that interference with these systems can impair normal functions and lower resistance to disease. Chiropractors think that misalignment or compression of the spinal nerves, for example, can alter many important body functions. Therefore, they attempt to alleviate pain and problems by manually manipulating or adjusting the spinal column and joints. In addition, therapy that includes massage and heat may be used. No drugs or surgery are used.

In 1999, 142,000 persons worked in the offices and clinics of chiropractors, up from 99,000 only three years earlier. About 70 percent of chiropractors are in private practice, with the remaining 30 percent in group practice or teaching at the nation's 17 accredited chiropractic schools.

Holistic Health Care

Holistic (or wholistic) health care stresses treatment of the whole person—medically, emotionally, and spiritually. It has evolved in reaction to the growth of medical specialization that has sometimes led to emphasizing only the diseased part of the body and not the whole organism. Holistic health care is an attempt to combine scientific treatment of medical problems with the treatment of psychological and spiritual problems.

Homeopathy

Homeopathy is a form of medical practice in which the practitioner (homeopathist) administers remedies that cause reactions in the patient that are similar to the symptoms of the illness. The homeopathist usually prescribes a minute quantity of an agent similar to, but not identical to, the cause of the disease. An example would be to give a small amount of a laxative to treat diarrhea.

Naturopathy

Naturopathy is a therapeutic system that dates back to the 1890s. This system emphasizes the use of natural forces to maintain health and to prevent disease. Naturopathists rely on sun, water, heat, and air to treat illness. Their remedies include sunbathing, diet (with an emphasis on a high intake of vegetables and a ban on salt and stimulants), steam baths, and exercise.

Herbalism

Herbalists use plants both to treat and prevent disease and to relieve pain. For example, garlic is used as a germ killer, aloe vera is used to fight infection and relieve arthritis pain, and rosemary serves as an insect repellant.

Many centuries ago, herbs were the only available medications. Today, the modern pharmacy stocks many examples of purified herbs in the form of pills and liquids. Herbalists use the barks, leaves, stalks, roots, flowers, and seeds of a wide variety of plants. Herbal medicine is the most common form of alternative treatment.

CHAPTER 6
HEALTH CARE INSTITUTIONS

HOSPITALS

The first hospitals in the United States were established well over two hundred years ago. No records of hospitals in the early colonies exist, but almshouses, which sheltered the poor, also cared for those who were ill. Started in 1751, the Pennsylvania Hospital was the first American institution devoted entirely to the sick.

Until the late 1800s, American hospitals had a bad reputation. The upper classes saw hospitals as places for the poor who could not afford home care. The poor saw hospitalization as a humiliating signal of personal economic failure. All classes thought hospitals were places to go to die.

TYPES OF HOSPITALS

Hospitals are described as short-stay or long-term, depending on the amount of time a patient spends before discharge. Short-stay facilities include community, teaching, and public hospitals. Long-term hospitals are usually psychiatric hospitals or hospitals for the treatment of tuberculosis or other respiratory diseases.

Community (General) Hospitals

The most common type of hospital in America is the community, or general, hospital. General hospitals, where most people receive care, are typically small, with anywhere from 50 to 500 beds. These hospitals normally provide good care for everyday medical and surgical problems. In the 1990s many smaller hospitals closed because they were not profitable. The larger ones, usually found in cities, are often equipped with a full complement of medical and surgical personnel and up-to-date equipment.

Some community hospitals are nonprofit corporations, supported by local funding. These include hospitals supported by religious, cooperative, or osteopathic

organizations. Increasing numbers of community hospitals have become proprietary hospitals, which are owned and operated on a for-profit basis by corporations. Many nonprofit hospitals have been joining investor-owned corporations because they need financial resources to maintain their existence in an increasingly competitive industry. Often, the investor-owned corporations acquire nonprofit hospitals to build market share, expand their provider networks, and penetrate new health care markets.

Teaching Hospitals

A teaching hospital, which provides clinical training for medical students and other medical professionals, is usually part of a major medical school and may have several hundred beds. Most of the physicians on staff at the hospital also hold teaching positions at the university affiliated with the hospital, in addition to doing a great deal of their teaching at the bedside of the patients. Patients in teaching hospitals understand that they may be examined by medical students, interns, and residents in addition to their primary "attending" physicians.

An advantage of obtaining care at a teaching hospital is that the patient receives treatment from highly qualified physicians who can use the latest technical equipment. A disadvantage is the inconvenience and invasion of privacy related to being examined by numerous students. While some teaching hospitals have a reputation for being very impersonal, patients usually receive the best treatment at a teaching hospital if their health problems are complex, unusual, or difficult.

Public Hospitals

Public hospitals are owned and operated by federal, state, or city governments. Many have a continuing tradition of caring for the poor. They are usually located in the inner cities and are often in precarious financial situ-

TABLE 6.1

Number and rate of discharges from short-stay hospitals and days of care, with average length of stay, by sex, age, and geographic region: 1998

Sex, age, and region	Discharges		Days of care		Average length of stay in days
	Number in thousands	Rate per 1,000 population	Number in thousands	Rate per 1,000 population	
Both sexes					
All ages:					
United States	31,827	116.5	160,914	589.2	5.1
Northeast	6,818	130.9	39,426	756.7	5.8
Midwest	7,366	116.5	34,959	553.0	4.7
South	12,022	124.5	60,939	631.0	5.1
West	5,621	91.8	25,590	417.9	4.6
Male					
All ages:					
United States	12,469	93.5	69,027	517.5	5.5
Northeast	2,855	113.2	17,493	693.9	6.1
Midwest	2,924	94.8	14,891	482.8	5.1
South	4,552	97.3	25,620	547.5	5.6
West	2,139	70.0	11,023	360.8	5.2
Female					
All ages:					
United States	19,358	138.5	91,886	657.6	4.7
Northeast	3,964	147.4	21,933	815.6	5.5
Midwest	4,442	137.2	20,068	619.9	4.5
South	7,470	150.0	35,318	709.4	4.7
West	3,482	113.5	14,567	474.8	4.2

SOURCE: Jennifer R. Popvic and Lola Jean Kozak, "National Hospital Discharge Survey: Annual Summary, 1998," *Vital and Health Statistics*, Series 13, no. 148, National Center for Health Statistics, September 2000

ations because many of their patients are unable to pay for services. These hospitals depend heavily on Medicaid payments supplied by local, state, and federal agencies or on grants from local governments. Well-known public hospitals include Bellevue Hospital Center (New York City), Parkland Memorial Hospital (Dallas, Texas), Truman Medical Center (Kansas City, Missouri), University of Southern California Medical Center (Los Angeles, California), and Temple University Hospital (Philadelphia, Pennsylvania). The last two are also teaching hospitals.

TREATING SOCIETY'S WEAKEST MEMBERS. Increasingly, public hospitals must bear the burden of the weaknesses in the nation's health system. The major problems in American society are usually apparent in the emergency rooms and corridors of public hospitals—poverty, drug and alcohol abuse, street violence, and infectious diseases such as AIDS and tuberculosis.

LOSING MONEY. The typical public hospital provides millions of dollars in health care for which it is not reimbursed by private insurance, Medicare, or Medicaid. The National Association of Public Hospitals (NAPH) estimated that nearly half of all public hospital charges are not ultimately paid. This figure has grown sharply as the

number of uninsured Americans has grown. State and local governments provide subsidies to help pay for these expenses, but even with the subsidies public hospitals are not paid for billions of dollars' worth of care.

PROVIDING A NUMBER OF SERVICES. The NAPH believes that the mission of public hospitals is to respond to the needs of their communities. As a result, most provide a broad spectrum of services. Although the need for trauma care exists for all socioeconomic levels, the American Hospital Association reported that NAPH members are twice as likely to have trauma centers as do community hospitals in general.

Almost half of NAPH member hospitals provide prison services. Some of these hospitals have dedicated ward beds for prisoners. County and city revenues provide most, if not all, of the funds available for prison services. Many of the NAPH member hospitals are also major academic centers, training medical and dental residents.

MORE THAN THEY CAN HANDLE. For many Americans, the public hospital emergency room has replaced the doctor's office. With no insurance and little money, many people go to the only place that will take them without question. Insurance companies estimate that half of all emergency room visits are for nonemergency treatment.

Public hospitals are usually underfunded and understaffed, and service is generally slow. All-day waits in the emergency room for initial treatment are not uncommon. An NAPH survey found that the average wait to get a bed upon admission from the emergency room was 5.6 hours, although waits of three to four days were not unusual. Seriously ill patients could wait an average of 3.2 hours to get into intensive care units.

EFFECTS OF VIOLENCE. Many urban public hospitals are located in inner cities and are often the only resource for 24-hour standby emergency and trauma care. As a result, they care for a disproportionate number of victims of violence. Between 1983 and 1999, 10 of the original 23 hospitals with designated trauma centers in Los Angeles closed their trauma units, causing severe overcrowding in the ones that remained. During the 1992 Los Angeles riots, King Drew Medical Center treated 94 lacerations, 54 gunshot wounds, 87 assaults, and 19 stab wounds over the course of six days.

REASONS FOR HOSPITALIZATION

In 1998 an estimated 31.8 million inpatients were discharged from short-stay nonfederal hospitals. These inpatients included an estimated 12.5 million males and 19.4 million females. The overall discharge rate for 1998 was 116.5 discharges per 1,000 civilian population. The rate per 1,000 population for females was 138.5, well above the 93.5 discharge rate for males. (See Table 6.1.) These numbers were higher for females primarily because women are hospitalized for childbirth and pregnancy-related conditions.

By Diagnosis

Heart disease is the number-one killer of Americans (see Chapter 7 for details). In 1998 diseases of the circulatory system, which include heart disease, ranked first among diagnoses for patients discharged from nonfederal short-stay hospitals, accounting for an estimated 6.3 million discharges.

The leading specific diagnoses included 4.3 million discharges for heart disease, 4 million for women delivering babies, and 1.2 million for malignant neoplasms (cancers). Approximately 1.3 million each were discharged for psychoses and pneumonia, and almost 1 million went to the hospital for treatment of broken bones. (See Table 6.2.) For patients 15 to 44 years of age, the most frequent diagnoses were deliveries (females only), mental disorders, and injuries. For patients aged 45 to 64 years and 65 years and over, heart disease, malignant neoplasms, mental disorders, and pneumonia were some of the major causes of hospitalization. (See Table 6.3.)

The average length of stay was 5.1 days in 1998, ranging from 2.5 days for childbirth to 9.2 days for perinatal (around the time of birth) conditions. Other long stays included 8.8 days for malignant neoplasms of the large intestine and rectum, 8.7 days to treat incidents of psychoses, 7.6 days to treat septicemia (blood infections), and 6.8 days for the treatment of fractures in the neck or the femur (the long thighbone). (See Table 6.4.)

By Procedures

In 1998, 41.5 million surgical and nonsurgical procedures were performed on patients discharged from short-stay hospitals. More than four of five (81.4 percent, or 33.8 million) of all procedures fell into just five categories: obstetrical procedures (more than 6.6 million); operations on the digestive system (5.1 million); operations on the cardiovascular system (5.8 million); operations on the musculoskeletal system (3.3 million); and the largest category, miscellaneous diagnostic and therapeutic procedures (13 million). The latter category included computerized axial tomography (usually referred to as a CAT or CT scan), arteriography and angiocardiography, diagnostic ultrasounds, and respiratory therapy. (See Table 6.5.)

In 1998, 16.2 million American males and 25.3 million American females underwent hospital procedures. The most frequent procedures for males included arteriography and angiocardiography, cardiac catheterization, diagnostic ultrasound, respiratory therapy, and CAT scans. Most common for women were various obstetrical procedures, such as episiotomy (usually an incision made in the vaginal area to make the birth process easier for both mother and infant), repair of vaginal laceration (tearing), and Cesarean sections. A large number of women also underwent arteriography and angiocardiography procedures. (See Table 6.5.)

The rate of procedures by age per 10,000 population ranged from 333.9 for patients under 15 years of age to 4,469.1 for patients 65 years of age and over. For patients under age 15, some of the most commonly performed procedures included respiratory therapy, spinal tap, and appendectomy. For patients between the ages of 15 and 44 years (not including obstetrical procedures), the most common procedures were bilateral destruction or occlusion of the fallopian tubes (female sterilization for birth control purposes). Other common procedures included oophorectomy and salpingo-oophorectomy (removal of the ovaries and operations on the ovaries and fallopian tubes), diagnostic ultrasound, hysterectomy, and CAT scans. (See Table 6.6.)

For patients aged 45 to 64 years, arteriography and angiocardiography, cardiac catheterization, and diagnostic ultrasound were most frequent. For elderly patients aged 65 years and over, arteriography and angiocardiography, diagnostic ultrasound, respiratory therapy, and cardiac catheterization were most common. (See Table 6.6.)

Organ Transplants

Organ transplants have become a viable means of saving lives in hospitals across the country. The United Network for Organ Sharing (UNOS) maintains data on organ transplants, distributes organ donor cards, and keeps a registry of patients awaiting organ transplants. UNOS reported that, in 1998, 54,500 Americans were waiting for transplants. More than 4,000 people die each year while waiting for an organ transplant. According to UNOS, the wait in some regions of the country is longer than in others. For example, in 1995, the wait for a liver transplant in Indiana, Michigan, and Ohio was 370 days, while in the region that includes Alabama, Florida, Georgia, Louisiana, and Mississippi, the wait was only 96 days.

In March 1998, the Clinton administration ordered UNOS to change its organ allocation policy. Under the previous system, when an organ became available in a local area, that organ was offered to the sickest patient in that area. If no local patient needed the organ, then it was offered regionally, then nationally. The government wanted organs to be given to the sickest patients first, regardless of where they lived.

The new regulations changed the allocation of organs from a regional system to a national system in which medical necessity, rather than geography, was the

TABLE 6.2

Number of discharges from short-stay hospitals by sex and first-listed diagnosis: 1998
[Discharges of inpatients from non-Federal hospitals. Excludes newborn infants.]

Category of first-listed diagnosis	Both sexes	Male	Female
		Number in thousands	
All conditions	31,827	12,469	19,358
Infectious and parasitic diseases	866	419	447
Septicemia	347	154	194
Neoplasms	1,706	644	1,062
Malignant neoplasms	1,266	575	691
Malignant neoplasm of large intestine and rectum	169	81	88
Malignant neoplasm of trachea, bronchus, and lung	165	95	69
Malignant neoplasm of breast	124	*	123
Benign neoplasms	389	44	345
Endocrine, nutritional and metabolic diseases, and immunity disorders	1,332	551	780
Diabetes mellitus	513	251	261
Volume depletion	448	170	278
Diseases of the blood and blood-forming organs	358	155	203
Mental disorders	1,974	1,015	958
Psychoses	1,253	592	661
Alcohol dependence syndrome	179	134	45
Diseases of the nervous system and sense organs	511	224	287
Diseases of the circulatory system	6,272	3,139	3,133
Heart disease	4,335	2,242	2,093
Acute myocardial infarction	783	463	320
Coronary atherosclerosis	1,094	669	426
Other ischemic heart disease	308	135	173
Cardiac dysrhythmias	670	322	348
Congestive heart failure	978	438	540
Cerebrovascular disease	1,010	457	553
Diseases of the respiratory system	3,403	1,574	1,829
Acute bronchitis and bronchiolitis	219	109	110
Pneumonia	1,328	638	690
Chronic bronchitis	498	218	280
Asthma	423	168	255
Diseases of the digestive system	3,046	1,339	1,706
Appendicitis	249	152	97
Noninfectious enteritis and colitis	275	106	169
Diverticula of intestine	230	91	139
Cholelithiasis	358	105	253
Diseases of the genitourinary system	1,720	534	1,186
Calculus of kidney and ureter	177	103	74
Complications of pregnancy, childbirth, and the puerperium	512	. . .	512
Diseases of the skin and subcutaneous tissue	517	264	252
Cellulitis and abscess	364	190	174
Diseases of the musculoskeletal system and connective tissue	1,534	658	876
Osteoarthrosis and allied disorders	435	161	274
Intervertebral disc disorders	352	187	165
Congenital anomalies	197	115	82
Certain conditions originating in the perinatal period	150	87	64
Symptoms, signs, and ill-defined conditions	297	135	162
Injury and poisoning	2,540	1,236	1,304
Fractures, all sites	966	414	552
Fracture of neck or femur	329	96	232
Poisonings	198	86	112
Supplementary classifications	4,892	378	4,514
Females with deliveries	4,000	. . .	4,000

* Figure does not meet standard of reliability or precision.
. . . Category not applicable.

SOURCE: Jennifer R. Popvic and Lola Jean Kozak, "National Hospital Discharge Survey: Annual Summary, 1998," *Vital and Health Statistics*, Series 13, no. 148, National Center for Health Statistics, September 2000

primary factor determining who received organs. The new rules have met with great resistance in Congress. Some members felt that the government should have no role in deciding life and death issues, and others insisted that a national program would result in the closure of smaller transplant centers, forcing some transplant recipients to travel great distances for life-saving care. UNOS also bitterly opposed the regulations, arguing that the new system would obstruct their ability to supply donated organs.

TABLE 6.3

Number of discharges from short-stay hospitals by age and first-listed diagnosis: 1998

[Discharges of inpatients from non-Federal hospitals. Excludes newborn infants.]

Category of first-listed diagnosis	All ages	Under 15 years	15–44 years	45–64 years	65 years and over
			Number in thousands		
All conditions	31,827	2,299	10,376	6,696	12,456
Infectious and parasitic diseases	866	178	209	145	335
Septicemia	347	17	34	62	234
Neoplasms	1,706	34	302	579	790
Malignant neoplasms	1,266	23	124	410	708
Malignant neoplasm of large intestine and rectum	169	*	*	41	120
Malignant neoplasm of trachea, bronchus, and lung	165	*	9	55	99
Malignant neoplasm of breast	124	*	13	55	56
Benign neoplasms	389	*	169	157	53
Endocrine, nutritional and metabolic diseases, and immunity disorders	1,332	139	272	329	592
Diabetes mellitus	513	22	131	161	200
Volume depletion	448	92	60	69	228
Diseases of the blood and blood-forming organs	358	49	99	62	148
Mental disorders	1,974	111	1,162	423	277
Psychoses	1,253	46	711	267	229
Alcohol dependence syndrome	179	*	112	55	11
Diseases of the nervous system and sense organs	511	83	122	112	193
Diseases of the circulatory system	6,272	30	395	1,753	4,094
Heart disease	4,335	17	241	1,248	2,829
Acute myocardial infarction	783	*	42	239	500
Coronary atherosclerosis	1,094	*	48	428	618
Other ischemic heart disease	308	*	21	115	172
Cardiac dysrhythmias	670	5	48	153	464
Congestive heart failure	978	*	25	175	773
Cerebrovascular disease	1,010	*5	41	218	746
Diseases of the respiratory system	3,403	632	396	653	1,721
Acute bronchitis and bronchiolitis	219	136	14	20	49
Pneumonia	1,328	211	131	226	760
Chronic bronchitis	498	*	18	138	342
Asthma	423	166	104	92	60
Diseases of the digestive system	3,046	210	771	798	1,266
Appendicitis	249	57	142	37	13
Noninfectious enteritis and colitis	275	62	80	47	86
Diverticula of intestine	230	*	19	67	144
Cholelithiasis	358	*	120	100	136
Diseases of the genitourinary system	1,720	70	577	419	653
Calculus of kidney and ureter	177	*	81	63	30
Complications of pregnancy, childbirth, and the puerperium	512	*	510	*	...
Diseases of the skin and subcutaneous tissue	517	62	137	130	188
Cellulitis and abscess	364	31	101	99	133
Diseases of the musculoskeletal system and connective tissue	1,534	42	349	476	667
Osteoarthrosis and allied disorders	435	*	10	130	295
Intervertebral disc disorders	352	*	158	140	53
Congenital anomalies	197	136	33	20	8
Certain conditions originating in the perinatal period	150	150	*	*	*
Symptoms, signs, and ill-defined conditions	297	56	105	70	66
Injury and poisoning	2,540	234	792	524	991
Fractures, all sites	966	76	231	151	508
Fracture of neck or femur	329	*	8	23	294
Poisonings	198	23	122	32	21
Supplementary classifications	4,892	80	4,145	202	466
Females with deliveries	4,000	7	3,990	*3	...

* Figure does not meet standard of reliability or precision.
... Category not applicable.

SOURCE: Jennifer R. Popvic and Lola Jean Kozak, "National Hospital Discharge Survey: Annual Summary, 1998," *Vital and Health Statistics*, Series 13, no. 148, National Center for Health Statistics, September 2000

The proposed changes were to take effect in July 1998, but opponents in Congress were able to block the implementation of the rules until March 2000. In September 2000, UNOS signed a new three-year contract with the government that compelled the network to put the new rules into effect. There was still a chance, however, that Congress would ultimately pass legislation overturning the rules.

TABLE 6.4

Average length of stay for discharges from short-stay hospitals by age and first-listed diagnosis: 1998

[Discharges of inpatients from non-Federal hospitals. Excludes newborn infants.]

Category of first-listed diagnosis	All ages	Under 15 years	15–44 years	45–64 years	65 years and over
			Average length of stay in days		
All conditions	5.1	4.6	3.7	5.1	6.2
Infectious and parasitic diseases	6.3	3.8	6.4	7.3	7.1
Septicemia	7.6	4.4	9.3	7.8	7.6
Neoplasms	6.4	7.0	4.5	5.6	7.6
Malignant neoplasms	7.2	8.8	6.3	6.5	7.7
Malignant neoplasm of large intestine and rectum	8.8	*	*9.0	7.4	9.2
Malignant neoplasm of trachea, bronchus, and lung	8.0	*	7.7	7.9	8.2
Malignant neoplasm of breast	2.7	*	3.1	2.8	2.6
Benign neoplasms	3.5	2.3	3.1	3.3	5.9
Endocrine, nutritional and metabolic diseases, and immunity disorders	4.8	3.3	4.6	4.6	5.3
Diabetes mellitus	5.2	2.9	4.2	5.6	5.7
Volume depletion	4.3	2.9	3.5	4.3	5.1
Diseases of the blood and blood-forming organs	4.6	3.8	5.0	4.7	4.4
Mental disorders	7.6	11.6	6.8	7.3	9.9
Psychoses	8.7	11.5	7.8	8.8	10.7
Alcohol dependence syndrome	5.7	*	5.6	5.9	6.6
Diseases of the nervous system and sense organs	5.2	3.8	4.4	4.8	6.6
Diseases of the circulatory system	5.2	6.9	4.3	4.8	5.4
Heart disease	4.9	5.5	3.8	4.6	5.2
Acute myocardial infarction	5.9	*	4.5	5.2	6.3
Coronary atherosclerosis	4.1	*	3.0	3.6	4.5
Other ischemic heart disease	3.2	*	2.2	3.4	3.1
Cardiac dysrhythmias	4.0	2.6	2.9	3.6	4.2
Congestive heart failure	5.9	*3.8	5.1	6.4	5.8
Cerebrovascular disease	5.9	*5.6	6.4	6.0	5.9
Diseases of the respiratory system	5.6	3.3	4.5	5.7	6.8
Acute bronchitis and bronchiolitis	3.7	3.2	3.1	3.9	5.1
Pneumonia	6.0	3.5	4.8	6.2	6.9
Chronic bronchitis	5.8	*	6.2	5.7	5.9
Asthma	3.3	2.3	3.2	3.8	5.4
Diseases of the digestive system	4.8	3.6	3.8	4.8	5.7
Appendicitis	3.5	3.8	2.9	4.3	6.6
Noninfectious enteritis and colitis	4.3	2.5	3.9	4.3	5.8
Diverticula of intestine	5.4	*	*	5.4	5.1
Cholelithiasis	3.7	*	2.8	3.2	4.8
Diseases of the genitourinary system	3.8	3.7	2.8	3.5	4.9
Calculus of kidney and ureter	2.2	*	1.9	2.1	3.3
Complications of pregnancy, childbirth, and the puerperium	2.5	*	2.5	*	...
Diseases of the skin and subcutaneous tissue	5.7	4.8	4.8	5.4	6.8
Cellulitis and abscess	4.9	2.9	4.0	4.9	6.1
Diseases of the musculoskeletal system and connective tissue	4.3	5.2	3.1	4.0	5.0
Osteoarthrosis and allied disorders	4.5	*	3.4	4.1	4.7
Intervertebral disc disorders	2.9	*	2.5	2.6	4.6
Congenital anomalies	4.9	5.2	3.6	5.0	5.6
Certain conditions originating in the perinatal period	9.2	9.2	*	*	*
Symptoms, signs, and ill-defined conditions	2.7	2.1	2.1	2.1	4.9
Injury and poisoning	5.4	4.4	4.3	5.4	6.4
Fractures, all sites	5.8	3.5	4.8	5.4	6.6
Fracture of neck or femur	6.8	*	5.7	6.1	7.0
Poisonings	3.0	1.8	2.5	*	4.0
Supplementary classifications	3.8	5.7	2.6	8.2	11.6
Females with deliveries	2.5	2.2	2.5	*3.0	...

* Figure does not meet standard of reliability or precision.
... Category not applicable.

SOURCE: Jennifer R. Popvic and Lola Jean Kozak, "National Hospital Discharge Survey: Annual Summary, 1998," *Vital and Health Statistics,* Series 13, no. 148, National Center for Health Statistics, September 2000

SURGICENTERS AND URGICENTERS

Ambulatory surgery centers, often called surgicenters, are equipped to perform routine surgical procedures that do not require an overnight stay. A surgicenter requires less sophisticated and expensive equipment than a hospital operating room. Minor surgery, such as biopsies, abortions, hernia repair, and some cosmetic surgery are typical procedures performed at surgicenters. Most

TABLE 6.5

Number of all-listed procedures from short-stay hospitals by sex and procedure category: 1998

[Discharges of inpatients from non-Federal hospitals. Excludes newborn infants.]

Procedure category	Both sexes	Male	Female
	Number in thousands		
All procedures	41,500	16,188	25,312
Operations on the nervous system	1,062	485	577
Spinal tap	321	157	164
Operations on the endocrine system	96	32	64
Operations on the eye	122	66	56
Operations on the ear	57	34	23
Operations on the nose, mouth, and pharynx	288	161	126
Operations on the respiratory system	1,004	544	460
Bronchoscopy with or without biopsy	264	145	119
Operations on the cardiovascular system	5,791	3,364	2,427
Removal of coronary artery obstruction and insertion of stent(s)	926	594	332
Coronary artery bypass graft	553	396	158
Cardiac catheterization	1,202	716	486
Insertion, replacement, removal, and revision of pacemaker leads or device	364	178	185
Hemodialysis	425	219	205
Operations on the hemic and lymphatic system	334	166	167
Operations on the digestive system	5,116	2,178	2,938
Endoscopy of small intestine with or without biopsy	892	414	478
Endoscopy of large intestine with or without biopsy	531	215	316
Partial excision of large intestine	242	112	130
Appendectomy, excluding incidental	278	156	122
Cholecystectomy	439	128	311
Lysis of peritoneal adhesions	310	59	250
Operations on the urinary system	946	470	476
Cystoscopy with or without biopsy	194	121	73
Operations on the male genital organs	298	298	...
Prostatectomy	203	203	...
Operations on the female genital organs	2,187	...	2,187
Oophorectomy and salpingo-oophorectomy	491	...	491
Bilateral destruction or occlusion of fallopian tubes	364	...	364
Hysterectomy	645	...	645
Obstetrical procedures	6,640	...	6,640
Episiotomy with or without forceps or vacuum extraction	1,220	...	1,220
Artificial rupture of membranes	815	...	815
Cesarean section	900	...	900
Repair of current obstetric laceration	1,093	...	1,093
Operations on the musculoskeletal system	3,257	1,552	1,705
Partial excision of bone	260	130	130
Reduction of fracture	610	282	328
Open reduction of fracture with internal fixation	416	177	239
Excision or destruction of intervertebral disc	312	163	149
Total hip replacement	160	68	92
Total knee replacement	266	99	167
Operations on the integumentary system	1,325	577	748
Debridement of wound, infection, or burn	335	195	140
Miscellaneous diagnostic and therapeutic procedures	12,977	6,261	6,716
Computerized axial tomography	986	462	524
Arteriography and angiocardiography using contrast material	1,961	1,115	845
Diagnostic ultrasound	1,123	488	635
Respiratory therapy	1,109	564	545
Insertion of endotracheal tube	399	200	199
Injection or infusion of cancer chemotherapeutic substance	254	121	134

... Category not applicable.

SOURCE: Jennifer R. Popvic and Lola Jean Kozak, "National Hospital Discharge Survey: Annual Summary, 1998," *Vital and Health Statistics,* Series 13, no. 148, National Center for Health Statistics, September 2000

procedures are done under a local anesthetic, and the patient goes home the same day.

Emergency centers, or urgicenters, usually run by private for-profit organizations, provide up to 24-hour care on a drop-in basis. These centers fill several special needs in a community. They provide quick help in an emergency when the nearest hospital is miles away, they are normally open during the hours that most doctors' offices are closed, and they man-

TABLE 6.6

Rate of all-listed procedures for discharge from short-stay hospitals by age and procedure category: 1998

[Discharges of inpatients from non-Federal hospitals. Excludes newborn infants.]

Procedure category	All ages	Under 15 years	15–44 years	45–64 years	65 years and over
			Rate per 10,000 population		
All procedures	1,519.4	333.9	1,188.1	1,710.5	4,469.1
Operations on the nervous system	38.9	34.9	29.5	39.8	77.6
Spinal tap	11.8	23.6	6.7	7.0	17.1
Operations on the endocrine system	3.5	*0.4	2.5	7.1	6.4
Operations on the eye	4.5	1.8	2.3	4.9	16.2
Operations on the ear	2.1	5.2	0.8	*	*1.5
Operations on the nose, mouth, and pharynx	10.5	11.1	8.3	10.2	18.3
Operations on the respiratory system	36.7	10.6	14.4	49.0	142.1
Bronchoscopy with or without biopsy	9.7	3.0	3.1	13.8	38.1
Operations on the cardiovascular system	212.0	28.5	44.9	356.2	891.5
Removal of coronary artery obstruction and insertion of stent(s)	33.9	*	4.9	71.8	133.8
Coronary artery bypass graft	20.3	*	1.2	41.0	89.3
Cardiac catheterization	44.0	1.9	7.5	88.1	175.0
Insertion, replacement, removal, and revision of pacemaker leads or device	13.3	*	*0.6	7.9	90.7
Hemodialysis	15.5	*	5.8	27.3	57.5
Operations on the hemic and lymphatic system	12.2	3.2	4.8	19.2	43.1
Operations on the digestive system	187.3	37.9	95.6	232.0	703.6
Endoscopy of small intestine with or without biopsy	32.7	2.7	10.4	37.8	156.4
Endoscopy of large intestine with or without biopsy	19.4	1.5	4.8	20.0	102.5
Partial excision of large intestine	8.9	*	2.2	11.5	42.9
Appendectomy, excluding incidental	10.2	10.6	13.0	6.9	4.8
Cholecystectomy	16.1	*	11.8	22.2	48.3
Lysis of peritoneal adhesion	11.3	1.0	11.1	14.8	24.6
Operations on the urinary system	34.6	7.5	17.0	51.9	116.6
Cystoscopy with or without biopsy	7.1	1.1	2.4	9.0	31.3
Operations on the male genital organs	10.9	4.1	1.2	11.3	57.1
Prostatectomy	7.4	*	*	8.4	45.2
Operations on the female genital organs	80.1	1.4	103.8	109.9	83.5
Oophorectomy and salpingo-oophorectomy	18.0	*	17.2	37.9	18.8
Bilateral destruction or occlusion of fallopian tubes	13.3	*	29.8	*	*
Hysterectomy	23.6	*	26.9	42.8	21.3
Obstetrical procedures	243.1	2.0	542.8	*1.1	...
Episiotomy with or without forceps or vacuum extraction	44.7	*	99.8	*	...
Artificial rupture of membranes	29.8	*	66.6	*	...
Cesarean section	32.9	*	73.6	*	...
Repair of current obstetric laceration	40.0	*	89.4	*	...
Operations on the musculoskeletal system	119.3	29.2	75.7	160.3	364.8
Partial excision of bone	9.5	1.8	7.4	16.9	18.5
Reduction of fracture	22.3	9.0	15.6	20.6	72.6
Open reduction of fracture with internal fixation	15.2	2.8	10.4	15.5	54.1
Excision or destruction of intervertebral disc	11.4	*	11.1	23.0	13.0
Total hip replacement	5.9	*	0.7	8.0	30.9
Total knee replacement	9.7	*	*0.4	14.2	52.7
Operations on the integumentary system	48.5	*	30.6	66.9	129.9
Debridement of wound, infection, or burn	12.3	3.1	7.6	16.8	37.5
Miscellaneous diagnostic and therapeutic procedures	475.1	135.1	214.0	588.9	1,816.7
Computerized axial tomography	36.1	7.2	17.8	41.9	142.8
Arteriography and angiocardiography using contrast material	71.8	3.0	13.7	139.1	287.8
Diagnostic ultrasound	41.1	7.9	17.6	48.5	171.3
Respiratory therapy	40.6	30.8	12.4	42.1	156.4
Insertion of endotracheal tube	14.6	5.6	4.9	16.1	62.8
Injection or infusion of cancer chemotherapeutic substance	9.3	6.8	4.6	14.7	21.7

* Figure does not meet standard of reliability or precision.

... Category not applicable.

SOURCE: Jennifer R. Popvic and Lola Jean Kozak, "National Hospital Discharge Survey: Annual Summary, 1998," *Vital and Health Statistics,* Series 13, no. 148, National Center for Health Statistics, September 2000

age to cut costs because they do not provide hospital beds. They usually deal with such problems as cuts that require sutures, sprains and bruises from accidents, and various infections. Many provide inexpensive vaccinations for influenza. They tend to be more expensive than a visit to the family doctor, but less expensive than a trip to a traditional hospital emergency room.

TABLE 6.7

Nursing homes, beds, occupancy, and residents: 1995–98

[Data are based on a census of certified nursing facilities]

	Nursing homes				Beds			
	1995	1996	1997	1998	1995	1996	1997	1998
United States	16,389	16,706	17,121	17,259	1,751,302	1,780,772	1,827,615	1,812,056

	Occupancy rate[1]				Resident rate[2]			
United States	84.5	83.1	82.2	83.5	404.5	393.3	388.3	373.6

[1] Percent of beds occupied.
[2] Number of nursing home residents (all ages) per 1,000 resident population 85 years of age and over.

SOURCE: *Health, United States, 2000*, National Center for Health Statistics, Hyattsville, MD, 2000

NURSING HOMES

Families are still the major caretakers of older, dependent, and disabled members of our society. The number of people aged 65 and older living in nursing homes, however, is rising because the population in this age group is increasing rapidly. Even though many older people now live longer, healthier lives, the increase in overall length of life has increased the need for long-term care in facilities such as nursing homes.

Types of Nursing Homes

Nursing homes fall into three broad categories: residential care facilities, intermediate care establishments, and skilled nursing facilities. Each provides various services:

- A residential care facility (RCF) normally provides meals and housekeeping for its residents, plus some basic medical monitoring, such as administering medications. This type of home is for a person who is fairly independent and does not need constant medical attention but does need help with tasks such as laundry and cleaning. Many RCFs also provide social and recreational programs for their residents.

- An intermediate care facility (ICF) offers room and board and nursing care as necessary for persons who can no longer live independently. As in the RCF, exercise and social programs are provided, and some ICFs have physical therapy and rehabilitation programs as well.

- A skilled nursing facility (SNF) provides around-the-clock nursing care, plus physician coverage. The SNF is for patients who need intensive care, plus such services as occupational therapy, physical therapy, and rehabilitation.

Number of Nursing Home Residents Rising

In 1998 the National Center for Health Statistics (NCHS) counted 17,259 nursing homes, containing more than 1.8 million beds, with 83.5 percent of those beds occupied. (See Table 6.7.)

In 1996, 92 percent of all nursing homes were privately owned. Most (66.1 percent) nursing homes were company-owned and operated on a for-profit basis. Another 25.7 percent were operated by nonprofit, volunteer organizations, and only 8.2 percent were operated by governmental agencies. About 7 in 10 (73 percent) were certified (approved for payment) by both Medicare and Medicaid.

Most residents of nursing homes are the "oldest old." Of the 1.5 million elderly nursing home residents in 1997, only 198,400 (13.5 percent) were between 65 and 74 years of age, 36 percent (528,300) were aged 75 to 84, and more than half (738,300, or 50.3 percent) of residents were 85 years old and older. People aged 85 and older (the so-called oldest old) are a fast-growing segment of the population. Notice, however, that even among the oldest old, fewer than one in five was living in a nursing home in 1997. (See Table 6.8.)

Among nursing home residents in 1997, women (1.1 million) outnumbered men (372,100) by almost three to one. (See Table 6.8.) Females have a considerably longer life expectancy than males. For persons born in 1997, the estimated average life expectancy at birth for females was 79.4 years, compared to 73.6 years for males. (See Table 1.6 in Chapter 1.)

In nursing home surveys, taken in 1973–74 and 1985, the ratio of nursing home residents over age 65 remained stable; almost 50 of every 1,000 persons aged 65 and over lived in nursing homes. In 1998, however, only 43.4 persons per 1,000 population resided in nursing homes. These data indicate that elderly persons are not moving into nursing homes at the same rate as before. One reason may be the rapid growth in the home health care industry (see below).

High Costs of Nursing Home Care

With the elderly population growing rapidly, the problems of long-term care and its costs have become

TABLE 6.8

Nursing home residents 65 years of age and over according to age, sex, and race: 1973–74, 1985, 1995, 1997

[Data are based on a sample of nursing home residents]

Age, sex, and race	Residents				Residents per 1,000 population			
	1973–74	1985	1995	1997	1973–74	1985	1995	1997
Age								
65 years and over, age adjusted[1]	...	...	...	...	58.5	54.0	45.9	45.3
65 years and over, crude	961,500	1,318,300	1,422,600	1,465,000	44.7	46.2	42.4	43.4
65–74 years	163,100	212,100	190,200	198,400	12.3	12.5	10.1	10.8
75–84 years	384,900	509,000	511,900	528,300	57.7	57.7	45.9	45.5
85 years and over	413,600	597,300	720,400	738,300	257.3	220.3	198.6	192.0
Male								
65 years and over, age adjusted[1]	...	...	...	...	42.5	38.8	32.8	32.0
65 years and over, crude	265,700	334,400	356,800	372,100	30.0	29.0	26.1	26.7
65–74 years	65,100	80,600	79,300	80,800	11.3	10.8	9.5	9.8
75–84 years	102,300	141,300	144,300	159,300	39.9	43.0	33.3	34.6
85 years and over	98,300	112,600	133,100	132,000	182.7	145.7	130.8	119.0
Female								
65 years and over, age adjusted[1]	...	...	...	...	67.5	61.5	52.3	51.9
65 years and over, crude	695,800	983,900	1,065,800	1,092,900	54.9	57.9	53.7	55.1
65–74 years	98,000	131,500	110,900	117,700	13.1	13.8	10.6	11.6
75–84 years	282,600	367,700	367,600	368,900	68.9	66.4	53.9	52.7
85 years and over	315,300	484,700	587,300	606,300	294.9	250.1	224.9	221.6
White								
65 years and over, age adjusted[1]	...	...	...	...	61.2	55.5	45.4	44.5
65 years and over, crude	920,600	1,227,400	1,271,200	1,294,900	46.9	47.7	42.3	43.0
65–74 years	150,100	187,800	154,400	160,800	12.5	12.3	9.3	10.0
75–84 years	369,700	473,600	453,800	464,400	60.3	59.1	44.9	44.2
85 years and over	400,800	566,000	663,000	669,700	270.8	228.7	200.7	192.4
Black								
65 years and over, age adjusted[1]	...	...	...	...	28.2	41.5	50.4	54.4
65 years and over, crude	37,700	82,000	122,900	137,400	22.0	35.0	45.2	49.4
65–74 years	12,200	22,500	29,700	31,400	11.1	15.4	18.4	19.2
75–84 years	13,400	30,600	47,300	51,900	26.7	45.3	57.2	60.6
85 years and over	12,100	29,000	45,800	54,100	105.7	141.5	167.1	186.0

... Category not applicable.
[1] Age adjusted by the direct method to the year 2000 population standard using the following three age groups: 65–74 years, 75–84 years, and 85 years and over.

Notes: Excludes residents in personal care or domiciliary care homes. Age refers to age at time of interview. Rates are based on the resident population as of July 1.

SOURCE: *Health, United States, 2000*, National Center for Health Statistics, Hyattsville, MD, 2000

explosive public issues. Nursing home care costs an average of $40,000 per year, and in some homes the costs can be more than $80,000 a year. Medicare does not cover routine nursing home care, and Medicaid is intended to cover expenses only for the poor.

To be eligible for Medicaid, a person must have no more than $2,500 in assets. (In the case of a married couple where only one spouse is in a nursing home, the remaining spouse can retain a house, a car, up to $75,000 in assets, and $2,000 in monthly income.) Many elderly persons must deplete their entire life savings before qualifying for Medicaid assistance.

Although the Medigap policies available through private insurers pay for some costs not covered by Medicare, most of these policies do not cover the average nursing home stay. Many elderly people are eager to buy private insurance policies for long-term care. The average policy, covering two years of care after a one-hundred-day waiting period, costs about $300 a month for a couple in which the husband is in his early seventies and the wife in her late sixties.

Coverage by these private policies varies widely. Some insurers refuse to pay for the first 20 days in a nursing home, and others require a waiting period of 100 days before they will pay. Some will allow coverage for only one year; others allow longer stays. Because of the variations and limitations on coverage, some policyholders have found that their claims have been denied or their policies canceled. The purchasers of such policies must be very careful to understand what they are getting in terms of benefits.

Diversification of Nursing Homes

As a means of staying competitive with home care and the increasing array of alternative services for the elderly, many nursing homes began to offer alternative services and programs. New services include adult day care and visiting nurse care to people who still live at home. Other programs include respite plans that allow people who need to go away on business or vacation to leave an elderly relative in the nursing home temporarily.

TABLE 6.9

Number and percent distribution of home health and hospice care current patients and selected agency characteristics according to type of care received: 1996

Agency characteristic	All patients	Type of care		All patients	Type of care	
		Home health	Hospice		Home health	Hospice
		Number			Percent distribution	
Total	2,486,800	2,427,500	59,400	100.0	100.0	100.0
Ownership						
Proprietary	1,017,500	1,010,900	6,500	40.9	41.6	11
Voluntary nonprofit	1,240,100	1,190,000	50,200	49.9	49.0	84.6
Government and other	229,200	226,600	*2,600	9.2	9.3*	*4.4
Certification						
Certified by Medicare[1]	2,299,800	2,242,300	57,500	92.5	92.4	96.8
As a home health agency	2,259,300	2,229,700	29,600	90.9	91.9	49.8
As a hospice	652,100	596,000	56,100	26.2	24.6	94.4
Certified by Medicaid[1]	2,326,700	2,271,000	55,700	93.6	93.6	93.8
As a home health agency	2,293,700	2,264,800	28,800	92.2	93.3	48.6
As a hospice	579,200	526,600	52,600	23.3	21.7	88.5
Not certified	*104,300	*102,900	1,400	*4.2	*4.2	2.3
Affiliation						
Affiliated[1,2]	1,570,200	1,540,300	29,900	63.1	63.5	50.4
Part of group or chain	1,053,000	1,032,000	21,000	42.3	42.5	35.4
Operated by a hospital	844,900	828,660	16,300	34.0	34.1	27.4
Not affiliated	916,700	887,200	29,500	36.9	36.5	49.6
Geographic region						
Northeast	651,700	642,700	8,900	26.2	26.5	15.0
Midwest	668,100	646,900	21,300	26.9	26.6	35.9
South	811,300	792,300	19,000	32.6	32.6	32.0
West	355,700	345,600	10,100	14.3	14.2	7.1
Location of agency						
In a metropolitan statistical area	1,999,600	1,951,400	48,100	80.4	80.4	81.l
Not in a metropolitan statistical area	487,300	476,000	11,200	19.6	19.6	18.9

* Figure does not meet standard of reliability or precision.
[1] Numbers may add to more than totals since an agency may be listed in more than one category.
[2] Includes a small number of patients that were served by agencies that are operated by a nursing home or health maintenance organization.
Notes: Numbers may not add to totals because of rounding. Percents are based on the unrounded figures.
SOURCE: Barbara J. Haupt, *Advance Data from Vital and Health Statistics,* no. 297, National Center for Health Statistics, Hyattsville, MD, 1998

One of the most popular nontraditional services is subacute care, which is comprehensive inpatient treatment for people recovering from acute illnesses such as pneumonia, injuries such as a broken hip, and chronic diseases such as arthritis that do not require hospital-level treatment. This new approach also allows nursing homes to offer services to younger patients.

HOME HEALTH CARE

Home health care grew faster in the early 1990s than any other segment of health services. In many cases, caring for a patient at home is preferable to and more cost-effective than care provided in a hospital, nursing home, or some other residential facility. For one thing, elderly persons are often more comfortable and much happier living in their own homes or with family members. Disabled persons may also be able to function better at home with limited assistance than in a residential setting with full-time monitoring ("Home Health Care," *Family Economics and Nutrition Review,* vol. 9, no. 2, 1996).

Home health care agencies provide a wide variety of services. The types of services range from helping with activities of daily living, such as bathing, light housekeeping, and meals, to skilled nursing care, such as the care needed by AIDS or cancer patients. About 20 percent of the staffs of home health agencies are registered nurses, another 7 percent are licensed practical nurses, and 13 percent are nursing aides. Other personnel include physical therapists, social workers, speech therapists, and those with other specialized skills.

The NCHS reported that more than 2.4 million persons received home health care in 1996. Of these, the largest proportion (1.2 million) received care through voluntary nonprofit agencies, 1 million were cared for by proprietary for-profit agencies, and government or other agencies assisted 229,200. About 92.4 percent of recipients were receiving care from agencies certified for Medicare coverage, and 93.6 percent were with agencies also certified for Medicaid (note that agencies may be certified by both Medicare and Medicaid). (See Table 6.9.)

HOSPICES

Hospice is a philosophy, an approach to dying, rather than a physical facility. A hospice may be a free-standing institution, a special wing of a hospital, or a service that cares for dying patients in their homes or in nursing homes. The purpose of hospice care, also known as palliative (to relieve without curing) care, is to provide support and care for terminally ill people in the final stages of their diseases so that they can live as comfortably and fully as possible. A hospice offers services for both patients and their families so they can make the necessary preparations for death.

In 1996, 59,400 persons were receiving hospice care, the majority through voluntary agencies. Medicare-certified agencies served about 96.8 percent of the patients, and Medicaid-certified agencies helped 93.8 percent. (See Table 6.9.)

What Makes Hospice Unique?

The hospice concept is special because it focuses on care, not cure. Hospices try to minimize the two greatest fears associated with dying: fear of isolation and fear of pain. Medications are offered to any patient in pain, with the goal of controlling pain without impairing alertness so that the patient can be as comfortable as possible.

Hospice care also emphasizes living life to its fullest. Patients are encouraged to stay active for as long as possible, to do things they enjoy, and to learn something new. Quality of life, rather than length of life, is the focus. In addition, whenever it is possible, family and friends are urged to be the primary caregivers in the home. Care at home helps both patients and family members enrich their lives and face death together.

Hospice organizations also treat the patient and family members as a unit. The programs provide relief at any time to families who are occasionally overwhelmed and may be neglecting their own needs. Finally, hospice programs work to prepare relatives and friends for the loss of their loved one. Hospice workers offer support groups and counseling to help deal with grief and may even help with funeral arrangements.

MANAGED CARE ORGANIZATIONS

Managed care, which has a primary purpose of controlling costs, represents a rapidly growing segment of the health care industry. The beneficiaries of employer-funded health plans, as well as Medicare and Medicaid recipients, often find themselves in this type of health care program. The term "managed care" covers several types of health care delivery systems, such as health maintenance organizations, preferred provider organizations, and "utilization review" groups that oversee diagnoses,

recommend treatments, and control costs for their beneficiaries.

Health Maintenance Organizations

Health maintenance organizations (HMOs) began to grow in the 1970s as an alternative to traditional health insurance, which was becoming more and more expensive. The federal government has been promoting HMOs since the Nixon administration, maintaining that groups of doctors following certain rules of practice could slow rising medical costs and improve health care.

HMOs are group practices organized to provide complete coverage for subscribers' health needs at negotiated prices. The patients (and/or their employers) pay a set amount each month; in turn, the HMO group provides, at no extra charge or at a very minimal charge, preventive care, such as routine checkups and immunizations, and care for any illness or accident. Hospitalization and referral services that the HMO group cannot provide are also covered by the monthly fee, often at a discounted price. Members are usually "locked into" the plan for a specified period—usually one year. If the necessary service is available within the HMO, patients normally must use an HMO doctor. There are several types of HMOs:

- Staff model—the HMO delivers services through physicians, nurses, and technicians who are employed by the HMO and who provide services in a clinic-type facility.

- Group model—the HMO contracts with a group of multispecialty health providers.

- Network model—the HMO contracts with two or more groups of health providers that agree to provide health care at negotiated prices to all members enrolled in the HMO.

- Independent practice association model—the HMO contracts with individuals or groups who then provide medical care to HMO members at their own offices. The individual doctors agree to follow the practices and procedures of the HMO in caring for the HMO members.

An HMO may offer an open-ended or point-of-service option that allows members to choose their own doctors and hospitals, either within or outside the HMO. A member who chooses an outside provider, however, will generally have to pay a larger portion of the expenses.

The number of people enrolled in HMOs more than tripled between 1980 and 1990. In 1980 HMOs covered only 9.1 million people. By 1990, 33 million Americans were enrolled in HMOs. Enrollment continued to explode through the 1990s, and by 1999, there were 643 HMOs covering 81.3 million persons—over one-fourth (29 percent) of the American population. (See Table 6.10.)

TABLE 6.10

Health maintenance organizations (HMO's) and enrollment, according to model type, geographic region, and federal program: selected years 1976–99

[Data are based on a census of health maintenance organizations]

Plans and enrollment	1976	1980	1985[1]	1990	1993	1994[2]	1995[2]	1996[2]	1997[2]	1998[2]	1999[2]
Plans						Number					
All plans	174	235	478	572	551	543	562	630	652	651	643
Model type:[3]											
Individual practice association[4]	41	97	244	360	332	321	332	367	284	317	309
Group[5]	122	138	234	212	150	118	108	122	98	116	123
Mixed	- - -	- - -	- - -	- - -	69	104	122	141	258	212	208
Geographic region:											
Northeast	29	55	81	115	102	101	100	111	110	107	110
Midwest	52	72	157	160	169	159	157	182	184	185	179
South	23	45	141	176	167	173	196	218	236	237	239
West	70	63	99	121	113	110	109	119	121	122	115
Enrollment						Number of persons in millions					
Total	6.0	9.1	21.0	33.0	38.4	45.1	50.9	59.1	66.8	76.6	81.3
Model type:[3]											
Individual practice association[4]	0.4	1.7	6.4	13.7	15.3	17.8	20.1	26.0	26.7	32.6	32.8
Group[5]	5.6	7.4	14.6	19.3	15.4	13.9	13.3	14.1	11.0	13.8	15.9
Mixed	- - -	- - -	- - -	- - -	7.7	13.4	17.6	19.0	29.0	30.1	32.6
Federal program:[6]											
Medicaid[7]	- - -	0.3	0.6	1.2	1.7	2.6	3.5	4.7	5.6	7.8	10.4
Medicare	- - -	0.4	1.1	1.8	2.2	2.5	2.9	3.7	4.8	5.7	6.5
						Percent of HMO enrollees					
Model type:[3]											
Individual practice association[4]	6.6	18.7	30.4	41.6	39.8	39.4	39.4	44.1	39.9	42.6	40.3
Group[5]	93.4	81.3	69.6	58.4	40.1	30.7	26.0	23.7	16.5	18.0	19.6
Mixed	- - -	- - -	- - -	- - -	20.1	29.9	34.5	32.2	43.4	39.2	40.1
Federal program:[6]											
Medicaid[7]	- - -	2.9	2.7	3.5	4.4	5.8	6.9	8.0	8.2	10.2	12.7
Medicare	- - -	4.3	5.1	5.4	5.7	5.5	5.7	6.3	7.2	7.4	8.0
						Percent of population enrolled in HMO's					
Total	2.8	4.0	8.9	13.4	15.1	17.3	19.4	22.3	25.2	28.6	30.1
Geographic region:											
Northeast	2.0	3.1	7.9	14.6	18.0	20.8	24.4	25.9	32.4	37.8	36.7
Midwest	1.5	2.8	9.7	12.6	13.2	15.2	16.4	18.8	19.5	22.7	23.3
South	0.4	0.8	3.8	7.1	8.4	10.2	12.4	15.2	17.9	21.0	23.9
West	9.7	12.2	17.3	23.2	25.1	27.4	28.6	33.2	36.4	39.1	41.4

- - - Data not available.
[1] Increases partly due to changes in reporting methods.
[2] Open-ended enrollment in HMO plans, amounting to 8.9 million on Jan. 1, 1999, is included from 1994 onwards.
[3] In 1976, 11 HMO's with 35,000 enrollment did not report model type. In 1997, 11 HMO's with 153,000 enrollment did not report model type. In 1998, 6 HMO's with 109,000 enrollment did not report model type. In 1999, 3 HMO's with 18,000 enrollment did not report model type.
[4] An HMO operating under an individual practice association model contracts with an association of physicians from various settings (a mixture of solo and group practices) to provide health services.
[5] Group includes staff, group, and network model types.
[6] Federal program enrollment in HMO's refers to enrollment by Medicaid or Medicare beneficiaries, where the Medicaid or Medicare program contracts directly with the HMO to pay the appropriate annual premium.
[7] Data for 1990 and later include enrollment in managed care health insuring organizations.

Notes: Data as of June 30 in 1976–80, December 31 in 1985, and January 1 in 1990–99. Medicaid enrollment in 1990 is as of June 30. HMO's in Guam are included starting in 1994; HMO's in Puerto Rico, starting in 1998. In 1999 HMO enrollment in Guam was 93,000 and in Puerto Rico, 1,354,000.

SOURCE: *Health, United States, 2000*, National Center for Health Statistics, Hyattsville, MD, 2000

HMOs have been the subject of considerable debate. Many physicians feel HMOs interfere in the doctor-patient relationship and do not let them effectively practice medicine. These physicians claim they know their patients' conditions and are, therefore, in the best situation to recommend treatment. The doctors resent being overruled by insurance administrators. (Physicians can recommend what treatment they believe is best, but if the insurance company will not cover the costs, patients may be unwilling to undergo the treatment.)

The HMO industry counters that its judgments are based upon the experiences of many thousands of doctors and, therefore, it knows best what is most likely to be successful. The industry generally claims that, in the past, physicians have not tested their diagnoses scientifically, and so do not really know how effective the treatments are.

Many doctors also resent that, with a few exceptions, HMOs are not financially liable for their decisions. If a doctor chooses to forgo a certain procedure and is wrong,

TABLE 6.11

Inpatient and residential mental health organizations and beds, according to type of organization: selected years 1984–94

[Data are based on inventories of mental health organizations]

Type of organization	1984	1986	1988	1990	1992	1994
	Number of mental health organizations					
All organizations	2,849	3,039	3,231	3,430	3,415	3,319
State and county mental hospitals	277	285	285	273	273	256
Private psychiatric hospitals	220	314	444	462	475	430
Non-Federal general hospital psychiatric services	1,259	1,287	1,425	1,571	1,517	1,531
Department of Veterans Affairs psychiatric services[1]	124	124	125	130	133	135
Residential treatment centers for emotionally disturbed children	322	437	440	501	497	459
All other[2]	647	592	512	493	520	508
	Number of beds					
All organizations	262,673	267,613	271,923	272,253	270,867	252,333
State and county mental hospitals	130,411	119,033	107,109	98,789	93,058	79,294
Private psychiatric hospitals	21,474	30,201	42,255	44,871	43,684	41,195
Non-Federal general hospital psychiatric services	46,045	45,808	48,421	53,479	52,059	52,984
Department of Veterans Affairs psychiatric services[1]	23,546	26,874	25,742	21,712	22,466	21,146
Residential treatment centers for emotionally disturbed children	16,745	24,547	25,173	29,756	30,089	32,110
All other[2]	24,452	21,150	23,223	23,646	29,511	25,604
	Beds per 100,000 civilian population					
All organizations	112.9	111.7	111.4	111.6	107.4	97.5
State and county mental hospitals	56.1	49.7	44.0	40.5	36.9	30.6
Private psychiatric hospitals	9.2	12.6	17.3	18.4	17.3	15.9
Non-Federal general hospital psychiatric services	19.8	19.1	19.8	21.9	20.7	20.5
Department of Veterans Affairs psychiatric services[1]	10.1	11.2	10.5	8.9	8.9	8.2
Residential treatment centers for emotionally disturbed children	7.2	10.3	10.3	12.2	11.9	12.4
All other[2]	10.5	8.8	9.5	9.7	11.7	9.9

[1] Includes Department of Veterans Affairs neuropsychiatric hospitals and general hospital psychiatric services.
[2] Includes other multiservice mental health organizations with inpatient and residential treatment services that are not elsewhere classified.

SOURCE: *Health, United States, 2000,* National Center for Health Statistics, Hyattsville, MD, 2000

he or she may well be held legally accountable. If an HMO informs a doctor that it will not cover a recommended procedure and it is wrong, it cannot be held directly liable. Many doctors claim that because HMOs make such choices, they are practicing medicine, and should, therefore, be held accountable. The HMOs counter that these are administrative decisions, and they are not practicing medicine.

The legal climate, however, was beginning to change for HMOs. Both the Third Circuit Federal Court of Appeals in *Dukes v. U.S. Healthcare* (64 LW 2007, 1995) and the Tenth Circuit Federal Court of Appeals in *PacifiCare of Oklahoma, Inc., v. Burrage* (59 F.3rd 151, 1995) agreed that HMOs were liable for malpractice and negligence claims against the HMO and HMO physicians. In *Frappier Estate v. Wishnov* (Florida District Court of Appeals, Fourth District, No. 95-0669, May 8, 1996), the Florida court agreed with the earlier findings. In addition, both houses of Congress passed legislation (the "Patients' Bill of Rights") giving patients more recourse to contest the decisions of HMOs, although the House of Representatives and the Senate disagree about what those specific rights should be. Because of this disagreement, the bill never made it into law in the 1999–2000 Congress, but it was high on the agenda for 2001–2002.

The HMO industry pointed to the slower increase in health care expenses as an indicator of its management success. Industry spokespersons noted that any major change in how the industry is run would lead to increasing costs. They claimed that HMOs and managed care were bringing a more rational approach to the industry while maintaining a high level of health care and controlling costs.

Preferred Provider Organizations

In the 1990s, in response to HMOs and other efforts by insurance groups to cut costs, physicians began forming or joining preferred provider organizations (PPOs). A PPO obtains discounted rates from participating doctors; in return, the health insurer refers its members, usually with the incentive of lower out-of-pocket payments, to the PPO group. Members of the insured group may use other doctors, but they usually have to pay a higher proportion of the costs.

MENTAL HEALTH FACILITIES

In earlier centuries, mental illness was often considered a sign of possession by the devil or, at best, moral weakness. A change in these attitudes began in the late eighteenth century, when mental illness began to be perceived as a treatable condition. It was then that the concept of "asylums" was developed, not simply to lock the mentally ill away, but also to provide them with "relief" from the conditions they found troubling.

Who Are the Mentally Ill?

Providers of mental health care distinguish between people who are severely mentally ill (defined by diagnosis), those who are mentally disabled (defined by level of disability), and those who are chronic mental patients (defined by duration of hospitalization). These three dimensions—diagnosis, disability, and duration—are the models used to describe the mentally ill population in the United States.

The Public Health Service uses this definition:

The chronically mentally ill population includes persons who suffer from emotional disorders that interfere with their functional capacities in relation to such primary aspects of daily life as self-care, interpersonal relationships, and work or schooling, and that may often necessitate prolonged mental health care.

Where Are the Mentally Ill?

The chronically mentally ill may be found either in mental hospitals or in community settings, such as with families, in boarding homes, in single-room-occupancy hotels (usually a cheap hotel or boardinghouse), in jail, or even on the streets as part of the homeless population.

The institutionalized mentally ill are those people with any psychiatric diagnosis who have lived in mental hospitals for more than one year or those with a diagnosed mental condition who are living in nursing homes.

Between 1970 and 1990, the number of patients housed in mental health institutions dropped dramatically. In 1970 there were 524,878 beds available in all types of mental institutions. By 1990 this number had dropped to 272,253. In 1994 there were only 252,333 beds available. Between 1990 and 1994, the number of beds available per 1,000 nonmilitary Americans dropped from 111.6 to 97.5. (See Table 6.11.) This is not necessarily a result of better treatment for the mentally ill, but rather a consequence of reduced funding for those institutions and individuals. Unfortunately, many patients who were once housed in mental institutions now fend for themselves on the streets or in prisons. (For more information on mental health, see Chapter 11.)

CHAPTER 7

CHRONIC DISEASES: CAUSES, TREATMENT, AND PREVENTION

The Centers for Disease Control and Prevention (CDC) defines chronic diseases as prolonged illnesses that do not resolve spontaneously and are rarely cured completely. According to the CDC, illnesses such as cardiovascular disease, cancer, respiratory disease, and diabetes account for 70 percent of all deaths in the United States and one-third of the years of potential life lost before age 65 (*The Robert Wood Johnson Foundation, Annual Report 1994; Health, United States,* 1994).

CARDIOVASCULAR DISEASES

Cardiovascular disease, which includes coronary heart diseases, arrhythmias, diseases of the arteries, congestive heart failure, rheumatic heart disease, congenital heart defects, and stroke (cerebrovascular disease), is the number-one cause of death in the United States. In 1998 heart (724,269) and cerebrovascular (158,060) disease killed almost as many Americans as cancer, lung disease, accidents, pneumonia, influenza, and diabetes combined. (See Table 7.1.)

Of the approximately 280 million people in the United States, about 58 million (1 in 4.8 Americans) suffer from cardiovascular disease. Almost half of all Americans will eventually die from heart disease. The American Heart Association (AHA) reported that more than 2,600 Americans died each day in 1995 from cardiovascular diseases. In 1998 cardiovascular disease accounted for 37.7 percent of all deaths, or 1 of every 2.6 deaths.

TABLE 7.1

Deaths and death rates for the 10 leading causes of death for all ages: preliminary 1998

[Data are based on a continuous file of records received from the States. Rates per 100,000 population in specified group. Figures are based on weighted data rounded to the nearest individual, so categories may not add to totals]

Rank [1]	Cause of death and age (Based on Ninth Revision, International Classification of Diseases, 1975)	Number	Rate
All ages [2]			
...	All causes	2,338,075	865.0
1	Diseases of heart	724,269	268.0
2	Malignant neoplasms, including neoplasms of lymphatic and hematopoietic tissues	538,947	199.4
3	Cerebrovascular diseases	158,060	58.5
4	Chronic obstructive pulmonary diseases and allied conditions	114,381	42.3
5	Pneumonia and influenza	94,828	35.1
6	Accidents and adverse effects	93,207	34.5
...	Motor vehicle accidents	41,826	15.5
...	All other accidents and adverse effects	51,382	19.0
7	Diabetes mellitus	64,574	23.9
8	Suicide	29,264	10.8
9	Nephritis, nephrotic syndrome, and nephrosis	26,295	9.7
10	Chronic liver disease and cirrhosis	24,936	9.2
...	All other causes	469,314	173.6

. . . Category not applicable.
[1] Rank based on number of deaths.
[2] Includes deaths under 1 year of age.

Note: Data are subject to sampling and/or random variation.

SOURCE: Joyce A. Martin et al., "Births and Deaths: Preliminary Data for 1998," *National Vital Statistics Report,* vol. 47, no. 25, October 5, 1999

Heart Attack and Angina Pectoris

A heart attack, or myocardial infarction, occurs when the blood supply to the heart muscle (the myocardium) is cut off or reduced. This happens when one of the major arteries that supply blood to the heart is blocked by some kind of obstruction, usually a blood clot. When the blood supply is reduced drastically or continuously, the heart's muscle cells are injured and die. Disability or death can result, depending on how much of the heart muscle has been damaged.

Angina pectoris is not a disease; it is the name for pain that occurs when the muscular wall of the heart becomes temporarily short of oxygen. A common condition, angina is usually a warning of the risk of heart attack. Its dull, constricting pain typically occurs when a person is physically active or excited but fades when activity ceases. In men, angina usually occurs after the age of 30 and is almost always caused by diseases or blockage of the arteries supplying the heart. In women, angina tends to begin later in life. In 1995 an estimated 7.2 million persons in the United States suffered from angina. According to the *Framingham Heart Study*—a famous study of heart disease in the residents of Framingham, Massachusetts, over the course of a half-century—about 350,000 new cases of angina occur annually.

WARNING SIGNALS OF A HEART ATTACK. The AHA lists several warning signs of a heart attack:

- An uncomfortable pressure, squeezing, fullness, or pain in the center of the chest behind the breastbone.

- Pain that spreads to the shoulders, neck, or arms.

- Chest discomfort accompanied by sweating, nausea, shortness of breath, or a feeling of weakness.

PROMPT CARE IS CRUCIAL. Prompt care dramatically improves the odds of surviving a heart attack. A Harvard Medical School study examining invasive heart surgeries discovered that patients who received intensive emergency care in the first 24 hours after a heart attack had a better chance of survival after four years. The researchers believed that more heart attack patients would benefit from early intensive treatment available at specialized centers, such as better monitoring of their condition and aggressive use of drug therapy, including new "clot-busting" medications.

Coronary Artery Bypass Surgery

Heart disease can be treated in various ways. Coronary bypass operations can improve blood flow to the heart, relieve chest pains, and make the heart pump more efficiently. Generally, a segment of large healthy vein, usually from the patient's leg or stomach, is spliced between the aorta (the main vessel carrying blood from the left side of the heart to all the arteries of the body and limbs) and the blocked coronary arteries. The coronary bypass operation thus supplies blood to the area of the heart that had a deficient blood supply. During the operation, the patient is placed on a heart-lung machine that takes over the functions of the heart and lungs while the surgery is proceeding. Usually, the patient spends two or three days in the intensive care unit and another week in the hospital following the surgery.

NEW REFINEMENTS. Heart surgeons have developed a procedure called "minimally invasive direct coronary bypass" surgery. In this procedure, the surgeon makes one or more small incisions (about 3 inches long) in the chest wall and works directly on the clogged artery while the heart is beating. Some surgeons use fiber-optic techniques similar to those used in gallbladder and other procedures. Anesthesiologists can slow the heartbeat with drugs such as calcium channel blockers and beta blockers to allow surgeons more control. Another technique under development actually stops the heartbeat and uses a modified heart-lung machine connected to a large artery in the groin while the doctor operates through small incisions using a video camera and long-handled instruments.

The expected benefits of these new refinements include reduced costs, shorter recovery times, and the possibility of combining the new procedure with angioplasty or other procedures. To date, however, there are no data to substantiate these benefits. Also, the long-term success of the procedures will depend on increased survival rates for patients and on how acceptable surgeons find the procedure.

Percutaneous Transluminal Coronary Angioplasty

Some patients may qualify for a much simpler procedure, performed under a local anesthetic, called percutaneous transluminal coronary angioplasty, or balloon angioplasty. A doctor inserts a balloon-tipped catheter into an artery in the patient's groin, and the tip of the catheter is slowly fed through the arterial system and positioned in the coronary artery at the point of the blockage. The small, sausage-shaped balloon on the end of the catheter is then inflated, flattening the fatty plaque and widening the artery. The balloon is sometimes inflated and deflated several times to clear the artery.

Balloon angioplasty has several obvious advantages over bypass surgery. First, it is performed under a local rather than a general anesthetic and does not involve opening the chest or using a heart-lung machine. Also, it is less expensive, and the patient is usually out of the hospital and recovering in a few days. As technology advances, devices such as fiber optics and laser methods may replace angioplasty as the treatment of choice. Some doctors are also using a tiny cutting blade attached to the end of a fiber-optic tube to remove accumulated plaque, although this method has not yet been proven to be more effective than the balloon angioplasty. Doctors are also experimenting with placing a wire mesh tube into the artery to prevent later collapse.

Less Surgery for the Elderly

In 1994 a Harvard Medical School study of more than 200,000 elderly heart attack patients found that invasive treatments such as bypass catheterization might not contribute to long-term survival. In fact, invasive cardiovascular procedures could be reduced by as much as 25 percent without a corresponding increase in mortality. The hundreds of millions of dollars saved by avoiding the expensive surgery would be put to better use, the study asserted, by aggressively improving care in the crucial 24-hour period after the onset of a heart attack.

It is particularly important, however, that elderly patients receive proper medications and treatment following heart attacks. A government study of Medicare patients found that many older patients were not treated with drugs that prolong life after a heart attack. Almost one-quarter of elderly heart attack survivors were not even encouraged to take regular doses of aspirin, although the widely available and inexpensive drug has been proven to prevent or postpone later heart attacks.

Risk Factors for Heart Disease

NONCHANGEABLE FACTORS. Four risk factors for heart disease that cannot be altered are heredity, race, gender, and increasing age. People whose parents suffer from cardiovascular diseases are more likely to develop them. Race is also a significant factor—African Americans, for instance, are twice as likely as whites to have high blood pressure, which elevates risk for heart disease. Men have a greater risk of heart attack than do women—while heart attacks are the leading cause of death among men over the age of 40, heart disease is not a major cause of death among women until they reach the age of 60. Heart attacks also increase with age. More than half of American heart attack victims are aged 65 or older. Of those who die from their attacks, more than 80 percent are over 65. (See Figure 7.1.)

CHANGEABLE FACTORS. Cigarette smoking doubles the risk of heart attack. A smoker who suffers a heart attack is more likely to die from it and more likely to die suddenly (within an hour) than a nonsmoker. Once people stop smoking, however, regardless of the length of time or the amount they have smoked, the risk of heart disease decreases dramatically.

High blood pressure, which usually has no symptoms or warning signs, is called the "silent killer." High blood pressure means that it is more difficult for blood to pump through the veins, which increases the heart's workload,

FIGURE 7.1

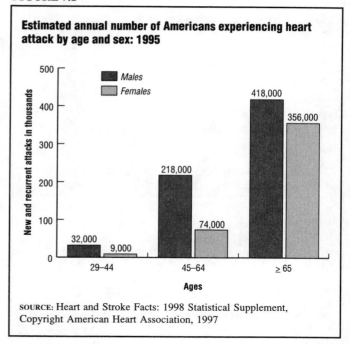

Estimated annual number of Americans experiencing heart attack by age and sex: 1995

SOURCE: Heart and Stroke Facts: 1998 Statistical Supplement, Copyright American Heart Association, 1997

causing it to weaken and enlarge over time. Generally, blood pressure rises with age. Men have a higher incidence of high blood pressure than women until about age 55; then the risks become equal for both sexes. High blood pressure is a major problem for older women; more than 50 percent of all women over age 65 have the disease. In most cases, high blood pressure can be controlled through diet, exercise, and medication.

High blood cholesterol levels increase the risk of coronary heart disease. Reduction of dietary fat, especially artery-clogging saturated fat, can lower blood cholesterol levels, as can exercise. Proper diet and exercise can also enhance the effectiveness of cholesterol-lowering drugs. Figure 7.2 shows the danger of heart attack within eight years when these factors (cigarettes, high blood cholesterol, and high blood pressure) are present.

Lack of physical exercise is also a risk factor for heart disease. The AHA recommends 30 to 60 minutes of aerobic exercise three or four times a week for maximum heart fitness. Even lower levels of regular activity, such as walking or gardening, can help to prevent heart and blood vessel disease.

Some researchers also link the risk of heart disease with stress levels, behavioral habits, and socioeconomic level. Many studies have indicated that the risk of death from heart disease is considerably greater for the least-educated persons than for the most-educated persons. There may be several reasons for this. For instance, people who are better educated usually have higher incomes, better access to health care, and greater knowledge of prevention techniques.

FIGURE 7.2

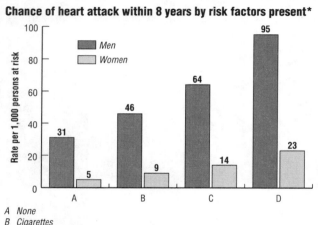

Chance of heart attack within 8 years by risk factors present*

A None
B Cigarettes
C Cigarettes and high blood cholesterol
D Cigarettes, high blood cholesterol, and high blood pressure
(Average probability of heart attack in 8 years is 47/1,000 in men and 8/1,000 in women)

This chart shows how a combination of three major risk factors can increase the likelihood of heart attack. **This chart uses an abnormal blood pressure level of 150 mmHg systolic and a cholesterol level of 260 mg/dL in a 55-year-old male and female.**

*Risk ratios for males in the Framingham Heart Study, where the average is equal to 100 are 66 for men with no major risk factors; 98 for men who smoke cigarettes; 136 for men who smoke cigarettes and have elevated blood cholesterol; and 202 for men who smoke cigarettes, have elevated blood cholesterol and have high blood pressure. For females, comparable ratios are 63, 113, 175 and 288, respectively.

SOURCE: *Heart and Stroke Facts: 1998 Statistical Supplement, 1997*
Copyright American Heart Association

CONTRIBUTING FACTORS. Diabetes, or high blood sugar, affects cholesterol and triglyceride levels (fats made by the body). The disease can sharply increase the risk of heart attack. In fact, more than 80 percent of diabetics die from some form of heart or blood vessel disease.

Obesity is also a contributing factor to heart disease. Research has shown that the location of fat in the body may significantly affect one's risk of suffering a heart attack. Men who have a waist measurement that exceeds their hip measurement and women whose waistline measurement is more than 80 percent of their hip dimension are at greater risk. Being overweight to any degree adds strain on the heart.

Prevalence of Heart Disease

In 1998, 724,269 people in the United States died from heart disease, the leading cause of death in America. The CDC, however, reported that from 1980 to 1998 the age-adjusted death rate from heart disease declined by 37.3 percent. In 1980, 202 Americans out of every 100,000 died of heart disease. By 1998 that number had dropped to 126.6. Table 7.2 shows that, in 1998, the age-adjusted death rate for heart disease was highest among black males (231.8 per 100,000) and white males (162.3 per 100,000) and lowest among Asian/Pacific Islander females (47.7 per 100,000) and Hispanic females (63.4

per 100,000). The death rate for white females was 88.1 per 100,000, while black females had a death rate of 146.8 per 100,000.

Between 1980 and 1998, the death rate declined 41.5 percent for white males and 34.5 percent for white females. Deaths dropped at a lower rate for black males (29.1 percent) and black females (27 percent). Consequently, between 1980 and 1998, the race differential in heart disease mortality widened. (See Table 7.2.)

Based on the *Framingham Heart Study,* the AHA reported that while heart attacks are most prevalent among older persons, they also occur in younger persons; 5 percent of all heart attacks occur in persons younger than age 40, and 45 percent occur in those under age 65. Nevertheless, about four of five people (83 percent) who die of heart attacks are over age 65.

The AHA estimated that the direct and indirect cost of cardiovascular diseases and stroke in 2001 would be $299.2 billion. Direct costs include expenditures for physician and nursing services, hospital expenses, nursing home care, home health care, and medications. Indirect costs include the loss of productivity that results from these diseases. The estimation for the cost of heart disease alone was $193.8 billion in 2001.

Women and Heart Disease

Until recently, almost all research on heart disease was carried out on middle-aged men. When a woman enters menopause, however, she begins to lose the protection provided by the hormones that appear to lower the risk of heart disease. One in three women over age 65 suffers from heart or blood vessel disease. Today, women are almost 50 percent more likely to die from a heart attack than men are; 44 percent of women who have heart attacks die within the first year, compared to 27 percent of men. The occurrence of a second attack during the six years following the initial attack is 31 percent for women and only 23 percent for men. Among black women 35 to 74 years of age, the death rate from coronary heart disease is about 71 percent higher than it is for white women.

Women are more seriously affected by heart disease than men are because their arteries are smaller, they frequently wait longer to get care, and they are generally older (typically by 10 years) when heart disease strikes. Another reason may be that women's early symptoms of heart disease are not taken as seriously by their health care providers as are those of men. Women also undergo fewer cardiac procedures than do men. The American Heart Association estimated in 1998 that men had almost twice as many angioplasties and nearly three times as many bypass operations as women did. Finally, research has shown that anticlotting drugs have been formulated for men and that women benefit less from these drugs.

TABLE 7.2

Death rates for diseases of heart, according to sex, detailed race, Hispanic origin, and age: selected years 1950–98

[Data are based on the National Vital Statistics System]

Sex, race, Hispanic origin, and age	1950[1]	1960[1]	1970	1980	1985	1990	1995	1996	1997	1998	1996–98[2]
All persons						Deaths per 100,000 resident population					
All ages, age adjusted	307.2	286.2	253.6	202.0	181.4	152.0	138.3	134.5	130.5	126.6	130.5
All ages, crude	355.5	369.0	362.0	336.0	324.1	289.5	280.7	276.4	271.6	268.2	272.1
Under 1 year	3.5	6.6	13.1	22.8	25.0	20.1	17.1	16.6	16.4	16.1	16.4
1–4 years	1.3	1.3	1.7	2.6	2.2	1.9	1.6	1.4	1.4	1.4	1.4
5–14 years	2.1	1.3	0.8	0.9	1.0	0.9	0.8	0.9	0.8	0.8	0.8
15–24 years	6.8	4.0	3.0	2.9	2.8	2.5	2.9	2.7	3.0	2.8	2.8
25–34 years	19.4	15.6	11.4	8.3	8.3	7.6	8.5	8.3	8.3	8.3	8.3
35–44 years	86.4	74.6	66.7	44.6	38.1	31.4	32.0	30.5	30.1	30.5	30.4
45–54 years	308.6	271.8	238.4	180.2	153.8	120.5	111.0	108.2	104.9	101.4	104.8
55–64 years	808.1	737.9	652.3	494.1	443.0	367.3	322.9	315.2	302.4	286.9	301.2
65–74 years	1,839.8	1,740.5	1,558.2	1,218.6	1,089.8	894.3	799.9	776.2	753.7	735.5	755.2
75–84 years	4,310.1	4,089.4	3,683.8	2,993.1	2,693.1	2,295.7	2,064.7	2,010.2	1,943.6	1,897.3	1,949.5
85 years and over	9,150.6	9,317.8	7,891.3	7,777.1	7,384.1	6,739.9	6,484.1	6,314.5	6,198.9	6,009.6	6,170.4
Male											
All ages, age adjusted	383.8	375.5	348.5	280.4	250.1	206.7	184.9	178.8	173.1	166.9	172.9
All ages, crude	423.4	439.5	422.5	368.6	344.1	297.6	282.7	277.4	272.2	268.0	272.5
Under 1 year	4.0	7.8	15.1	25.5	27.8	21.9	17.5	17.4	18.0	16.2	17.2
1–4 years	1.4	1.4	1.9	2.8	2.2	1.9	1.7	1.4	1.5	1.5	1.5
5–14 years	2.0	1.4	0.9	1.0	0.9	0.9	0.8	0.9	0.9	1.0	0.9
15–24 years	6.8	4.2	3.7	3.7	3.5	3.1	3.6	3.3	3.6	3.5	3.5
25–34 years	22.9	20.1	15.2	11.4	11.6	10.3	11.4	11.0	10.8	10.8	10.9
35–44 years	118.4	112.7	103.2	68.7	58.6	48.1	47.2	44.2	43.7	44.0	44.0
45–54 years	440.5	420.4	376.4	282.6	237.8	183.0	168.6	161.8	157.7	152.2	157.1
55–64 years	1,104.5	1,066.9	987.2	746.8	659.1	537.3	465.4	453.8	434.6	411.1	432.7
65–74 years	2,292.3	2,291.3	2,170.3	1,728.0	1,535.8	1,250.0	1,102.3	1,065.0	1,031.1	997.3	1,031.2
75–84 years	4,825.0	4,742.4	4,534.8	3,834.3	3,496.9	2,968.2	2,615.0	2,529.4	2,443.6	2,377.2	2,448.6
85 years and over	9,659.8	9,788.9	8,426.2	8,752.7	8,251.8	7,418.4	7,039.6	6,834.0	6,658.5	6,330.6	6,598.6
Female											
All ages, age adjusted	233.9	205.7	175.2	140.3	127.4	108.9	100.4	98.2	95.4	93.3	95.6
All ages, crude	288.4	300.6	304.5	305.1	305.2	281.8	278.8	275.5	271.1	268.3	271.6
Under 1 year	2.9	5.4	10.9	20.0	22.0	18.3	16.7	15.7	14.7	16.1	15.5
1–4 years	1.2	1.1	1.6	2.5	2.2	1.9	1.5	1.4	1.2	1.3	1.3
5–14 years	2.2	1.2	0.8	0.9	1.0	0.8	0.7	0.8	0.7	0.7	0.7
15–24 years	6.7	3.7	2.3	2.1	2.1	1.8	2.2	2.0	2.4	2.1	2.2
25–34 years	16.2	11.3	7.7	5.3	5.0	5.0	5.6	5.6	5.8	5.8	5.7
35–44 years	55.1	38.2	32.2	21.4	18.3	15.1	17.1	16.8	16.5	17.3	16.9
45–54 years	177.2	127.5	109.9	84.5	74.4	61.0	56.0	56.9	54.3	52.8	54.6
55–64 years	510.0	429.4	351.6	272.1	252.1	215.7	193.9	189.3	182.1	173.9	181.6
65–74 years	1,419.3	1,261.3	1,082.7	828.6	746.1	616.8	557.8	543.8	529.4	522.6	532.0
75–84 years	3,872.0	3,582.7	3,120.8	2,497.0	2,220.4	1,893.8	1,715.2	1,674.7	1,616.6	1,579.5	1,623.1
85 years and over	8,796.1	9,016.8	7,591.8	7,350.5	7,037.6	6,478.1	6,267.8	6,108.0	6,013.7	5,876.6	5,997.0
White male											
All ages, age adjusted	381.1	375.4	347.6	277.5	246.2	202.0	179.7	174.5	168.7	162.3	168.3
All ages, crude	433.0	454.6	438.3	384.0	360.3	312.7	297.9	293.3	287.7	283.1	288.0
45–54 years	423.6	413.2	365.7	269.8	225.5	170.6	155.7	149.8	145.4	140.2	145.0
55–64 years	1,081.7	1,056.0	979.3	730.6	640.1	516.7	443.0	431.8	411.2	388.1	409.9
65–74 years	2,308.3	2,297.9	2,177.2	1,729.7	1,522.7	1,230.5	1,080.5	1,049.5	1,015.1	981.3	1,015.5
75–84 years	4,907.3	4,839.9	4,617.6	3,883.2	3,527.0	2,983.4	2,616.1	2,536.0	2,453.7	2,381.5	2,455.6
85 years and over	9,950.5	10,135.8	8,818.0	8,958.0	8,481.7	7,558.7	7,165.5	7,014.5	6,829.7	6,478.8	6,764.6
Black male											
All ages, age adjusted	415.5	381.2	375.9	327.3	310.8	275.9	255.9	242.6	236.2	231.8	236.8
All ages, crude	348.4	330.6	330.3	301.0	288.6	256.8	244.2	234.8	230.8	230.5	232.0
45–54 years	624.1	514.0	512.8	433.4	385.2	328.9	317.1	297.7	293.7	282.7	291.1
55–64 years	1,434.0	1,236.8	1,135.4	987.2	935.3	824.0	757.8	740.9	727.8	699.9	722.5
65–74 years	2,140.1	2,281.4	2,237.8	1,847.2	1,839.2	1,632.9	1,482.9	1,381.3	1,335.4	1,312.7	1,342.9
75–84 years	- - -	3,533.6	3,783.4	3,578.8	3,436.6	3,107.1	2,881.4	2,762.0	2,641.6	2,649.3	2,683.3
85 years and over	- - -	6,037.9	5,367.6	6,819.5	6,393.5	6,479.6	5,985.7	5,675.4	5,538.7	5,446.7	5,550.8

Stroke

Stroke (cerebrovascular disease) is a cardiovascular disease that affects the blood vessels of the central nervous system. When an artery bringing oxygen and nutrients to the brain bursts or becomes clogged with a blood clot, a part of the brain does not receive the oxygen it needs. Without the necessary oxygen, the affected nerve cells cannot function and die within moments. The parts of the body controlled by these nerve cells also become dysfunctional. Because dead brain cells cannot be replaced, the damage is often permanent.

A stroke affects different people in different ways. The extent of the damage depends on the type of stroke

TABLE 7.2

Death rates for diseases of heart, according to sex, detailed race, Hispanic origin, and age: selected years 1950–98 [CONTINUED]

[Data are based on the National Vital Statistics System]

Sex, race, Hispanic origin, and age	1950[1]	1960[1]	1970	1980	1985	1990	1995	1996	1997	1998	1996–98[2]
American Indian or Alaska Native male[3]					Deaths per 100,000 resident population						
All ages, age adjusted	---	---	---	180.9	162.2	144.6	136.7	131.6	136.5	128.7	132.1
All ages, crude	---	---	---	130.6	117.9	108.0	110.4	110.7	116.8	113.2	113.6
45–54 years	---	---	---	238.1	209.1	173.8	151.4	157.5	171.8	151.8	160.3
55–64 years	---	---	---	496.3	438.3	411.0	403.2	404.9	427.2	402.5	411.5
65–74 years	---	---	---	1,009.4	984.6	839.1	918.5	778.0	828.1	793.6	799.9
75–84 years	---	---	---	2,062.2	2,118.2	1,788.8	1,534.9	1,546.5	1,513.8	1,274.0	1,439.0
85 years and over	---	---	---	4,413.7	2,766.7	3,860.3	2,308.7	2,660.1	2,764.2	2,800.9	2,744.2
Asian or Pacific Islander male[4]											
All ages, age adjusted	---	---	---	136.7	123.4	102.6	106.2	98.1	95.9	92.3	95.3
All ages, crude	---	---	---	119.8	103.5	88.7	96.9	97.3	97.4	98.3	97.7
45–54 years	---	---	---	112.0	81.1	70.4	73.4	75.4	72.1	72.9	73.4
55–64 years	---	---	---	306.7	291.2	226.1	214.3	220.7	218.3	210.8	216.4
65–74 years	---	---	---	852.4	753.5	623.5	605.8	581.2	585.1	522.7	562.1
75–84 years	---	---	---	2,010.9	2,025.6	1,642.2	1,680.5	1,534.8	1,432.1	1,493.0	1,485.9
85 years and over	---	---	---	5,923.0	4,937.5	4,617.8	6,372.3	4,338.0	4,392.5	4,110.7	4,272.2
Hispanic male[5]											
All ages, age adjusted	---	---	---	---	152.3	136.3	121.9	117.6	113.4	109.3	113.2
All ages, crude	---	---	---	---	92.1	91.0	87.5	85.8	83.9	84.9	84.9
45–54 years	---	---	---	---	128.1	116.4	103.0	98.7	96.2	96.0	96.9
55–64 years	---	---	---	---	398.8	363.0	306.0	310.0	276.9	274.0	286.4
65–74 years	---	---	---	---	972.6	829.9	750.0	725.7	737.2	706.6	723.0
75–84 years	---	---	---	---	2,160.8	1,971.3	1,734.5	1,688.6	1,628.7	1,522.0	1,608.2
85 years and over	---	---	---	---	4,791.2	4,711.9	4,699.7	4,078.6	3,844.6	3,641.9	3,843.3
White, non-Hispanic male[5]											
All ages, age adjusted	---	---	---	---	240.3	204.1	181.2	176.2	171.1	164.6	170.5
All ages, crude	---	---	---	---	362.8	336.5	322.0	318.9	315.0	309.8	314.5
45–54 years	---	---	---	---	219.9	172.8	157.5	152.1	148.5	142.8	147.7
55–64 years	---	---	---	---	610.6	521.3	448.0	435.1	418.1	393.5	415.1
65–74 years	---	---	---	---	1,471.3	1,243.4	1,088.3	1,056.4	1,025.1	991.7	1,024.5
75–84 years	---	---	---	---	3,514.1	3,007.7	2,635.6	2,559.8	2,477.3	2,411.2	2,481.0
85 years and over	---	---	---	---	8,539.3	7,663.4	7,166.3	7,109.2	6,954.2	6,604.4	6,879.3
White female											
All ages, age adjusted	223.6	197.1	167.8	134.6	121.7	103.1	94.9	92.9	90.4	88.1	90.4
All ages, crude	289.4	306.5	313.8	319.2	321.8	298.4	297.4	294.2	289.8	286.8	290.3
45–54 years	141.9	103.4	91.4	71.2	62.5	50.2	45.9	46.9	44.9	43.4	45.0
55–64 years	460.2	383.0	317.7	248.1	227.1	192.4	173.1	167.8	162.5	153.9	161.3
65–74 years	1,400.9	1,229.8	1,044.0	796.7	713.3	583.6	526.3	515.1	500.7	493.8	503.3
75–84 years	3,925.2	3,629.7	3,143.5	2,493.6	2,207.5	1,874.3	1,689.8	1,652.9	1,595.9	1,556.3	1,601.2
85 years and over	9,084.7	9,280.8	7,839.9	7,501.6	7,170.0	6,563.4	6,352.6	6,211.4	6,108.0	5,971.4	6,094.5
Black female											
All ages, age adjusted	349.5	292.6	251.7	201.1	188.3	168.1	156.3	153.4	147.6	146.8	149.2
All ages, crude	289.9	268.5	261.0	249.7	250.3	237.0	231.1	229.0	224.2	224.6	225.9
45–54 years	526.8	360.7	290.9	202.4	176.2	155.3	143.1	144.7	134.8	132.9	137.3
55–64 years	1,210.7	952.3	710.5	530.1	510.7	442.0	384.9	388.4	364.8	361.5	371.4
65–74 years	1,659.4	1,680.5	1,553.2	1,210.3	1,149.9	1,017.5	933.7	890.0	871.6	858.8	873.4
75–84 years	---	2,926.9	2,964.1	2,707.2	2,533.4	2,250.9	2,163.1	2,097.7	2,030.5	2,044.8	2,057.4
85 years and over	---	5,650.0	5,003.8	5,796.5	5,686.5	5,766.1	5,614.8	5,493.6	5,542.5	5,373.1	5,468.1

and the area of the brain that has been damaged. The senses, speech, the ability to understand speech, behavioral patterns, thought, and memory are most frequently affected. The most common effect is for one side of the body to become paralyzed or severely weakened. A loss of feeling or vision due to the stroke can result in a loss of awareness, so many stroke victims may forget or "neglect" their weaker or paralyzed sides. This results in spills, bumping into objects, or dressing only one side of the body.

INCIDENCE OF STROKE DEATHS IS DECLINING. Stroke is the third-largest cause of death in America, following heart disease and cancer. About one-half million people

suffer a new or recurrent stroke each year, and an estimated 158,060 Americans died of stroke in 1998. (See Table 7.1.) About 31 percent of those who have a stroke die within the first year.

The age-adjusted death rate for stroke declined 38.5 percent between 1980 and 1998. The drop in the number of stroke victims has occurred at about the same rate for both sexes and both major racial groups. Nevertheless, Table 7.3 shows that in 1998 the age-adjusted death rate for stroke was almost twice as high among black males (46.8 per 100,000) as among white males (24.5 per 100,000). Black women died of stroke at a rate of 37.2 per

TABLE 7.2

Death rates for diseases of heart, according to sex, detailed race, Hispanic origin, and age: selected years 1950–98 [CONTINUED]

[Data are based on the National Vital Statistics System]

Sex, race, Hispanic origin, and age	1950[1]	1960[1]	1970	1980	1985	1990	1995	1996	1997	1998	1996–98[2]
American Indian or Alaska Native female[3]					Deaths per 100,000 resident population						
All ages, age adjusted	- - -	- - -	- - -	88.4	83.7	76.6	77.3	74.9	73.9	70.0	72.9
All ages, crude	- - -	- - -	- - -	80.3	84.3	77.5	87.0	86.7	88.6	89.0	88.1
45–54 years	- - -	- - -	- - -	65.2	59.2	62.0	69.2	61.1	59.7	49.4	56.6
55–64 years	- - -	- - -	- - -	193.5	230.8	197.0	210.2	192.5	172.8	183.3	182.8
65–74 years	- - -	- - -	- - -	577.2	472.7	492.8	503.3	512.8	473.8	440.3	475.1
75–84 years	- - -	- - -	- - -	1,364.3	1,258.8	1,050.3	1,045.6	1,030.0	1,115.2	1,019.8	1,054.7
85 years and over	- - -	- - -	- - -	2,893.3	3,180.0	2,868.7	2,209.8	2,108.8	2,019.5	2,348.9	2,163.9
Asian or Pacific Islander female[4]											
All ages, age adjusted	- - -	- - -	- - -	55.8	59.6	58.3	57.7	50.9	49.3	47.7	49.2
All ages, crude	- - -	- - -	- - -	57.0	60.3	62.0	68.2	66.8	66.9	67.3	67.0
45–54 years	- - -	- - -	- - -	28.6	23.8	17.5	21.6	17.2	18.8	18.4	18.2
55–64 years	- - -	- - -	- - -	92.9	103.0	99.0	93.0	82.3	80.5	70.5	77.6
65–74 years	- - -	- - -	- - -	313.3	341.0	323.9	294.9	282.0	272.8	282.9	279.2
75–84 years	- - -	- - -	- - -	1,053.2	1,056.5	1,130.9	1,063.0	1,009.8	944.0	880.9	941.3
85 years and over	- - -	- - -	- - -	3,211.0	4,208.3	4,161.2	4,717.9	3,394.7	3,326.2	3,385.5	3,368.7
Hispanic female[5]											
All ages, age adjusted	- - -	- - -	- - -	- - -	86.5	76.0	68.1	64.7	64.7	63.4	64.2
All ages, crude	- - -	- - -	- - -	- - -	75.0	79.4	78.9	77.0	78.3	77.7	77.7
45–54 years	- - -	- - -	- - -	- - -	46.6	43.5	32.0	31.3	31.5	31.0	31.3
55–64 years	- - -	- - -	- - -	- - -	184.8	153.2	137.3	125.1	129.5	122.4	125.6
65–74 years	- - -	- - -	- - -	- - -	534.0	460.4	402.4	387.6	391.9	399.8	393.3
75–84 years	- - -	- - -	- - -	- - -	1,456.5	1,259.7	1,150.1	1,152.8	1,102.4	1,071.1	1,107.2
85 years and over	- - -	- - -	- - -	- - -	4,523.4	4,440.3	4,243.9	3,673.8	3,748.7	3,499.1	3,634.7
White, non-Hispanic female[5]											
All ages, age adjusted	- - -	- - -	- - -	- - -	120.2	103.7	95.4	93.6	91.3	89.1	91.3
All ages, crude	- - -	- - -	- - -	- - -	334.2	320.0	321.4	318.9	315.6	313.6	316.0
45–54 years	- - -	- - -	- - -	- - -	61.3	50.2	46.6	47.5	45.7	44.2	45.7
55–64 years	- - -	- - -	- - -	- - -	219.6	193.6	173.6	169.0	163.9	155.3	162.6
65–74 years	- - -	- - -	- - -	- - -	700.4	584.7	529.1	518.0	504.0	496.2	506.1
75–84 years	- - -	- - -	- - -	- - -	2,201.5	1,890.2	1,697.8	1,663.5	1,609.4	1,571.1	1,614.0
85 years and over	- - -	- - -	- - -	- - -	7,164.7	6,615.2	6,384.5	6,285.4	6,176.4	6,054.4	6,169.3

- - - Data not available.

[1] Includes deaths of persons who were not residents of the 50 States and the District of Columbia.

[2] Average annual death rate.

[3] Interpretation of trends should take into account that population estimates for American Indians increased by 45 percent between 1980 and 1990, partly due to better enumeration techniques in the 1990 decennial census and to the increased tendency for people to identify themselves as American Indian in 1990.

[4] Interpretation of trends should take into account that the Asian population in the United States more than doubled between 1980 and 1990, primarily due to immigration.

[5] Excludes data from States lacking an Hispanic-origin item on their death certificates.

Notes: Rates are age adjusted to the 1940 U.S. standard million population. Age groups were selected to minimize the presentation of unstable age-specific death rates based on small numbers of deaths and for consistency among comparison groups. The race groups, white, black, Asian or Pacific Islander, and American Indian or Alaska Native, include persons of Hispanic and non-Hispanic origin. Conversely, persons of Hispanic origin may be of any race. Bias in death rates results from inconsistent race identification between the death certificate (source of data for numerator of death rates) and data from the Census Bureau (denominator); and from undercounts of some population groups in the census. The net effects of misclassification and under coverage result in death rates estimated to be overstated by 1 percent for the white population and 5 percent for the black population; and death rates estimated to be understated by 21 percent for American Indians, 11 percent for Asians, and 2 percent for Hispanics (Rosenberg HM, Maurer JD, Sorlie PD, Johnson NJ, et al. Quality of death rates by race and Hispanic origin: A summary of current research, 1999. National Center for Health Statistics. Vital Health Stat 2(128). 1999).

SOURCE: *Health, United States, 2000*, National Center for Health Statistics, Hyattsville, MD, 2000

100,000, much higher than the death rate of 22 per 100,000 for white females.

Warfarin, a blood thinner, is often used to reduce the chance of blood clot, although government studies have found that some doctors are reluctant to use it because of potential bleeding problems. Clinical trials have shown that the drug is safe if its use is monitored. Another drug, tissue plasminogen activator (tPA), is the only medication approved specifically for fighting strokes. TPA, which became available in 1996, must be administered within three hours after the onset of a stroke. The drug works to stop the swift advance of damage caused by clots shutting off blood flow to the brain, which accounts for four-fifths of strokes. Early detection and immediate treatment is vital if tPA is to work.

REHABILITATION FOR STROKE SURVIVORS. The AHA estimated that stroke accounts for more than half of all patients hospitalized for acute brain diseases. Of victims who survive an initial stroke, two-thirds survive the first year, and half are alive seven years later. Many survivors lose mental and physical abilities and need expensive, lengthy, and intensive rehabilitation to regain their independence, if they can. The stroke can affect virtually all their senses dealing with perception and everyday life.

TABLE 7.3

Death rates for cerebrovascular diseases, according to sex, detailed race, Hispanic origin, and age: selected years 1950–98

[Data are based on the National Vital Statistics System]

Sex, race, Hispanic origin, and age	1950[1]	1960[1]	1970	1980	1985	1990	1995	1996	1997	1998	1996–98[2]
All persons						Deaths per 100,000 resident population					
All ages, age adjusted	88.8	79.7	66.3	40.8	32.5	27.7	26.7	26.4	25.9	25.1	25.8
All ages, crude	104.0	108.0	101.9	75.1	64.3	57.9	60.1	60.3	59.7	58.6	59.5
Under 1 year	5.1	4.1	5.0	4.4	3.7	3.8	5.8	6.2	7.0	7.8	7.0
1–4 years	0.9	0.8	1.0	0.5	0.3	0.3	0.4	0.3	0.4	0.4	0.4
5–14 years	0.5	0.7	0.7	0.3	0.2	0.2	0.2	0.2	0.2	0.2	0.2
15–24 years	1.6	1.8	1.6	1.0	0.8	0.6	0.5	0.5	0.5	0.5	0.5
25–34 years	4.2	4.7	4.5	2.6	2.2	2.2	1.8	1.8	1.7	1.7	1.7
35–44 years	18.7	14.7	15.6	8.5	7.2	6.5	6.5	6.3	6.3	6.0	6.2
45–54 years	70.4	49.2	41.6	25.2	21.3	18.7	17.6	17.9	16.9	16.5	17.1
55–64 years	194.2	147.3	115.8	65.2	54.8	48.0	46.1	45.3	44.4	42.6	44.0
65–74 years	554.7	469.2	384.1	219.5	172.8	144.4	137.2	135.5	134.8	130.0	133.5
75–84 years	1,499.6	1,491.3	1,254.2	788.6	601.5	499.3	481.4	477.0	462.0	455.4	464.6
85 years and over	2,990.1	3,680.5	3,014.3	2,288.9	1,865.1	1,633.9	1,636.5	1,612.7	1,584.6	1,500.0	1,564.3
Male											
All ages, age adjusted	91.9	85.4	73.2	44.9	35.5	30.2	28.9	28.5	27.9	26.6	27.7
All ages, crude	102.5	104.5	94.5	63.6	52.5	46.8	48.0	48.1	47.8	46.3	47.4
Under 1 year	6.4	5.0	5.8	5.0	4.6	4.4	6.3	6.5	7.6	9.0	7.7
1–4 years	1.1	0.9	1.2	0.4	0.4	0.3	0.4	0.3	0.5	0.3	0.4
5–14 years	0.5	0.7	0.8	0.3	0.2	0.2	0.2	0.2	0.2	0.2	0.2
15–24 years	1.8	1.9	1.8	1.1	0.7	0.7	0.5	0.5	0.6	0.6	0.6
25–34 years	4.2	4.5	4.4	2.6	2.2	2.1	1.9	1.7	1.7	1.7	1.7
35–44 years	17.5	14.6	15.7	8.7	7.4	6.8	7.1	6.7	6.5	6.2	6.5
45–54 years	67.9	52.2	44.4	27.3	23.2	20.5	19.8	20.0	19.2	18.5	19.2
55–64 years	205.2	163.8	138.7	74.7	63.5	54.4	53.4	52.5	51.4	49.5	51.1
65–74 years	589.6	530.7	449.5	259.2	201.4	166.8	155.9	154.7	153.1	145.7	151.2
75–84 years	1,543.6	1,555.9	1,361.6	868.3	661.2	552.7	517.1	508.7	488.7	474.7	490.4
85 years and over	3,048.6	3,643.1	2,895.2	2,199.2	1,730.1	1,533.2	1,537.7	1,512.7	1,500.7	1,347.2	1,450.4
Female											
All ages, age adjusted	86.0	74.7	60.8	37.6	30.0	25.7	24.8	24.6	24.2	23.6	24.1
All ages, crude	105.6	111.4	109.0	86.1	75.5	68.6	71.7	71.9	71.2	70.4	71.2
Under 1 year	3.7	3.2	4.0	3.8	2.7	3.1	5.2	5.9	6.3	6.6	6.3
1–4 years	0.7	0.7	0.7	0.5	0.3	0.3	0.3	0.3	0.3	0.4	0.3
5–14 years	0.4	0.6	0.6	0.3	0.3	0.2	0.2	0.2	0.2	0.2	0.2
15–24 years	1.5	1.6	1.4	0.8	0.8	0.6	0.4	0.4	0.5	0.4	0.4
25–34 years	4.3	4.9	4.7	2.6	2.1	2.2	1.7	1.8	1.7	1.8	1.8
35–44 years	19.9	14.8	15.6	8.4	6.9	6.1	6.0	5.9	6.2	5.7	5.9
45–54 years	72.9	46.3	39.0	23.3	19.4	17.0	15.5	15.9	14.8	14.6	15.1
55–64 years	183.1	131.8	95.3	56.9	47.2	42.2	39.4	38.8	37.9	36.3	37.7
65–74 years	522.1	415.7	333.3	189.0	150.7	126.9	122.2	120.1	120.1	117.2	119.1
75–84 years	1,462.2	1,441.1	1,183.1	741.6	566.3	467.4	458.7	456.5	444.4	442.6	447.8
85 years and over	2,949.4	3,704.4	3,081.0	2,328.2	1,918.9	1,672.7	1,675.0	1,652.4	1,618.4	1,563.3	1,610.4
White male											
All ages, age adjusted	87.0	80.3	68.8	41.9	33.0	27.7	26.5	26.3	25.7	24.5	25.5
All ages, crude	100.5	102.7	93.5	63.3	52.7	47.0	48.6	49.1	48.8	47.3	48.4
45–54 years	53.7	40.9	35.6	21.7	18.1	15.4	14.8	15.2	14.6	14.2	14.7
55–64 years	182.2	139.0	119.9	64.2	54.6	45.8	44.7	43.4	42.3	40.8	42.2
65–74 years	569.7	501.0	420.0	240.4	186.4	153.2	143.5	142.0	141.8	134.9	139.6
75–84 years	1,556.3	1,564.8	1,361.6	854.8	650.0	540.7	503.1	500.1	480.3	464.9	481.4
85 years and over	3,127.1	3,734.8	3,018.1	2,236.9	1,765.6	1,549.8	1,550.0	1,537.7	1,530.6	1,365.9	1,474.8
Black male											
All ages, age adjusted	146.2	141.2	122.5	77.5	62.7	56.1	52.2	50.9	48.6	46.8	48.7
All ages, crude	122.0	122.9	108.8	73.1	59.2	53.1	51.0	50.1	48.3	47.5	48.7
45–54 years	211.9	166.1	136.1	82.1	71.1	68.4	64.1	62.1	59.8	55.7	59.1
55–64 years	522.8	439.9	343.4	189.8	160.7	141.8	134.1	137.5	135.5	129.2	134.0
65–74 years	783.6	899.2	780.1	472.8	379.7	327.2	291.5	292.2	274.3	255.8	274.0
75–84 years	- - -	1,475.2	1,445.7	1,067.6	814.4	723.7	700.2	653.0	600.5	621.3	624.7
85 years and over.	- - -	2,700.0	1,963.1	1,873.2	1,429.0	1,430.5	1,393.9	1,329.5	1,281.6	1,243.1	1,283.7

Victims may be unable to recognize or understand familiar objects or people. The simplest activities become difficult, and depression is a common problem, as stroke patients feel that they are now less than "whole."

In the *Framingham Heart Study* of cardiovascular disease, 31 percent of stroke survivors needed help in taking care of themselves, 20 percent required help in walking, and 71 percent had some type of impaired vocational ability when examined seven years after the occurrence of their stroke. Sixteen percent needed to be institutionalized.

Spontaneous recovery in the initial 30 days after a stroke probably accounts for the highest levels of regained functional

TABLE 7.3

Death rates for cerebrovascular diseases, according to sex, detailed race, Hispanic origin, and age: selected years 1950–98 [CONTINUED]

[Data are based on the National Vital Statistics System]

Sex, race, Hispanic origin, and age	1950[1]	1960[1]	1970	1980	1985	1990	1995	1996	1997	1998	1996–98[2]
					Deaths per 100,000 resident population						
American Indian or Alaska Native male[3]											
All ages, age adjusted	---	---	---	30.7	24.9	20.5	23.5	21.4	20.1	18.5	20.0
All ages, crude	---	---	---	23.2	18.5	16.0	20.1	18.7	18.5	16.6	17.9
45–54 years	---	---	---	*	*	*	28.4	19.9	*	17.6	17.4
55–64 years	---	---	---	72.0	*	39.8	45.7	42.9	49.4	53.5	48.7
65–74 years	---	---	---	170.5	200.0	120.3	153.1	139.1	112.5	109.8	120.3
75–84 years	---	---	---	535.1	372.7	325.9	290.1	319.4	324.0	257.8	299.0
85 years and over	---	---	---	1,384.7	733.3	949.8	748.8	550.4	707.9	450.2	569.6
Asian or Pacific Islander male[4]											
All ages, age adjusted	---	---	---	32.3	28.0	26.9	31.2	26.9	28.3	26.5	27.2
All ages, crude	---	---	---	28.7	24.0	23.4	28.6	27.0	28.8	28.1	28.0
45–54 years	---	---	---	17.0	13.9	15.6	17.3	19.5	18.3	16.9	18.2
55–64 years	---	---	---	59.9	48.8	51.8	62.1	55.6	58.0	56.0	56.5
65–74 years	---	---	---	197.9	155.6	167.9	162.3	161.4	160.9	160.9	161.1
75–84 years	---	---	---	619.5	583.7	485.7	571.8	430.0	524.0	456.5	470.4
85 years and over	---	---	---	1,399.0	1,387.5	1,196.6	1,808.5	1,348.7	1,219.4	1,149.6	1,233.4
Hispanic male[5]											
All ages, age adjusted	---	---	---	---	27.7	22.7	23.1	22.3	22.1	21.8	22.0
All ages, crude	---	---	---	---	17.2	15.6	17.1	16.8	16.7	17.4	16.9
45–54 years	---	---	---	---	23.6	20.0	20.5	23.1	20.4	22.3	21.9
55–64 years	---	---	---	---	63.9	49.4	46.1	50.7	52.7	53.0	52.2
65–74 years	---	---	---	---	163.5	126.4	132.2	114.8	134.9	124.0	124.7
75–84 years	---	---	---	---	396.7	356.6	349.9	348.6	304.2	296.0	314.8
85 years and over	---	---	---	---	1,152.1	866.3	996.3	866.3	787.8	795.7	814.9
White, non-Hispanic male[5]											
All ages, age adjusted	---	---	---	---	31.6	27.9	26.3	26.1	25.6	24.3	25.4
All ages, crude	---	---	---	---	52.2	50.7	52.3	53.0	53.1	51.3	52.5
45–54 years	---	---	---	---	16.0	14.9	14.1	14.2	13.9	13.2	13.8
55–64 years	---	---	---	---	50.5	45.2	43.9	42.0	41.1	39.4	40.8
65–74 years	---	---	---	---	178.5	154.8	143.1	142.0	141.1	134.7	139.3
75–84 years	---	---	---	---	637.0	548.8	507.4	505.1	486.0	471.1	487.0
85 years and over	---	---	---	---	1,735.1	1,583.6	1,552.4	1,560.6	1,562.9	1,391.9	1,501.7
White female											
All ages, age adjusted	79.7	68.7	56.2	35.2	27.9	23.8	23.1	22.9	22.5	22.0	22.5
All ages, crude	103.3	110.1	109.8	88.8	78.4	71.8	76.0	76.3	75.7	75.0	75.7
45–54 years	55.0	33.8	30.5	18.7	15.5	13.5	12.7	12.8	11.6	11.3	11.9
55–64 years	156.9	103.0	78.1	48.7	40.0	35.8	33.6	33.3	31.8	31.3	32.1
65–74 years	498.1	383.3	303.2	172.8	137.9	116.3	112.6	110.2	111.4	108.6	110.1
75–84 years	1,471.3	1,444.7	1,176.8	730.3	552.9	457.6	449.5	446.7	437.5	434.2	439.4
85 years and over	3,017.9	3,795.7	3,167.6	2,367.8	1,944.9	1,691.4	1,690.0	1,679.3	1,645.8	1,589.6	1,637.3
Black female											
All ages, age adjusted	155.6	139.5	107.9	61.7	50.6	42.7	39.6	39.2	37.9	37.2	38.1
All ages, crude	128.3	127.7	112.2	77.9	68.6	60.7	60.4	59.7	58.0	57.9	58.5
45–54 years	248.9	166.2	119.4	61.9	50.8	44.1	36.4	38.6	38.6	39.9	39.1
55–64 years	567.7	452.0	272.4	138.7	113.6	97.0	85.5	82.9	84.0	76.5	81.1
65–74 years	754.4	830.5	673.5	362.2	285.6	236.8	221.2	216.4	204.8	197.3	206.1
75–84 years	---	1,413.1	1,338.3	918.6	753.8	596.0	583.2	586.5	540.0	560.0	562.0
85 years and over	---	2,578.9	2,210.5	1,896.3	1,657.1	1,496.5	1,568.8	1,443.6	1,433.1	1,398.4	1,424.5

ability. Rehabilitation, however, to reduce dependency and improve physical ability is also vital. The patient's attitude, the skills of the rehabilitation team, and support and understanding from the patient's family all affect the quality of recovery.

NATIONAL COSTS OF STROKE. The costs of stroke are high. The AHA estimated that $45.4 billion would be spent on treating stroke victims in 2001, including the costs of hospitalization, nursing home service, doctors' and nurses' services, medications, and lost productivity. The overwhelming proportion of that money is spent on health care facilities, because so many victims are disabled following their strokes.

High Blood Pressure

Blood pressure is a combination of two forces: the heart pumping blood into the arteries, and the resistance of small arteries called arterioles to the flow of blood. The greater the resistance, the greater the pressure needed by the heart to keep the blood moving. The walls of the arterioles are elastic enough to allow for the expansion and contraction called for by the constantly changing rate of blood flow, thus allowing for a steady blood pressure in normal bodies. If the arterioles stay contracted or lose their elasticity, however, they increase the resistance of the blood flow, and high blood pressure results.

TABLE 7.3

Death rates for diseases of heart, according to sex, detailed race, Hispanic origin, and age: selected years 1950–98 [CONTINUED]

[Data are based on the National Vital Statistics System]

Sex, race, Hispanic origin, and age	1950[1]	1960[1]	1970	1980	1985	1990	1995	1996	1997	1998	1996–98[2]
American Indian or Alaska Native female[3]				Deaths per 100,000 resident population							
All ages, age adjusted	---	---	---	88.4	83.7	76.6	77.3	74.9	73.9	70.0	72.9
All ages, crude	---	---	---	80.3	84.3	77.5	87.0	86.7	88.6	89.0	88.1
45–54 years	---	---	---	65.2	59.2	62.0	69.2	61.1	59.7	49.4	56.6
55–64 years	---	---	---	193.5	230.8	197.0	210.2	192.5	172.8	183.3	182.8
65–74 years	---	---	---	577.2	472.7	492.8	503.3	512.8	473.8	440.3	475.1
75–84 years	---	---	---	1,364.3	1,258.8	1,050.3	1,045.6	1,030.0	1,115.2	1,019.8	1,054.7
85 years and over	---	---	---	2,893.3	3,180.0	2,868.7	2,209.8	2,108.8	2,019.5	2,348.9	2,163.9
Asian or Pacific Islander female[4]											
All ages, age adjusted	---	---	---	55.8	59.6	58.3	57.7	50.9	49.3	47.7	49.2
All ages, crude	---	---	---	57.0	60.3	62.0	68.2	66.8	66.9	67.3	67.0
45–54 years	---	---	---	28.6	23.8	17.5	21.6	17.2	18.8	18.4	18.2
55–64 years	---	---	---	92.9	103.0	99.0	93.0	82.3	80.5	70.5	77.6
65–74 years	---	---	---	313.3	341.0	323.9	294.9	282.0	272.8	282.9	279.2
75–84 years	---	---	---	1,053.2	1,056.5	1,130.9	1,063.0	1,009.8	944.0	880.9	941.3
85 years and over	---	---	---	3,211.0	4,208.3	4,161.2	4,717.9	3,394.7	3,326.2	3,385.5	3,368.7
Hispanic female[5]											
All ages, age adjusted	---	---	---	---	86.5	76.0	68.1	64.7	64.7	63.4	64.2
All ages, crude	---	---	---	---	75.0	79.4	78.9	77.0	78.3	77.7	77.7
45–54 years	---	---	---	---	46.6	43.5	32.0	31.3	31.5	31.0	31.3
55–64 years	---	---	---	---	184.8	153.2	137.3	125.1	129.5	122.4	125.6
65–74 years	---	---	---	---	534.0	460.4	402.4	387.6	391.9	399.8	393.3
75–84 years	---	---	---	---	1,456.5	1,259.7	1,150.1	1,152.8	1,102.4	1,071.1	1,107.2
85 years and over	---	---	---	---	4,523.4	4,440.3	4,243.9	3,673.8	3,748.7	3,499.1	3,634.7
White, non-Hispanic female[5]											
All ages, age adjusted	---	---	---	---	120.2	103.7	95.4	93.6	91.3	89.1	91.3
All ages, crude	---	---	---	---	334.2	320.0	321.4	318.9	315.6	313.6	316.0
45–54 years	---	---	---	---	61.3	50.2	46.6	47.5	45.7	44.2	45.7
55–64 years	---	---	---	---	219.6	193.6	173.6	169.0	163.9	155.3	162.6
65–74 years	---	---	---	---	700.4	584.7	529.1	518.0	504.0	496.2	506.1
75–84 years	---	---	---	---	2,201.5	1,890.2	1,697.8	1,663.5	1,609.4	1,571.1	1,614.0
85 years and over	---	---	---	---	7,164.7	6,615.2	6,384.5	6,285.4	6,176.4	6,054.4	6,169.3

- - - Data not available.
[1] Includes deaths of persons who were not residents of the 50 States and the District of Columbia.
[2] Average annual death rate.
[3] Interpretation of trends should take into account that population estimates for American Indians increased by 45 percent between 1980 and 1990, partly due to better enumeration techniques in the 1990 decennial census and to the increased tendency for people to identify themselves as American Indian in 1990.
[4] Interpretation of trends should take into account that the Asian population in the United States more than doubled between 1980 and 1990, primarily due to immigration.
[5] Excludes data from States lacking an Hispanic-origin item on their death certificates.
Notes: Rates are age adjusted to the 1940 U.S. standard million population. Age groups were selected to minimize the presentation of unstable age-specific death rates based on small numbers of deaths and for consistency among comparison groups. The race groups, white, black, Asian or Pacific Islander, and American Indian or Alaska Native, include persons of Hispanic and non-Hispanic origin. Conversely, persons of Hispanic origin may be of any race. Bias in death rates results from inconsistent race identification between the death certificate (source of data for numerator of death rates) and data from the Census Bureau (denominator); and from undercounts of some population groups in the census. The net effects of misclassification and under coverage result in death rates estimated to be overstated by 1 percent for the white population and 5 percent for the black population; and death rates estimated to be understated by 21 percent for American Indians, 11 percent for Asians, and 2 percent for Hispanics (Rosenberg HM, Maurer JD, Sorlie PD, Johnson NJ, et al. Quality of death rates by race and Hispanic origin: A summary of current research, 1999. National Center for Health Statistics. Vital Health Stat 2(128). 1999).

SOURCE: *Health, United States, 2000*, National Center for Health Statistics, Hyattsville, MD, 2000

Blood pressure is measured in millimeters (mm) of mercury (Hg) by an instrument known as a sphygmomanometer. The sphygmomanometer produces two values: the systolic pressure is a measurement of the maximum pressure of the blood flow when the heart contracts (beats), and the diastolic pressure is the minimum pressure of the blood flow between beats. A typical "normal" range of values may vary, but the harder it is for the blood to flow, the higher the reading will be. High blood pressure (hypertension) for adults is defined as a systolic pressure equal to or greater than 140 mm Hg and/or a diastolic pressure equal to or greater than 90 mm Hg.

Elevated blood pressure—also known as hypertension—is an indication that the heart is working harder than normal and the arteries are under a strain that might contribute to a heart attack, stroke, and atherosclerosis (hardening of the arteries). When the heart works too hard, it can become enlarged and eventually will be unable to function at maximum capacity.

PREVALENCE OF HYPERTENSION. As many as 50 million Americans, including children as young as age six, have high blood pressure. Persons with lower educational and income levels tend to have higher levels of blood pres-

TABLE 7.4

Hypertension among persons 20 years of age and over, according to sex, age, race, and Hispanic origin: United States, 1960–62, 1971–74, 1976–80, and 1988–94

[Data are based on physical examinations of a sample of the civilian noninstitutionalized population]

Sex, age, race, and Hispanic origin[1]	1960–62	1971–74	1976–80[2]	1988–94
20–74 years, age adjusted		Percent of population		
Both sexes[3]	36.9	38.3	39.0	23.1
Male	40.0	42.4	44.0	25.3
Female[3]	33.7	34.3	34.0	20.8
White male	39.3	41.7	43.5	24.3
White female[3]	31.7	32.4	32.3	19.3
Black male	48.1	51.8	48.7	34.9
Black female[3]	50.8	50.3	47.5	33.8
White, non-Hispanic male	- - -	- - -	43.9	24.4
White, non-Hispanic female[3]	- - -	- - -	32.1	19.3
Black, non-Hispanic male	- - -	- - -	48.7	35.0
Black, non-Hispanic female[3]	- - -	- - -	47.6	34.2
Mexican male	- - -	- - -	25.0	25.2
Mexican female[3]	- - -	- - -	21.8	22.0
20–74 years, crude				
Both sexes[3]	39.0	39.7	39.7	23.1
Male	41.7	43.3	44.0	24.7
Female[3]	36.6	36.5	35.6	21.5
White male	41.0	42.8	43.8	24.3
White female[3]	34.9	34.9	34.2	20.4
Black male	50.5	52.1	47.4	31.5
Black female[3]	52.0	50.2	46.1	30.6
White, non-Hispanic male	- - -	- - -	44.3	25.0
White, non-Hispanic female[3]	- - -	- - -	34.4	20.9
Black, non-Hispanic male	- - -	- - -	47.5	31.6
Black, non-Hispanic female[3]	- - -	- - -	46.1	31.2
Mexican male	- - -	- - -	18.8	18.0
Mexican female[3]	- - -	- - -	16.7	15.8
Male				
20–34 years	22.8	24.8	28.9	8.6
35–44 years	37.7	39.1	40.5	20.9
45–54 years	47.6	55.0	53.6	34.1
55–64 years	60.3	62.5	61.8	42.9
65–74 years	68.8	67.2	67.1	57.3
75 years and over	- - -	- - -	- - -	64.2
Female[3]				
20–34 years	9.3	11.2	11.1	3.4
35–44 years	24.0	28.2	28.8	12.7
45–54 years	43.4	43.6	47.1	25.1
55–64 years	66.4	62.5	61.1	44.2
65–74 years	81.5	78.3	71.8	60.8
75 years and over	- - -	- - -	- - -	77.3

- - - Data not available.
[1] The race groups, white and black, include persons of Hispanic and non-Hispanic origin. Conversely, persons of Hispanic origin may be of any race.
[2] Data for Mexicans are for 1982–84.
[3] Excludes pregnant women.

Notes: A person with hypertension is defined by either having elevated blood pressure (systolic pressure of at least 140 mmHg or diastolic pressure of at least 90 mmHg) or taking antihypertensive medication. Percents are based on a single measurement of blood pressure to provide comparable data across the 4 time periods. In 1976–80, 31.3 percent of persons 20–74 years of age had hypertension, based on the average of 3 blood pressure measurements, in contrast to 39.7 percent when a single measurement is used.

SOURCE: *Health, United States, 2000*, National Center for Health Statistics, Hyattsville, MD, 2000

sure. The cause of hypertension is unknown in 90 to 95 percent of the cases and is called essential hypertension. The remaining cases are called secondary because the hypertension is an identified symptom of another condition, such as an abnormality in the kidneys, adrenal gland, or aorta.

The AHA reported that blacks, Puerto Ricans, and Cuban and Mexican Americans were more likely to suffer from hypertension than whites. Table 7.4 shows data from the CDC on the presence of hypertension among persons 20 years of age and over by race and Hispanic origin. Both

black males and black females have a higher incidence of high blood pressure than white or Mexican American males and females. A far smaller number of Asian/Pacific Islander Americans suffer from hypertension.

In 1995 hypertension killed 39,981 Americans and contributed to the deaths of thousands more. As many as 30 percent of all deaths among hypertensive black men and 20 percent of all deaths among hypertensive black women can be attributed to high blood pressure. Nonetheless, death rates from this disease have declined dramatically.

TREATMENT. In many cases, hypertension is treatable. Numerous medications, including diuretics, which rid the body of excess fluids and salt, can lower blood pressure.

Diet and change of habit are also essential to control hypertension. Some people with only mildly elevated blood pressure need only reduce or eliminate salt in their diets. Blood pressure in obese persons often declines when they lose weight. Heavy drinkers often see improved blood pressure when they drink less. Some patients find exercise and relaxation therapy helpful. When people are aware of the problem and follow the prescribed treatment, high blood pressure can be controlled and need not be fatal. Patients, however, often cease to take high blood pressure medication once their hypertension is controlled. This poses a serious danger; it is essential that patients continue to take the medication even though they might feel perfectly well.

CANCER

Cancer is a large group of diseases characterized by the uncontrolled growth and spread of abnormal cells. These cells may grow into masses of tissue called tumors. Tumors made up of cells that are not cancerous are called benign tumors. The tumors consisting of cancer cells are called malignant tumors. The dangerous aspect of cancer is that cancer cells invade and destroy normal tissue.

The spread of cancer cells occurs either by growth of the tumor or by some of the cells becoming detached and traveling through the blood and lymph systems to other parts of the body. Metastasis (the spread of cancer cells) may be confined to a region of the body, but if left untreated (and often despite treatment), the cancer cells can spread throughout the entire body, causing death. It is perhaps the rapid, invasive, and destructive nature of cancer that makes it, arguably, the most feared of all diseases, even though it is second to heart disease as the leading cause of death in the United States.

What Causes Cancer? Who Gets Cancer? Who Survives?

Cancer can be caused by both external (chemicals, radiation, and viruses) and internal (hormones, immune conditions, and inherited mutations) factors. These factors may act together or in sequence to begin or promote cancer.

No one is immune to cancer. Because the incidence increases with age, most cases are found among adults in mid-life or older. As noted in Chapter 1, however, cancer is the second-leading cause of death in the United States among children aged 5 to 14.

The American Cancer Society (ACS) estimated that more than 1.2 million people were diagnosed with cancer in 1998. That same year an estimated 538,947 people died of cancer, about 1,500 patients per day, or about one person every minute. (See Table 7.1.) The death rates for most forms of cancer have remained fairly steady since the 1930s. Three exceptions are lung, stomach, and uterine cancer. In the 1930s stomach cancer and uterine cancer had some of the highest death rates, but they have since declined to some of the lowest. Meanwhile, the lung cancer death rate rose dramatically from 1930 up until 1990, especially for men, then began to decline.

Many cancer patients do survive. In 1998 about 491,400 Americans, or nearly 5 of 10 patients diagnosed with cancer had survived for at least five years after cancer treatment. In contrast, fewer than 1 in 4 patients treated 50 years ago was still living after five years. Approximately 8 million Americans have a history of cancer. Most of those can be considered "cured," meaning that there is no evidence of the disease and survivors have the same life expectancy as someone who has never had cancer.

Could More Americans Be Saved?

The ACS estimated that even more lives could be saved with early detection and treatment. Regular screening and self-exams can detect cancers of the breast, tongue, mouth, colon, rectum, cervix, prostate, testis, and skin at an early stage when treatment is more likely to be successful. These cancer sites include approximately half of all new cases. Of these types of cancer, about 80 percent of all patients currently survive five years or more. With early detection, more than 95 percent could survive. In addition, staying out of the sun or using sun protection could prevent many of the 1 million skin cancers found annually. All cancers caused by smoking and heavy drinking are also preventable.

Cancer among African Americans

African Americans are diagnosed with cancer at a higher rate than whites—430.9 out of every 100,000, as opposed to 387.3 of every 100,000 whites. Blacks have considerably higher incidence for cancers of the esophagus, uterus, cervix, stomach, liver, prostate, and larynx than other minorities. Mortality (death) rates are also higher for blacks. The difference in death rates is attributed to the fact that more whites than blacks had their cancers diagnosed at an earlier, localized stage when the chances for survival are best. Part of the problem is public awareness and the use of cancer testing. Other factors, such as a lack of health insurance or transportation, can also prevent or delay testing and treatment.

Gender and Cancer

In 1996 the overall cancer incidence rate for men was significantly higher than that for women—cancer was found in 454.6 of every 100,000 men, while only 342 of every 100,000 women were diagnosed with cancer. Men and women are more prone to certain types of cancer—most obviously, the cancers of the reproductive system such as ovarian and cervical cancer in women and prostate or testicular cancer in men. Breast cancer also occurs mainly in women, although some men do die from breast cancer as well. Men also suffer from higher rates of pancreatic, colorectal, and bladder cancer than do women. Women suffer from higher rates of malignant melanoma, the most aggressive type of skin cancer. (See Table 7.5.)

While diagnoses of lung cancer were still higher among men in 1996 (70 per 100,000) than women (42.3 per 100,000), incidences of lung cancer among women more than doubled between 1973 and 1996, from 18.2 cases per 100,000 in 1973 to 42.3 cases in 1996. Lung cancer incidences in men declined during that same period from 73.2 cases per 100,000 to 70. (See Table 7.5.)

The Seven Warning Signals

The ACS lists the following seven symptoms or changes as possible signals of cancer and indications to see a physician:

- Change in bowel or bladder habits.
- A sore that does not heal.
- Unusual bleeding or discharge.
- Thickening or lump in breast or elsewhere.
- Indigestion or difficulty swallowing.
- Obvious change in wart or mole.
- Nagging cough or hoarseness.

Lung Cancer

Lung cancer is the most common form of cancer in the United States, accounting for an estimated 171,500 new cases and 160,100 deaths in 1998. (See Table 7.6.) While the number of cases among men has begun to decline, the incidence of lung cancer among women continued to rise until 1994, when it reached a high of 43.4 per 100,000. That number dropped to 42.3 in 1996. (See Table 7.5.) Each year since 1987, more women have died of lung cancer than breast cancer, which had been the leading cause of cancer death for women for over 40 years.

The five-year survival rate for lung cancer is low— only 14 percent—but if lung cancer is detected in the early stages when it is still localized, the survival rate is 49 percent. Unfortunately, only 15 percent of all cases of lung cancer are detected early.

The main risk factor for lung cancer is cigarette smoking, especially a long history of smoking (20 years or more). In addition, exposure to certain industrial substances, such as asbestos, organic chemicals, and radon can increase one's risk of the disease.

Involuntary smoking, or inhaling other people's smoke, also increases the risk for nonsmokers. Recent research has found that the risk to a nonsmoking woman who is married to a smoker is 30 percent greater than for a woman with a nonsmoking spouse. The Environmental Protection Agency (EPA) claimed that 3,000 nonsmokers a year died from secondhand smoke-induced lung cancer, and in 1993, the EPA added secondhand smoke to their list of known carcinogens.

Early diagnosis of lung cancer is difficult; by the time a tumor is visible on X rays, it is often in the advanced stages. If an individual, however, stops smoking before cellular changes occur, damaged tissues often return to normal. The treatment options for lung cancer include surgery, radiation therapy, and chemotherapy.

Colon and Rectal Cancer

In 1998 an estimated 131,600 cases—95,600 colon cancers and 36,000 rectal cancers—were diagnosed. An estimated 56,500 people died of the disease in 1998— 47,700 from colon cancer and 8,800 from rectal cancer. (See Table 7.6.)

When colon and rectal cancers are detected early, the five-year survival rates are 93 and 88 percent, respectively. If the malignancy has spread regionally, the rates drop to 67 and 55 percent, respectively.

Colon cancer occurs most often in persons who have a family history of polyps in the colon or rectum or who have suffered from ulcerative colitis and other diseases of the bowel. In addition, a significant factor may be a diet high in fat and low in fiber.

The ACS recommends three types of screening tests to detect bowel cancer in its early stages. A digital rectal exam, performed by a physician during a routine office visit, is recommended annually for those over 40. For persons over 50, a simple stool test for hidden blood is recommended. The third test, sigmoidoscopy, the examination of the lower colon and rectum using a hollow lighted tube, can be used for detection every three to five years for people over age 50. If any abnormalities are found during these procedures, more extensive exams, such as a colonoscopy (examination of the entire colon) and an X-ray procedure, can be performed.

The most common treatment for cancer of the bowel is surgery to remove the diseased area, in combination with radiation. A colostomy (an opening in the abdomen to allow for waste elimination) is seldom necessary for colon cancer patients and even rarer for rectal cancer patients. The ACS reported that only about 15 percent of all rectal cancer victims require a permanent colostomy if the cancer is detected in the early stages. Of those who do require a permanent colostomy, most go on to lead normal, active lives.

Breast Cancer

Breast cancer is the most common form of cancer among women, accounting for an estimated 178,700 new

TABLE 7.5

Age-adjusted cancer incidence rates for selected cancer sites, according to sex and race: Selected geographic areas, selected years 1973–96

[Data are based on the Surveillance, Epidemiology, and End Results Program's population-based registries in Atlanta, Detroit, Seattle-Puget Sound, San Francisco-Oakland, Connecticut, Iowa, New Mexico, Utah, and Hawaii]

Race, sex, and site	1973	1975	1980	1985	1990	1992	1993	1994	1995	1996
All races, both sexes					Number of new cases per 100,000 population[1]					
All sites	320.0	332.7	345.8	372.5	399.7	425.6	412.1	403.8	395.2	388.6
Oral cavity and pharynx	11.3	11.4	11.6	11.5	11.2	10.5	10.9	10.4	10.0	10.0
Esophagus	3.4	3.5	3.7	3.8	4.2	3.9	4.0	3.8	3.7	4.0
Stomach	10.2	9.2	8.9	8.1	7.4	7.4	7.2	7.2	6.6	6.6
Colon and rectum	46.4	47.4	50.4	52.8	48.3	46.4	45.3	44.3	42.9	42.7
Colon	31.7	32.6	35.5	37.7	34.6	33.3	32.8	32.1	31.1	30.3
Rectum	14.7	14.8	14.9	15.1	13.7	13.1	12.5	12.3	11.8	12.5
Pancreas	10.0	9.5	9.3	9.6	9.0	9.3	8.7	9.0	8.7	8.6
Lung and bronchus	42.4	45.3	52.3	56.1	58.6	59.6	57.9	57.1	56.2	54.2
Urinary bladder	14.6	15.5	16.5	16.8	17.1	17.2	17.3	16.9	16.6	16.2
Non-Hodgkin's lymphoma	8.6	9.4	10.5	12.9	15.3	15.3	15.6	16.3	16.2	15.5
Leukemia	10.6	10.6	10.7	11.1	10.5	10.6	10.4	10.2	10.5	9.7
Male										
All sites	365.0	378.8	409.2	431.4	479.6	536.3	510.0	483.5	464.9	454.6
Oral cavity and pharynx	17.5	18.0	17.4	17.1	17.0	16.1	16.5	15.7	14.7	14.8
Esophagus	5.5	5.8	5.9	6.3	7.1	6.7	6.6	6.5	6.0	6.8
Stomach	15.1	13.5	13.5	11.9	10.9	10.7	10.7	10.9	9.9	9.8
Colon and rectum	53.1	54.1	58.7	63.0	58.9	56.3	54.5	53.1	50.5	51.1
Colon	34.2	35.5	39.3	43.2	40.5	39.0	38.4	37.1	35.1	34.9
Rectum	18.9	18.6	19.4	19.7	18.4	17.3	16.1	16.0	15.3	16.1
Pancreas	12.9	12.5	11.4	11.3	10.4	10.7	10.0	10.6	9.9	10.0
Lung and bronchus	73.2	76.2	84.4	83.8	81.7	81.7	78.7	75.6	74.1	70.0
Prostate gland	64.2	70.6	79.8	88.3	132.5	190.8	171.1	148.4	139.3	135.7
Urinary bladder	25.6	27.1	29.4	28.9	29.8	29.7	29.9	29.2	28.4	27.7
Non-Hodgkin's lymphoma	10.0	11.0	12.4	15.2	18.9	18.9	19.3	20.3	20.5	19.2
Leukemia	13.8	13.7	14.2	14.4	13.9	14.0	13.3	13.0	13.5	12.3
Female										
All sites	293.5	307.6	307.1	337.3	348.7	349.3	343.2	347.8	346.3	342.0
Colon and rectum	41.6	42.7	44.5	45.3	40.5	38.9	38.2	37.6	37.0	36.2
Colon	30.2	30.8	33.0	33.6	30.3	29.1	28.5	28.2	28.0	26.6
Rectum	11.4	11.9	11.5	11.7	10.1	9.8	9.7	9.3	9.0	9.6
Pancreas	7.7	7.3	7.7	8.2	8.0	8.2	7.6	7.8	7.7	7.4
Lung and bronchus	18.2	21.5	28.1	35.3	41.5	43.2	42.3	43.4	42.7	42.3
Melanoma of skin	5.4	6.3	8.2	9.4	9.9	10.4	10.3	10.5	11.3	11.4
Breast	82.6	88.1	85.4	104.1	110.4	111.1	108.9	110.8	111.6	110.7
Cervix uteri	14.2	12.4	10.2	8.5	8.9	8.3	8.1	7.9	7.4	7.7
Corpus uteri	28.4	32.1	24.2	22.1	21.8	21.5	21.0	21.8	21.9	21.1
Ovary	14.1	14.1	13.3	14.3	15.2	15.0	15.0	14.5	14.5	14.1
Non-Hodgkin's lymphoma	7.4	8.0	8.9	10.9	12.3	12.2	12.4	13.0	12.4	12.2
White										
All sites	319.7	333.9	346.4	375.4	405.1	428.7	412.2	404.2	396.4	387.3
Oral cavity and pharynx	11.2	11.4	11.2	11.4	10.9	10.4	10.6	10.0	9.8	9.5
Esophagus	3.0	3.0	3.0	3.2	3.6	3.5	3.6	3.5	3.4	3.6
Stomach	9.5	8.4	8.1	7.1	6.3	6.4	6.1	6.1	5.8	5.6
Colon and rectum	46.9	47.8	50.4	53.3	48.2	46.2	44.9	44.0	42.5	42.2
Colon	32.0	32.9	35.4	37.9	34.4	33.1	32.3	31.8	30.7	29.9
Rectum	14.9	14.9	15.0	15.4	13.8	13.1	12.6	12.2	11.8	12.3
Pancreas	9.8	9.4	8.9	9.2	8.8	9.1	8.3	8.6	8.3	8.2
Lung and bronchus	41.6	45.1	51.2	55.5	58.8	59.1	57.9	57.2	56.4	54.2
Urinary bladder	15.4	16.3	17.4	17.9	18.3	18.5	18.5	18.3	18.0	17.4
Non-Hodgkin's lymphoma	8.8	9.8	10.8	13.5	16.0	16.0	16.2	16.9	16.6	15.9
Leukemia	10.8	10.9	11.0	11.4	10.9	10.9	10.6	10.6	11.0	9.8
Black										
All sites	353.1	356.6	390.7	408.6	427.1	470.9	471.8	465.4	442.4	430.9
Oral cavity and pharynx	10.9	11.7	15.3	14.1	14.2	13.3	14.2	14.6	12.2	13.5
Esophagus	9.0	9.6	11.1	11.3	11.3	9.3	8.9	8.2	7.5	8.3
Stomach	16.7	13.8	12.4	12.9	11.7	11.0	11.3	12.1	10.5	11.5
Colon and rectum	42.4	45.4	55.7	52.1	52.4	52.1	51.7	51.7	48.5	45.7
Colon	30.9	33.7	43.2	40.7	40.7	40.1	40.7	39.6	37.9	34.6
Rectum	11.5	11.8	12.5	11.5	11.7	12.0	11.0	12.0	10.6	11.2
Pancreas	13.6	13.5	14.8	14.7	12.1	14.1	13.6	14.2	14.2	13.1
Lung and bronchus	58.7	56.5	76.0	79.0	75.3	81.9	74.7	75.9	73.1	69.9
Urinary bladder	7.0	8.7	10.6	10.6	10.3	9.9	10.9	9.7	9.4	9.2
Non-Hodgkin's lymphoma	7.0	5.6	7.4	8.3	11.3	11.4	11.6	12.0	13.6	12.0
Leukemia	9.6	9.3	10.0	9.7	8.9	8.9	9.2	7.7	7.9	8.1

TABLE 7.5

Age-adjusted cancer incidence rates for selected cancer sites, according to sex and race: Selected geographic areas, selected years 1973–96 [CONTINUED]

[Data are based on the Surveillance, Epidemiology, and End Results Program's population-based registries in Atlanta, Detroit, Seattle-Puget Sound, San Francisco-Oakland, Connecticut, Iowa, New Mexico, Utah, and Hawaii]

Race, sex, and site	1973	1975	1980	1985	1990	1992	1993	1994	1995	1996
White male					Number of new cases per 100,000 population[1]					
All sites	364.3	379.7	407.5	431.4	483.0	535.6	502.6	476.7	458.1	445.8
Oral cavity and pharynx	17.6	18.3	17.0	16.8	16.4	15.7	16.0	14.8	14.3	14.0
Esophagus	4.8	4.8	4.9	5.3	6.1	6.2	5.9	6.0	5.5	6.2
Stomach	14.0	12.5	12.3	10.5	9.4	9.4	9.1	9.4	8.9	8.4
Colon and rectum	54.2	55.1	58.7	63.5	59.1	56.4	54.2	52.9	49.9	50.7
Colon	34.8	36.1	39.3	43.4	40.4	39.1	38.1	37.0	34.7	34.9
Rectum	19.5	19.0	19.4	20.1	18.7	17.3	16.1	15.8	15.2	15.8
Pancreas	12.8	12.5	11.1	10.7	10.1	10.4	9.6	9.8	9.5	9.5
Lung and bronchus	72.4	75.9	82.2	82.0	80.9	79.3	77.1	74.5	72.3	68.4
Prostate gland	62.6	69.0	78.8	87.2	133.4	188.7	163.9	141.0	132.3	127.8
Urinary bladder	27.3	28.8	31.5	31.2	32.4	31.9	32.0	31.7	30.8	29.9
Non-Hodgkin's lymphoma	10.4	11.5	12.6	15.9	19.7	19.6	20.0	20.7	20.9	19.7
Leukemia	14.3	14.3	14.6	14.8	14.5	14.7	13.8	13.5	14.1	12.4
Black male										
All sites	441.4	438.2	510.4	533.0	561.4	657.2	664.4	636.5	594.8	563.1
Oral cavity and pharynx	16.6	17.2	23.1	22.6	24.5	22.6	22.9	25.0	20.3	21.9
Esophagus	13.3	17.6	16.4	19.4	19.5	15.7	15.2	13.2	12.4	14.0
Stomach	25.9	19.9	21.4	18.8	17.8	15.9	18.5	19.4	14.6	17.6
Colon and rectum	42.8	47.6	63.7	60.8	58.1	61.8	62.0	59.6	54.6	50.9
Colon	31.7	34.7	46.0	47.0	45.0	46.7	47.1	44.2	41.4	36.7
Rectum	11.1	12.9	17.7	13.8	13.1	15.1	14.8	15.3	13.2	14.2
Pancreas	15.9	15.6	17.6	19.7	15.0	15.4	15.4	17.3	16.4	15.9
Lung and bronchus	104.6	101.0	131.0	131.3	115.9	127.6	114.8	112.8	115.2	101.4
Prostate gland	106.3	111.5	126.6	133.8	168.4	258.0	271.6	246.9	218.3	211.3
Urinary bladder	10.6	13.5	14.5	16.3	15.1	16.6	18.1	15.7	14.3	14.0
Non-Hodgkin's lymphoma	8.8	7.0	9.3	10.0	14.0	15.3	15.7	17.7	19.1	15.0
Leukemia	12.0	12.5	13.1	13.0	11.7	11.4	12.2	9.8	10.2	10.1
White female										
All sites	295.1	310.6	311.3	343.9	356.9	356.3	349.6	354.5	354.5	347.1
Colon and rectum	41.7	42.9	44.7	46.0	40.2	38.4	37.7	36.9	36.7	35.5
Colon	30.3	30.9	32.9	34.0	30.1	28.7	27.9	27.7	27.6	25.9
Rectum	11.5	12.0	11.8	12.0	10.1	9.8	9.8	9.2	9.1	9.6
Pancreas	7.5	7.1	7.3	8.1	7.8	8.0	7.3	7.6	7.5	7.1
Lung and bronchus	17.8	21.8	28.2	35.9	42.6	44.3	43.8	44.4	44.5	43.7
Melanoma of skin	5.9	6.9	9.4	10.5	11.4	11.9	11.8	12.1	13.2	13.2
Breast	84.4	90.0	87.8	107.3	114.5	114.2	112.0	114.6	115.3	113.3
Cervix uteri	12.8	11.1	9.1	7.6	8.3	7.9	7.6	7.3	6.6	7.0
Corpus uteri	29.5	33.7	25.3	23.2	23.1	22.7	22.1	22.7	22.8	21.8
Ovary	14.6	14.4	14.0	15.1	16.1	15.8	15.7	15.0	15.4	15.3
Non-Hodgkin's lymphoma	7.6	8.5	9.2	11.4	12.9	12.9	12.8	13.5	12.8	12.7
Black female										
All sites	283.7	296.3	305.0	323.7	337.5	343.5	337.1	344.8	333.0	336.1
Colon and rectum	41.8	43.5	49.6	45.8	48.6	45.8	44.4	46.5	44.2	41.8
Colon	30.0	32.7	41.2	35.9	37.9	36.0	36.2	36.8	35.7	32.9
Rectum	11.8	10.8	8.5	9.9	10.7	9.8	8.2	9.7	8.5	8.9
Pancreas	11.6	11.6	13.0	11.3	10.0	12.8	12.0	11.9	12.4	10.8
Lung and bronchus	20.9	20.6	33.8	40.2	46.3	48.7	45.7	49.0	42.7	47.2
Breast	69.0	78.5	74.5	92.7	96.5	102.2	100.8	102.1	102.4	100.3
Cervix uteri	29.9	27.9	19.0	15.9	13.8	11.1	11.3	11.6	11.3	10.6
Corpus uteri	15.0	17.0	14.1	15.4	14.4	14.6	14.7	15.7	15.8	15.7
Ovary	10.5	10.1	10.1	10.1	10.1	10.6	11.1	12.4	9.9	8.5
Non-Hodgkin's lymphoma	5.5	4.2	6.0	7.0	9.2	8.2	8.1	7.2	9.1	9.5

[1] Age adjusted by the direct method to the 1970 U.S. population.

SOURCE: *Health, United States, 2000*, National Center for Health Statistics, Hyattsville, MD, 2000

cases in 1998. An estimated 43,900 deaths (400 of these deaths occurred among men) resulted from breast cancer in 1998. (See Table 7.6.)

Among white females, the incidence of breast cancer increased by 34.2 percent from 1973 to 1996. Among black females, the growth rate was 45.4 percent. (See Table 7.5.) A portion of the growth has probably been due to increased screening programs that detect tumors before they can be felt.

The survival rates for cancers of the breast are encouraging. If the cancer is localized, the survival rate is 97 percent. If the cancer, however, is undetected and has

TABLE 7.6

Estimated new cancer cases and deaths by sex for all sites, 1998

	Estimated new cases			Estimated deaths		
	Both sexes	Male	Female	Both sexes	Male	Female
All sites	1,228,600	627,900	600,700	564,800	294,200	270,600
Oral cavity & pharynx	30,300	20,600	9,700	8,000	5,300	2,700
Tongue	6,700	4,300	2,400	1,700	1,100	600
Mouth	10,800	6,500	4,300	2,300	1,300	1,000
Pharynx	8,600	6,500	2,100	2,100	1,500	600
Other oral cavity	4,200	3,300	900	1,900	1,400	500
Digestive system	227,700	119,200	108,500	130,300	69,400	60,900
Esophagus	12,300	9,300	3,000	11,900	9,100	2,800
Stomach	22,600	14,300	8,300	13,700	8,100	5,600
Small intestine	4,500	2,400	2,100	1,200	600	600
Colon	95,600	44,400	51,200	47,700	23,100	24,600
Rectum	36,000	20,200	15,800	8,800	4,800	4,000
Anus, anal canal, & anorectum	3,300	1,400	1,900	500	200	300
Liver	13,900	9,300	4,600	13,000	7,900	5,100
Gallbladder & other biliary	6,700	2,600	4,100	3,500	1,200	2,300
Pancreas	29,000	14,100	14,900	28,900	14,000	14,900
Other digestive organs	3,800	1,200	2,600	1,100	400	700
Respiratory system	187,900	104,500	83,400	165,600	97,200	68,400
Larynx	11,100	9,000	2,100	4,300	3,400	900
Lung	171,500	91,400	80,100	160,100	93,100	67,000
Other respiratory organs	5,300	4,100	1,200	1,200	700	500
Bones & joints	2,400	1,300	1,100	1,400	800	600
Soft tissue (including heart)	7,000	3,700	3,300	4,300	2,000	2,300
Skin (excluding basal & squamous)	53,100	33,800	19,300	9,200	5,800	3,400
Melanoma	41,600	24,300	17,300	7,300	4,600	2,700
Other nonepithelial skin	11,500	9,500	2,000	1,900	1,200	700
Breast	180,300	1,600	178,700	43,900	400	43,500
Reproductive organs	274,000	193,600	80,400	66,900	39,800	27,100
Cervix (uterus)	13,700	—	13,700	4,900	—	4,900
Endometrium (uterus)	36,100	—	36,100	6,300	—	6,300
Ovary	25,400	—	25,400	14,500	—	14,500
Vulva	3,200	—	3,200	800	—	800
Vagina & female genital	2,000	—	2,000	600	—	600
Prostate	184,500	184,500	—	39,200	39,200	—
Testis	7,600	7,600	—	400	400	—
Penis & male genital	1,500	1,500	—	200	200	—
Urinary system	86,300	58,400	27,900	24,700	15,800	8,900
Urinary bladder	54,400	39,500	14,900	12,500	8,400	4,100
Kidney	29,900	17,600	12,300	11,600	7,100	4,500
Ureter & other urinary organs	2,000	1,300	700	600	300	300
Eye & orbit	2,100	1,100	1,000	300	200	100
Brain	17,400	9,800	7,600	13,300	7,300	6,000
Endocrine system	18,800	5,500	13,300	2,000	800	1,200
Thyroid	17,200	4,700	12,500	1,200	400	800
Other endocrine	1,600	800	800	800	400	400
Lymphoma	62,500	34,800	27,700	26,300	13,700	12,600
Hodgkin's disease	7,100	3,700	3,400	1,400	700	700
Non-Hodgkin's lymphoma	55,400	31,100	24,300	24,900	13,000	11,900
Multiple myeloma	13,800	7,200	6,600	11,300	5,800	5,500
Leukemia	28,700	16,100	12,600	21,600	12,000	9,600
Acute lymphocytic leukemia	3,100	1,700	1,400	1,300	700	600
Chronic lymphocytic leukemia	7,300	4,100	3,200	4,800	2,800	2,000
Acute myeloid leukemia	9,400	4,700	4,700	6,600	3,600	3,000
Chronic myeloid leukemia	4,300	2,500	1,800	2,400	1,400	1,000
Other leukemia	4,600	3,100	1,500	6,500	3,500	3,000
Other & unspecified primary sites	36,300	16,700	19,600	35,700	17,900	17,800

* Excludes basal and squamous cell skin cancers and in situ carcinomas except urinary bladder. Carcinoma in situ of the breast accounts for about 36,900 new cases annually, and melanoma carcinoma in situ accounts for about 21,100 new cases annually. Estimates of new cases are based on incidence rates from the NCI SEER program 1979-1994.

SOURCE: *Cancer Facts and Figures—1998,* American Cancer Society, Atlanta, GA, 1998

spread regionally, the survival rate drops to 76 percent, and for women whose cancer has spread to distant parts of the body, the survival rate is only 21 percent.

The causes of breast cancer are still unknown. The disease, however, is most common in women over age 50, and the risks are higher among women with a family his-

tory of breast cancer, those who have never had children, and women who gave birth to their first baby after age 30.

As with other types of cancer, early detection is the key to cure and survival. The ACS recommends that all women aged 20 and over practice breast self-examination each month. In addition, mammography has become an invaluable screening and diagnostic tool in detecting cancers that are too small to be otherwise discovered. The ACS also recommends that women aged 35 to 39 have a baseline mammogram (an X ray that they can later compare to others), and those over age 40 should have routine mammograms each year.

CHOICES OF TREATMENT. Breast cancer treatment remains a subject of continuing medical debate. If a breast contains cancerous tissue, the patient and her doctor have several treatment options, depending on the location and size of the tumor. A small, contained tumor may be removed in a procedure commonly called a lumpectomy (removal of the tumor, or "lump"), followed by radiation therapy to the whole breast. If the cancer is more advanced and invasive, removing the breast (mastectomy) and usually the adjoining lymph nodes, combined with chemotherapy, may be the most effective treatment.

Two studies released in 1995 showed that both procedures were equally effective in appropriate cases. A 10-year study by the National Cancer Institute of 247 women who had been treated with lumpectomy and radiation for early cancers found that their survival and cancer recurrence rates were the same as those who had mastectomies. (The patients who had lumpectomies were also screened for lymph node cancer; if one or more nodes were cancerous, these women received combination chemotherapy in addition to radiation.) Ten years after treatment, more than 75 percent of the patients were still alive, and 70 percent had no recurrence of cancer. A 20-year study by the National Tumor Institute in Milan, Italy, found that of 386 women who had mastectomies followed by combination chemotherapy, 34 percent had fewer relapses and 26 percent fewer died than those treated by mastectomy alone.

A relatively new drug, tamoxifen, was expected to help prolong survival and recovery, especially for postmenopausal women with breast cancer. In April 1998, federal health officials declared tamoxifen to be the first drug ever shown to prevent breast cancer in women at high risk of developing the disease.

If the patient chooses a mastectomy, there are numerous support groups that can help women deal with breast cancer and its treatment. Also, new techniques have made breast reconstruction possible—sometimes during or immediately following surgery. Some health insurers, however, refuse to pay for breast reconstruction following mastectomy, considering it a cosmetic decision.

GENETIC RESEARCH. Doctors have known for some time that predisposition to some forms of breast cancer is inherited, and have been searching for the gene or genes responsible so that they could test patients and provide more careful monitoring for those at risk. In 1994 doctors identified the BRCA1 gene, and in late 1995 they also isolated the BRCA2 gene.

If a woman with a family history of breast cancer inherits a defective form of either BRCA1 or BRCA2, she has an estimated 80 to 90 percent risk of developing breast cancer. Researchers also think that the two genes are linked to ovarian, prostate, and colon cancer, and BRCA2 likely plays some role in breast cancer in men. Scientists suspect that the two genes may also participate in some way in the development of breast cancer in women with no family history of the disease.

A study completed in November 1996, headed by Dr. Stephen C. Rubin, a professor and chief of gynecological oncology (cancer of the female reproductive organs) at the University of Pennsylvania, reported a result that was totally unexpected by the researchers. The study found that women with defective BRCA1 genes who developed ovarian cancer survived longer than those without the mutated gene who developed ovarian cancer. Women with the defective gene lived an average of 77 months after diagnosis, while those without the mutated gene averaged only a 29-month survival. Doctors do not know if those with the defective gene had less deadly types of cancers or if their cancers responded better to treatment.

Another form of breast cancer, driven by multiple copies of a gene called HER-2, causes an estimated 30 percent of the approximately 180,000 new cases of the disease in the United States each year. HER-2/neu is an aggressive form of cancer that can cause death more quickly than other breast cancers, often within 10 to 18 months after the cancer spreads. The HER-2 gene produces a protein on the surface of cells that serves as a receiving point for growth-stimulating hormones.

A new drug, Herceptin, a genetically engineered antibody, increases the benefits of chemotherapy by shrinking tumors and slowing the progression of HER-2/neu. Herceptin became available in late 1998.

Skin Cancer

Skin cancer is a common form of malignancy, with an estimated 1 million new cases reported in 1998. The vast majority of these cancers are nonmelanoma types—usually basal or squamous cell cancers that can be easily cured. Malignant melanoma, which struck an estimated 41,600 people in 1998 (see Table 7.6), is the most serious form of skin cancer and has increased at a rate of 4 percent a year since 1973.

An estimated 9,200 people died of skin cancer in 1998, with most of the deaths (an estimated 7,300) resulting from malignant melanoma. (See Table 7.6.) Melanoma can spread to other parts of the body quickly, but if it is detected early and properly treated, it is highly curable. The five-year survival rate for a localized malignant melanoma is 95 percent, but once it has spread to distant parts of the body, the chances of survival plummet to 16 percent.

FIGURE 7.3

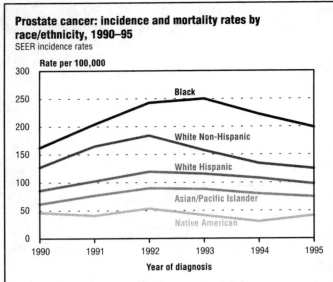

Prostate cancer: incidence and mortality rates by race/ethnicity, 1990–95
SEER incidence rates

Note: Rates are age-adjusted to the 1970 U.S. standard; incidence rates are based on data from 11 SEER registries. Mortality rates do not include data from Connecticut, Louisiana, New Hampshire, or Oklahoma.

SOURCE: J.L. Stanford et al., *Prostate Cancer Trends 1973–1995*, SEER Program, National Cancer Institute. NIH Pub. No. 99-4543. Bethesda, MD, 1999

Simple precautions can prevent most skin cancers. Avoiding the sun between 10 a.m. and 3 p.m. (when the ultraviolet rays are the strongest), using sunscreens, and wearing protective clothing decreases the risk of skin cancer considerably.

Prostate Cancer

An estimated 184,500 American men were diagnosed with prostate cancer in 1998, and approximately 39,200 died from the disease. (See Table 7.6.) A higher percentage of men over the age of 65 (77 percent) are found to have prostate cancer. Between the ages of 50 and 54 years of age, the rate is 82 cases per 100,000 males. For ages 60 to 64 years, the rate climbs to 518 cases per 100,000 males, and for men between 70 and 74 years of age, the rate is 1,326 per 100,000.

Incidences of prostate cancer and mortality rates vary among racial and ethnic groups. (See Figure 7.3.) Between 1980 and 1995, African American men were twice as likely to develop and die from prostate cancer than any other racial and ethnic group except white men.

In the late 1980s, prostate-specific antigen (PSA) screening became available to test men for the disease. This is a blood test that measures a protein made by prostate cells. PSA blood tests are reported in nanograms per milliliter (ng/mL). Results are considered normal if the reading is under 4 ng/mL; borderline results lie between 4 and 10 ng/mL; and any reading over 10ng/mL is high. The higher the reading, the more likely prostate cancer is present.

Prostate cancer may be treated in several ways. A radical prostatectomy is the removal of the prostate and some of the tissue surrounding the gland. This is done when the cancer has not spread outside the gland. Radiation therapy uses high-energy X rays to kill cancer cells and shrink tumors. It may be used before or after surgery. Impotence and urinary incontinence occur slightly more often when radiation is used following surgery. Radiation therapy can cause damage to the rectum.

Hormone therapy affects the hormone (testosterone) levels and is prescribed to limit cancer cell growth. Patients may be given drugs such as LHRH-agonists, which decrease the amount of testosterone in the body, or antiandrogens, which block the activity of testosterone. These cause cancer cells to shrink. (Testosterone may advance the growth of prostate cancer cells.)

Transurethral resection removes the cancerous section of the prostate gland. This procedure is often performed to relieve symptoms of urinary obstruction caused by the tumor. Chemotherapy is used to treat prostate cancer if it returns after other treatment. For men who have less aggressive tumors, are over 70 years of age, or have coexisting illnesses, many physicians watch and wait before suggesting further treatment.

RESPIRATORY DISEASES AND LUNG HEALTH

The American Lung Association (ALA) estimated that 73 million people suffer from some form of chronic respiratory disease. Eighteen million are victims of such lung diseases as emphysema, asthma, and chronic bronchitis. In 1998, 114,381 persons died from chronic obstructive pulmonary diseases (COPD). (See Table 7.1.) Children are especially sensitive to respiratory problems. Each year, more than 12,000 infants die of lung problems, and acute respiratory diseases account for more than half of all school absenteeism.

The number of COPD cases has increased dramatically since 1970, by 87.5 percent. Death rates from COPD have also increased sharply; in 1980 the age-adjusted death rate was 15.9 deaths per 100,000 resident population; by 1998 the rate had risen to 21.3 per 100,000, an increase of 34 percent. (See Table 7.7.)

The lungs are especially vulnerable to airborne particles, such as viruses, bacteria, tobacco smoke, pollen, fungi, and air pollution. Workers exposed to certain air hazards—cotton fibers; asbestos; and coal, metal, and silica dust—can also develop serious lung diseases. Pneumoconiosis is the general term for occupationally induced lung diseases.

Asthma

According to the CDC, asthma affects approximately 14 to 15 million Americans. It is the most common chron-

TABLE 7.7

Death rates for chronic obstructive pulmonary diseases, according to sex, detailed race, Hispanic origin, and age: selected years 1980–98

[Data are based on the National Vital Statistics System]

Sex, race, Hispanic origin, and age	1980	1985	1990	1992	1993	1994	1995	1996	1997	1998	1996–98[1]
All persons					Deaths per 100,000 resident population						
All ages, age adjusted	15.9	18.8	19.7	19.9	21.4	21.0	20.8	21.0	21.1	21.3	21.1
All ages, crude	24.7	31.4	34.9	36.0	39.2	39.0	39.2	40.0	40.7	41.7	40.8
Under 1 year	1.6	1.4	1.4	1.1	1.4	1.4	1.1	1.0	1.3	1.0	1.1
1–4 years	0.4	0.3	0.4	0.4	0.3	0.3	0.2	0.3	0.3	0.3	0.3
5–14 years	0.2	0.3	0.3	0.3	0.4	0.3	0.4	0.4	0.3	0.4	0.4
15–24 years	0.3	0.5	0.5	0.5	0.6	0.6	0.7	0.7	0.5	0.6	0.6
25–34 years	0.5	0.6	0.7	0.7	0.7	0.9	0.9	0.9	0.9	0.8	0.9
35–44 years	1.6	1.6	1.6	1.8	1.8	1.8	2.0	2.0	2.0	2.0	2.0
45–54 years	9.8	10.2	9.1	8.3	8.7	9.0	8.9	8.7	8.4	8.2	8.4
55–64 years	42.7	47.9	48.9	48.3	51.0	49.2	47.3	47.0	46.3	44.8	46.0
65–74 years	129.1	149.2	152.5	155.5	167.8	163.8	160.6	161.6	165.3	169.1	165.3
75–84 years	224.4	289.5	321.1	326.5	357.3	351.9	351.8	358.3	359.6	365.8	361.3
85 years and over	274.0	365.4	433.3	460.9	493.9	509.7	527.8	540.9	561.9	569.3	557.7

- - - Data not available.
[1] Average annual death rate.

Notes: Rates are age adjusted to the 1940 U.S. standard million population. Age groups were selected to minimize the presentation of unstable age-specific death rates based on small numbers of deaths and for consistency among comparison groups. The race groups, white, black, Asian or Pacific Islander, and American Indian or Alaska Native, include persons of Hispanic and non-Hispanic origin. Conversely, persons of Hispanic origin may be of any race. Bias in death rates results from inconsistent race identification between the death certificate (source of data for numerator of death rates) and data from the Census Bureau (denominator); and from undercounts of some population groups in the census. The net effects of misclassification and under coverage result in death rates estimated to be overstated by 1 percent for the white population and 5 percent for the black population; and death rates estimated to be understated by 21 percent for American Indians, 11 percent for Asians, and 2 percent for Hispanics (Rosenberg HM, Maurer JD, Sorlie PD, Johnson NJ, et al. Quality of death rates by race and Hispanic origin: A summary of current research, 1999. National Center for Health Statistics. Vital Health Stat 2(128). 1999).

SOURCE: *Health, United States, 2000,* National Center for Health Statistics, Hyattsville, MD, 2000

TABLE 7.8

Estimated average number of office visits for asthma as the first-listed diagnosis, by race, sex, and age group: 1975–95*

Category	1975	1980–1981	1985	1989	1990-1992	1993-1995
Race						
White	4,084,000	4,804,000	5,663,000	5,471,000	6,980,000	8,316,000
Black	463,000[†]	584,000[†]	702,000	893,000	1,196,000	1,373,000
Other	§	§	§	§	290,000	686,000
Sex						
Male	2,173,000	2,643,000	2,972,000	2,458,000	3,695,000	4,252,000
Female	2,460,000	2,830,000	3,531,000	4,364,000	4,866,000	6,122,000
Age group (yrs)						
0-4	429,000[†]	517,000[†]	556,000	626,000[†]	950,000	1,024,000
5-14	867,000	1,629,000	1,520,000	975,000	1,821,000	2,004,000
15-34	1,009,000	1,140,000	1,206,000	1,580,000	1,984,000	1,876,000
35-64	1,743,000	1,506,000	2,275,000	2,684,000	2,617,000	3,982,000
≥65	584,000	680,000	945,000	957,000	1,187,000	1,488,000
Total[¶]	**4,632,000**	**5,472,000**	**6,502,000**	**6,822,000**	**8,559,000**	**10,374,000**

* All relative standard errors are <30% (i.e., relative confidence interval <59%) unless otherwise indicated.
[†] Relative standard error of the estimate is 30%-50%; the estimate is unreliable.
§ Relative standard error of the estimate exceeds 50%.
[¶] Numbers for each variable may not add up to total because of rounding error and missing race for 1989 and 1990-1992.

SOURCE: "Surveillance for Asthma-United States, 1960-1995," *Morbidity and Mortality Weekly Report,* vol. 47, no SS-1, April 24, 1998

ic illness among children. Persons with asthma experience acute attacks of shortness of breath and difficulty in breathing because of a sudden narrowing of the bronchial tubes. While not always considered life threatening, asthma often limits activities and can be extremely serious for the very young and the very old.

The annual number of visits to doctors' offices for asthma more than doubled between 1975 and 1993–95, rising from 4.6 million to nearly 10.4 million. These statistics included persons of all races, ages, and both sexes. (See Table 7.8.) In 1995 more than 1.8 million persons visited an emergency room for treatment of asthma. Table

7.9 shows that in 1995 blacks (228.9 per 10,000) had far higher rates of emergency room usage than did whites (48.8 per 10,000). More females than males sought emergency room treatment, and more children through the age of four (120.7 per 10,000) visited the emergency room for treatment of asthma than any other age group.

In 1993 and 1994, 466,000 people were hospitalized for asthma. The hospitalization rates for blacks (35.5 per 10,000) were higher than for whites (10.9 per 10,000), and

the rates for very young children (49.7 per 10,000) were higher than for any other age group. (See Table 7.10.)

Deaths due to asthma decreased from 1960 to 1978, but gradually increased from 1979 to 1995. From 1993 to 1995, blacks (38.5 per 1 million) had higher death rates from asthma than whites (15.1 per 1 million). The death rates for persons aged 65 and older (89.8 per 1 million) were higher than for persons of any other age group. (See Table 7.11.) Between 1993 and 1995, 5,429 people died from asthma.

CAUSES OF ASTHMA ATTACKS. While the specific cause of asthma is not known, the disease seems to be associated with allergic reactions, heredity, and environment. Many environmental factors can trigger an asthma attack in susceptible individuals. While indoor and outdoor pollution does not cause the disease, pollutants such as ozone, sulfur dioxide, nitrogen dioxide, and tobacco smoke can set off an episode of asthma. Allergens such as pollen and dust mites can also trigger an attack.

Chronic Bronchitis

Bronchitis is an inflammation of the lining of the bronchial tubes, the bronchi, which connect the trachea (windpipe) to the lungs. When the bronchi are inflamed and infected, less air is able to flow to and from the lungs, and a heavy mucus forms and is coughed up. Acute bronchitis is usually brief in duration and follows the flu or a cold. Chronic bronchitis, however, lingers for months or even years and is characterized by a persistent mucus-producing cough. It is a long-term disease with symptoms of breathlessness and wheezing.

The ALA estimated that chronic bronchitis affects more than 5 percent of the total U.S. population. It is

TABLE 7.9

Estimated annual rate* of emergency room visits for asthma as the first-listed diagnosis, by race, sex, and age group: 1992–95[†]

Category	1992	1993	1994	1995
Race[§]				
White	46.8	50.3	46.1	48.8
Black	151.9	197.4	191.2	228.9
Other	28.6[¶]	23.7[¶]	21.9[¶]	33.1[¶]
Sex[§]				
Male	55.5	62.6	53.4	57.8
Female	61.4	69.7	65.9	82.3
Age group (yrs)				
0-4	143.5	164.3	145.5	120.7
5-14	77.1	82.8	80.3	81.3
15-34	52.9	59.0	62.8	69.2
35-64	39.6	50.7	41.8	64.4
≥ 65	27.7	22.6	23.5	29.5
Total[§]	**58.8**	**66.6**	**62.9**	**70.7**

* Per 10,000 population.
[†] All relative standard errors are <30% (i.e., relative confidence interval <59%) unless otherwise indicated.
[§] Age-adjusted to the 1970 U.S. population.
[¶] Relative standard error of the estimate is 30%-50%; the estimate is unreliable.

SOURCE: "Surveillance for Asthma-United States, 1960-1995," *Morbidity and Mortality Weekly Report*, vol. 47, no SS-1, April 24, 1998

TABLE 7.10

Estimated average rates* of hospitalization for asthma as the first-listed diagnosis, by race, sex, and age group: 1979–94[†]

Category	1979-1980	1981-1983	1984-1986	1987-1989	1990-1992	1993-1994
Race[§]						
White	14.2	16.2	15.9	14.1	11.9	10.9
Black	26.0	34.8	33.2	38.1	40.1	35.5
Other	28.2	30.6	32.7	33.6	24.4	23.0
Sex[§]						
Male	16.3	18.4	18.7	18.3	18.0	15.9
Female	18.7	21.4	21.8	21.0	20.8	20.0
Age group (yrs)						
0-4	34.3	42.8	48.5	52.2	58.3	49.7
5-14	15.9	19.2	18.9	18.7	20.6	18.0
15-34	8.7	9.5	9.5	9.5	9.3	10.0
35-64	18.2	20.3	19.0	16.7	15.4	15.2
≥ 65	31.5	33.6	37.5	35.2	29.7	25.6
Total[§]	**17.6**	**20.0**	**20.5**	**19.8**	**19.7**	**18.1**

* Per 10,000 population.
[†] All relative standard errors are <30% (i.e., relative confidence interval <59%).
[§] Age-adjusted to the 1970 U.S. population.

SOURCE: "Surveillance for Asthma-United States, 1960-1995," *Morbidity and Mortality Weekly Report*, vol. 47, no SS-1, April 24, 1998

TABLE 7.11

Rates* of death with asthma as the underlying cause of death diagnosis, by race, sex, and age group: 1960–95†

Category	1960-1962§	1963-1965	1966-1967	1968-1971§	1972-1974	1975-1978	1979-1980§	1981-1983	1984-1986	1987-1989	1990-1992	1993-1995
Race¶												
White	26.6	23.1	20.0	9.8	8.3	7.2	10.2	11.4	12.5	14.2	14.6	15.1
Black	42.0	40.8	38.0	28.4	20.7	17.3	22.2	26.7	30.0	36.1	35.6	38.5
Other	25.7	23.0	22.3	15.3	8.1	8.4	10.3	13.6	15.3	17.6	18.7	17.7
Sex¶												
Male	38.6	32.6	27.0	11.4	9.1	7.7	11.5	12.2	13.2	14.7	14.8	15.1
Female	19.5	18.7	17.7	12.3	10.0	8.8	11.6	13.8	15.5	18.2	18.9	20.0
Age group (yrs)												
0-4	4.3	4.0	3.4	3.0	1.9	1.3	1.6	1.6	1.6	1.5	2.1	1.8
5-14	2.1	2.4	2.6	1.8	1.3	1.1	1.5	2.2	2.6	2.9	3.0	3.7
15-34	5.6	5.2	4.9	4.3	3.0	2.4	2.8	3.9	4.1	4.9	5.3	6.3
35-64	36.9	33.9	30.8	17.5	13.8	10.9	13.8	16.0	17.0	19.0	18.5	19.6
≥65	141.5	118.8	98.1	43.6	38.7	37.6	58.6	63.0	72.3	85.0	89.0	89.8
Total¶	**28.2**	**24.9**	**21.8**	**11.8**	**9.5**	**8.2**	**11.5**	**13.1**	**14.4**	**16.6**	**17.1**	**17.9**

* Per 1,000,000 population.
† All relative standard errors are <30% (i.e., relative confidence interval <59%).
§ *International Classification of Diseases (ICD), Seventh Revision:* 1960-1967; *ICD, Eighth Revision (Adapted):* 1968-1978; *ICD, Ninth Revision:* 1979-1995.
¶ Age-adjusted to the 1970 U.S. population.

SOURCE: "Surveillance for Asthma-United States, 1960-1995," *Morbidity and Mortality Weekly Report,* vol. 47, no SS-1, April 24, 1998

responsible for about 7.5 million visits to physicians each year. In all age, sex, and race categories, people who smoke cigarettes are far more likely to develop chronic bronchitis than nonsmokers. Workers whose jobs involve inhaling large amounts of dust and irritating fumes are also more likely to get the disease. When air pollution becomes excessive, symptoms intensify.

Antibiotics and bronchodilator drugs are useful treatments, but even more important is the need to eliminate the sources of irritation to the respiratory system. This could mean quitting smoking or avoiding polluted air, fumes, and dust. Chronic bronchitis is often the forerunner of emphysema.

Emphysema

Emphysema is a severe disease of the lungs that usually develops gradually. The walls of the lungs' air sacs slowly lose their elasticity, and stale air becomes trapped in the lungs, which become overly inflated. This interferes with the normal exchange of oxygen and carbon dioxide. People with emphysema often feel as if they are drowning in a sea of air. Emphysema also affects the heart because the flow of blood from the lungs is disrupted by changes caused by emphysema, and the heart has to pump harder and can become enlarged. Death often results from heart failure.

DIABETES

Diabetes is a disease that affects the body's use of food, causing sugar levels in the blood to become too high. Normally, the body converts sugars, starches, and proteins into a form of sugar called glucose. The blood then carries glucose to all cells throughout the body. In the cells, with the help of the hormone insulin, the glucose is either changed into energy to be used immediately or stored for the future. Beta cells of the pancreas, a small organ located behind the stomach, manufacture the insulin. The process of turning food into energy via glucose (blood sugar) is important because the body depends on glucose for every function.

In diabetes, the body can convert food to glucose, but there is a problem with insulin. In one type of diabetes (Type I), the pancreas does not manufacture enough insulin, and in another type (Type II), the body cannot use the insulin effectively. When insulin is either absent or ineffective, glucose cannot get to the cells to be used for energy. Instead, the unused glucose builds up in the bloodstream and circulates through the kidneys. If a person's blood-glucose level rises high enough, the excess glucose "spills" over into the urine, causing frequent urination. This, in turn, leads to an increased feeling of thirst as the body tries to compensate for the fluid lost through urination.

Types of Diabetes

There are two distinct types of diabetes. Insulin-dependent diabetes (Type I, sometimes called juvenile diabetes), the most severe form of the disease, occurs most often in children and young adults. The pancreas stops manufacturing insulin, and the hormone must be injected daily. Non-insulin-dependent diabetes (Type II) is most often seen in adults. In this type, the pancreas produces insulin, but it is not used effectively and the body resists responding to it.

Warning Signs of Diabetes

The symptoms of Type I diabetes usually occur suddenly. These include excessive thirst, frequent urination, weight loss, weakness and fatigue, nausea and vomiting, and irritability. The symptoms of Type II diabetes generally appear more slowly. These may include any of the symptoms seen in Type I diabetes, plus recurring infections that are hard to heal, drowsiness, blurred vision, numbness in the hands or feet, and itching.

Prevalence of Diabetes

Approximately 15.7 million Americans (6 percent of the population) have diabetes. Of these, approximately one-third are undiagnosed. The individuals most at risk for Type II diabetes are usually overweight, over 40 years old, and have a family history of diabetes. Type II patients represent about 90 percent of diabetes patients. Type I patients account for only about 10 percent of diabetes sufferers.

In 1998 diabetes was the seventh-leading cause of death in the United States. The death rate was 23.9 per 100,000 population, for a total of 64,574 deaths. (See Table 7.1.)

Causes of Diabetes—a Mystery

The causes of both Type I and Type II diabetes are unknown, but a family history of diabetes increases the risk for both types, leading researchers to think there may be a genetic component. Some scientists believe that a flaw in the body's immune system may be a factor in Type I diabetes. Other researchers believe that poor cardiovascular fitness is a risk factor for developing diabetes.

In non-insulin-dependent diabetes, heredity may be a factor, but since the pancreas continues to produce insulin, the disease is considered more of a problem of insulin-resistance, in which the body is not using the hormone efficiently. In people prone to Type II diabetes, being overweight can set off the disease because excess fat prevents insulin from working correctly. Maintaining a normal weight and keeping physically fit can usually prevent non-insulin-dependent diabetes. So far, insulin-dependent diabetes (Type I) cannot be prevented.

Blacks are somewhat more likely to develop Type II diabetes than whites, while Hispanic Americans are much more likely to develop this type of the disease than the general population. Diabetes is also prevalent among many American Indians. The Pima Indians of southern Arizona, for example, have the highest incidence of Type II diabetes in the world (50 percent of those over age 35).

Complications of Diabetes

Because diabetes deprives body cells of the glucose needed to function properly, several complications can develop to further threaten the lives of victims. The heal-ing process of the body is slowed or impaired. Circulatory problems, especially in the legs, are often severe enough to require surgery or even amputation, and blindness is a constant fear for diabetics.

Diet and exercise are part of the treatment for dia-betes. Failure to follow the proper diet can be particularly dangerous to those who suffer from Type I diabetes.

CHAPTER 8
DEGENERATIVE DISEASES

Degenerative diseases are noninfectious disorders characterized by progressive disability in the patient. Victims can often live for years with their diseases. Sufferers may not die from degenerative diseases, but their symptoms usually grow more disabling and they often succumb to common complications of their disorders.

ARTHRITIS

The word "arthritis" literally means joint inflammation. The name applies to more than one hundred related diseases known as rheumatic diseases. A joint is any point where two bones meet. When a joint becomes inflamed, swelling, redness, pain, and loss of motion occur. In the most serious forms of the disease, the loss of motion can be a disabling physical problem.

Normally, inflammation is the body's response to an injury or a disease. Once the injury is healed or the disease is cured, the inflammation stops. In arthritis, however, the inflammation does not go away. Instead, it becomes part of the problem, damaging healthy tissues. This results in more inflammation, and more damage, and the painful cycle continues. The damage can change the shape of bones and other tissues of the joints, making movement difficult and painful.

Types of Arthritis

Over one hundred types of arthritis have been identified, but there are four major types that affect large numbers of Americans:

- Osteoarthritis—the most common type, generally affects people as they grow older. Sometimes called degenerative arthritis, it causes the breakdown of bones and cartilage and usually causes pain and stiffness in the fingers, knees, feet, hips, and back. This type affects about 20 million Americans, usually after age 45.

- Fibromyalgia—another common form, although it is often misdiagnosed. It affects the muscles and the tissues that connect them to the bones and causes widespread pain, as well as fatigue, sleeping problems, and stiffness. Fibromyalgia also causes "tender points" that are more sensitive to pain than other areas of the body. About 3.7 million persons, mostly women, suffer from this type.

- Rheumatoid arthritis—an inflammatory form of arthritis caused by a flaw in the body's immune system. The result is inflammation and swelling in the joint lining, followed by damage to bone and cartilage in the hands, wrists, feet, knees, ankles, shoulders, or elbows. About 2.1 million persons, mostly women, have this form of arthritis.

- Gout—an inflammation of a joint caused by a buildup of a natural substance, uric acid, in the joint, usually the big toe, a knee, or a wrist. The uric acid forms crystals in the affected joint, causing severe pain and swelling. This form affects more men than women, claiming about 1 million victims.

Prevalence

Arthritis is a very common problem. The Arthritis Foundation reported that more than 42 million Americans (one out of every six people) are affected by arthritis. Seven million of those arthritis sufferers are disabled by their disease. The total number was expected to increase to 60 million by 2020, with 11 million suffering from a disabling form of the disease.

Arthritis ranks second only to heart disease as a cause of disability payments. Rheumatic and musculoskeletal disorders are the most frequently reported cause of impairment in the adult population, the leading cause of limitation of mobility, and the second-leading cause of activity restriction. Lost wages and medical bills resulting from the effects of arthritis amount to more than $64 billion annually.

FIGURE 8.1

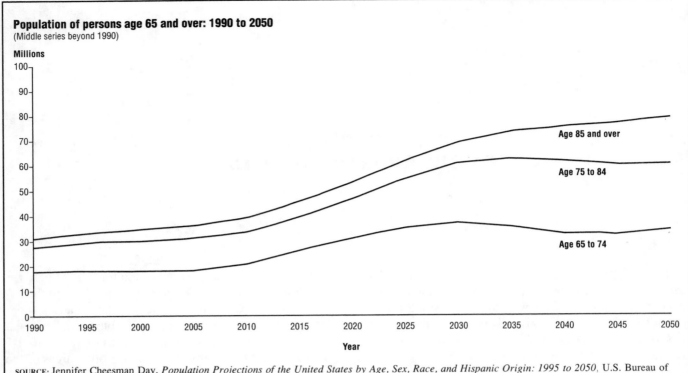

Population of persons age 65 and over: 1990 to 2050
(Middle series beyond 1990)

SOURCE: Jennifer Cheesman Day, *Population Projections of the United States by Age, Sex, Race, and Hispanic Origin: 1995 to 2050*, U.S. Bureau of the Census, Washington D.C., 1996

Almost half of all people over age 65 will experience some form of arthritis in their lifetimes. Although some think of it as only an older person's disease, nearly three of five arthritis sufferers are under age 65, and 29 percent of persons between the ages of 45 and 64 have arthritis. It can also affect children. An estimated 300,000 children and teenagers suffer from arthritis. Of these, approximately 71,000 suffer from rheumatoid arthritis, a potentially crippling disease that eventually destroys the joints.

In all age groups, women have a slightly higher likelihood of developing arthritis. In 1996 approximately 17 percent of all U.S. women suffered from arthritis, compared to 13 percent of men. As they age, women have an increasingly higher prevalence of arthritis than men do. Between the ages of 65 and 74, women have a 20 percent greater likelihood of developing arthritis than men; women aged 75 and older are 40 percent more likely to have the disease. Because of the expected increase in the proportion of persons aged 65 and older in the population, the number of arthritis victims is also expected to grow. By 2020 the population aged 65 and over will reach an estimated 53.2 million. (See Figure 8.1.)

Developments in Arthritis Research

As researchers learn more about inflammation and the body's immune system, they come closer to finding new drugs designed to relieve the pain of arthritis and to block the degenerative process of these diseases. Researchers are currently looking for ways to improve treatment by using the body's own biologic response modifiers (products that modify immune responses). They expect that these substances can be used to control the destructive processes of autoimmune diseases (in which the immune system attacks one's own cells) without weakening the whole immune system.

Among recent advances are more effective pain-relief drugs with fewer adverse side effects than those already on the market. One of the problems with nonsteroidal anti-inflammatory drugs (NSAIDs), the most widely used class of drugs for osteoarthritis, is the potential to irritate the stomach and even cause ulcers. Arthrotec, a new drug that received U.S. Food and Drug Administration (FDA) approval in 1997, encases the NSAID in a protective shell to decrease the gastrointestinal side effects. In addition, two new drugs known as COX-2 inhibitors were approved in 1998 and 1999. The drugs, known as Celebrex and Vioxx, reduce inflammation and relieve pain with far fewer gastrointestinal side effects than traditional arthritis drugs.

For rheumatoid arthritis sufferers, the FDA approved two new classes of drug. Arava (leflunomide) was approved in September 1998—the first drug for rheumatoid arthritis to become available in 10 years. It works by blocking the enzyme that increases the production of inflammation-causing cells. Arava is not a cure, but does ease pain and slow joint damage.

In 1999 the FDA also approved Enbrel, a drug that inhibits the function of the body's tumor necrosis factor receptors, which are believed to promote inflammation and are found in elevated levels in rheumatoid arthritis sufferers. In clinical trials, Enbrel reduced swollen or tender joints and disability by 20 percent or more.

Other scientists are studying how joints respond to different types of stresses. This may help in developing more effective exercises or new self-help devices. Researchers have found that regular exercise, weight control, and other self-help measures considerably lower the incidences and effects of the disease.

OSTEOPOROSIS

Osteoporosis literally means "porous bones." The bone-thinning and -weakening disease afflicts about 25 million Americans. Most of them are elderly, and 80 percent of them are women, according to the National Osteoporosis Foundation.

Bone density builds up during the growing years, reaching a peak in early adulthood. From that point on, bone loss gradually increases, outstripping the body's natural ability to replace bone. The denser a person's bones are during the growth years, the less likely he or she is to develop osteoporosis. Proper diet, especially the consumption of foods rich in calcium and vitamin D, taken long before the visible symptoms of osteoporosis appear, is vitally important.

About one-third of a person's risk of developing osteoporosis is hereditary. In 1994 an Australian research team identified a gene linked to bone density. There are two forms of the gene, B and b. Persons with two b genes, one from each parent, have the highest bone density and are least likely to develop osteoporosis, while those with one of each, the Bb genotype, have intermediate bone density. Persons with two B genes have the lowest bone density and the highest risk of osteoporosis. Women with the BB genotype may be four times as likely to experience hip fractures as those with the bb genotype.

The gene discovery was hailed as the most important finding in the osteoporosis field in a decade. Although much research remains to be done, researchers hope the identification of the gene will eventually lead to a simple test that can identify children at risk for osteoporosis in later life. The test would allow doctors to prescribe an increased intake of calcium and protein during the growth years for these individuals, thus preventing or delaying the onset of osteoporosis.

Osteoporosis worsens with age, leaving its victims at risk of broken hips or other bones, curvature of the spine, and other disabilities. An estimated 8 million women have a severe form of the disease, which causes many of them to experience spontaneous (without external causes) fractures, generally in the vertebrae of the spine.

Treatment of Osteoporosis

At the end of the twentieth century, the traditional treatment for postmenopausal women with osteoporosis, or those at risk of the disease, was hormone-replacement (estrogen) therapy, often combined with daily doses of calcium. This treatment slows the advance of the disease and helps to prevent fractures and disability. Because of the side effects of estrogen and the fear of increasing the risk of certain types of cancer, however, not all women take the replacement hormone.

In 1995 the FDA approved a new drug, marketed under the name Fosamax, that stops the accelerated breakdown or reabsorption of bone and allows the body's own bone-building mechanism to restore some of the bone mass already lost to the disease. Although the new drug is relatively expensive (about $600 per year), it offers hope for improvement to the victims of this disabling disease.

MULTIPLE SCLEROSIS

Multiple sclerosis (MS) is a chronic, degenerative, and often intermittent disease of the central nervous system. It eventually destroys the myelin protein sheath that surrounds and insulates nerve fibers in the brain and spinal cord. Myelin is a fatty substance that aids the flow of messages from the brain through the spinal cord. These nerve impulses control all conscious and unconscious movements. In MS, the myelin sheath disintegrates and is replaced by hard sclerotic plaques (scar tissue) that distort or prevent the flow of electrical impulses along the nerves to various parts of the body.

Multiple sclerosis usually appears in young adulthood and is common enough to have earned the title "the great crippler of young adults." Many problems and symptoms are associated with the disease, but the major problem is lost mobility. Symptoms can range from mild problems such as numbness and muscle weakness to uncontrollable tremors, slurred speech, loss of bowel and bladder control, memory lapses, and paralysis. Although almost all parts of the nervous system can become involved, the spinal cord is the most vulnerable. Wild mood swings, from euphoria to depression, are another manifestation of the disease. The disease is not fatal in itself, but it weakens its victims and makes them far more susceptible to infection. Life expectancies are six years shorter than normal among MS sufferers.

The disease is called "multiple" because it usually affects numerous parts of the nervous system and is often characterized by relapses followed by periods of partial and sometimes complete recovery. It is, therefore, multiple both in how it affects the body and in how often it strikes.

Prevalence

Multiple sclerosis affects between 250,000 and 300,000 people in the United States. Symptoms appear most often between ages 20 and 35. A possible clue to the cause of MS is that it is most common in cold, damp climates. In Europe it is found most often in the Scandinavian countries, the Baltic region, northern Germany, and Great Britain. It is rare in the Mediterranean countries, China, Japan, and among American Indians. It is also rare among American blacks. White females are affected twice as often as males. In the United States most cases are found in the northern areas, and it is more common in Canada than in the southern United States. The disease cannot be cured, however, by moving to a warmer climate.

Cause of Multiple Sclerosis

The cause of MS currently eludes researchers. Many theories about its cause have been proposed—a congenital or hereditary predisposition, an injury, exposure to heat or cold, vitamin deficiencies, allergies, and even psychological factors—but none have been proved. The most widely accepted theory is that infection by slow-acting viruses may initiate the MS process and trigger relapses. Many of these slow-acting viruses can stay inside the body for years before causing the disease to develop.

Scientists also think an immune reaction may play a role in initiating the onset of MS. The body's defense system can actually backfire and start attacking its own tissues. This is called an autoimmune reaction. MS could involve an autoimmune response in which the body mistakenly starts attacking its own cells. The cause may also be a combination of both a virus and an immune response.

Treatment of Multiple Sclerosis

There is no known specific treatment to stop the disease process. Once nerve fibers have been destroyed, they cannot recover their function. Antibiotics, vitamins, and muscle relaxants have been unsuccessful. Current methods of treatment include powerful immune-suppressant drugs that often leave the patient vulnerable to secondary infections. The best treatment seems to be to build general resistance and avoid fatigue and exposure to extremes in temperature. Physical therapy and psychotherapy are useful in helping patients and their families cope with the limitations caused by MS.

The National Multiple Sclerosis Society recommends that anyone who is diagnosed with the disease should start drug treatment immediately, before symptoms worsen. Although there are three drugs on the market that slow the progression of the disease, fewer than 50,000 of the 300,000 persons affected by the disease take the drugs. This is because many doctors are unfamiliar with the medications since they have been widely available only since 1993. Moreover, the drugs are expensive and may cause some discomfort. The society recommends the medication because it seems that patients who take the drugs will probably suffer fewer disabling symptoms than those who do not. The three multiple sclerosis drugs—Avonex, Betaseron, and Copaxone—work to trick the immune system into stopping or slowing the attack. Each of the medications costs about $1,000 per month and must be injected daily or weekly.

PARKINSON'S DISEASE

Parkinsonism refers not to a particular disease but to a condition marked by a characteristic set of symptoms believed to affect between 1 to 1.5 million people in the United States. The American Parkinson Disease Association estimated that 1 percent of the population over age 50 suffers from some manifestation of this disorder.

Parkinson's disease (PD) is caused by the death of about half a million brain cells small enough to fit on the head of a pin. These cells, in the basal ganglia of the brain, secrete dopamine, a neurotransmitter (chemical messenger). Dopamine's function is to allow nerve impulses to move smoothly from one nerve cell to another. These nerve cells, in turn, transmit messages to the muscles of the body to begin movement. When the normal supply of dopamine is reduced, the messages are not correctly sent, and the symptoms of PD appear.

The four early warning signs of Parkinson's disease are abnormal shaking, muscle stiffness, unusual slowness, and a stooped posture. Medications can control initial symptoms, but as time goes on, they become less effective. As the disease worsens, patients develop tremors, causing them to fall or jerk uncontrollably. At other times, rigidity sets in as hard as stone, rendering them unable to move. About one-third of patients also develop dementia, an impairment of thought processes.

Treatment of Parkinson's Disease

Management of PD is individualized and includes not only drug therapy but also a program that stresses daily exercise. Exercise can often lessen the rigidity of muscles, prevent weakness, and improve the ability to walk.

The main goal of drug treatment is to restore the chemical balance between dopamine and another neurotransmitter, acetylcholine. Most patients are given L-dopa, a compound that the body converts into dopamine. A number of drugs were approved in recent years to improve the efficacy of L-dopa or slow the destruction of dopamine in the nerve cells, including anticholinergics, COMT inhibitors, and Deprenyl.

In 1996 a study using rhesus monkeys reported that injections of a substance called glial-cell-line-derived neurotrophic factor (GDNF) into the brain relieved Parkinson-like symptoms. GDNF is found naturally in the brain; it makes brain cells produce more dopamine and, possibly, helps them regulate their release and retrieval of dopamine. While much more study of GDNF remains to be done, the first human tests were starting. Strangely enough, the injections did not increase the amount of dopamine in the parts of the brain that control movement. While GDNF reduced the problems of rigidity, slow movement, and poor balance by 25 percent, it had no significant effect on tremors. Researchers theorized that the tremors are produced by different brain circuits than the other symptoms.

In 1998 Dr. Jay S. Schneider and colleagues at the Jefferson Medical College of Thomas Jefferson University in Philadelphia, Pennsylvania, tested GM1 ganglioside, an experimental drug, in 45 patients. GM1, a naturally occurring substance, is a normal part of the cell membrane that plays an important role in cell growth, development, and repair. After 16 weeks, patients taking GM1 scored better on tests that measured stiffness and other physical variables than those who received a placebo. The patients also reported increased ability in performing basic daily tasks, such as getting dressed and using different utensils.

BAN ON HUMAN FETAL CELL IMPLANTS LIFTED. In 1993 President Bill Clinton lifted a 10-year federal ban on the use of federal funds to transplant tissue from aborted fetuses to the brains of Parkinson patients to try to correct the neurological damage. The Reagan administration had issued the ban for fear that this use of fetal tissue would encourage abortions, which the administration opposed. Prior to 1993, however, some researchers, adamant about the possibilities of the surgery, had proceeded without federal funds. Some patients, eagerly hoping for some relief, sought unproved therapies, traveling as far as Cuba and China for the surgery.

Dr. Curt Freed, a neurobiologist at the University of Colorado Health Sciences Center in Denver, conducted the first federal study on the effectiveness of fetal cell implants after the ban was lifted. Of the 40 Parkinson's patients in the five-year, $5.7 million trial, half of them received fetal tissues implants; the others received "placebo" operations, in which no fetal cells were implanted, as a control to determine the effectiveness of the real operation.

The placebo surgery, like the authentic surgery, involved cutting two oval holes in the skull and then closing the incision. During the surgery, which lasted about four hours, patients were awake; they were required to stay in the hospital for several days following the procedure. Those who had the placebo operation were given an opportunity for the real surgery the following year.

The concept of placebo surgeries caused some controversy. Parkinson Institute spokespeople defended the need

for the control group, and Dr. Freed claimed the procedure involved minimal risk. Still, some physicians wondered if even highly educated and informed patients could fully understand and appreciate the risks associated with any surgery and especially those involved in brain surgery.

In 1999 the Freed group released preliminary results from the study. One year after the surgeries, patients under 60 who received the fetal implants showed significant improvement in their symptoms, while those over 60 and those given the placebo surgery showed no improvement. None of the patients, however, perceived a benefit in terms of their everyday activities. The study will continue to follow the progress of all patients over five years.

The election of President George W. Bush in 2000 prompted great worry among fetal tissue researchers. President Bush had expressed his opposition to research on aborted fetuses throughout his campaign and through the early days of his presidency, and researchers expected him to reinstate the ban during his presidency.

FETAL PIG BRAIN IMPLANTS. In late 1995 a team from the Harvard Medical School reported that transplants of fetal pig brain cells into the brains of rats relieved Parkinson-like symptoms. Limited trials on human beings have also been successful. If future planned human trials are equally successful, the procedure could revolutionize the treatment of PD without raising the ethical and moral issues involved in human fetal tissue transplants.

ELECTRODE IMPLANTS. Another new procedure being tested is the use of electrical implants. Electrodes are surgically implanted in the brain and connected to a battery-operated device, also implanted in the body. The device allows patients to "turn off" the tremors that prevent such normal everyday activities as pouring a glass of milk and feeding themselves. One drawback is that the device's batteries must be surgically replaced every three to five years.

Researchers also plan to try this procedure on Huntington's disease victims. (See Chapter 9 for more about Huntington's disease.)

ALZHEIMER'S DISEASE

Alzheimer's disease (pronounced alz-hi-merz) is a progressive, degenerative disease that attacks the brain and results in severely impaired memory, thinking, and behavior. It affects an estimated 4 million American adults and is the most common form of dementia, or loss of intellectual function. The Centers for Disease Control and Prevention (CDC) reported that 22,638 persons died from Alzheimer's disease (AD) between July 1996 and June 1997. AD was the eleventh-leading cause of death in the United States. AD, however, contributes to many more deaths that are attributed to other causes, such as heart and respiratory failure.

TABLE 8.1

Projected estimates of any AD and moderate or severe AD for Americans 65 years of age or older: 1995–2015

Year	Any AD		Moderate or severe AD	
	Number	% change[a]	Number	% change[a]
1995	1,906,822	[b]	1,099,069	[b]
2000	2,141,772	+12	1,233,932	+12
2005	2,370,615	+24	1,365,085	+24
2010	2,605,231	+37	1,500,727	+37
2015	2,872,420	+51	1,656,046	+51

[a] All percentage changes are relative to the baseline number for 1995.
[b] Zero by definition,

SOURCE: *Alzheimer's Disease: Estimates of Prevalence in the United States,* U.S. General Accounting Office, Washington D.C., 1998

The disease, first described by the German physician Alois Alzheimer in 1907, knows no social or economic boundaries and affects men and women almost equally. While 90 percent of AD victims are over age 65, Alzheimer's can strike as early as the thirties, forties, and fifties. Most patients are cared for at home as long as possible, a situation that can be emotionally and physically devastating for the victims and their families.

The financial consequences of caring for Alzheimer's patients are also devastating. The costs of diagnosis, treatment, nursing home care, informal care, and lost wages is estimated at $90 billion each year. The federal government covers $4.4 billion and the states another $4.1 billion. The patients and their families pay most of the remaining costs. About 70 percent of the total care for AD victims is provided by their families at home. The cost to a family caring for an Alzheimer's patient at home averages approximately $20,000 each year. Eventually, 75 percent of AD victims become nursing home patients, spending about three years there. In the late 1990s, one year's stay in a nursing home averaged $40,000.

Tax relief is now available for families caring for AD patients. The Health Insurance Portability and Accountability Act of 1996 (PL 104-191) stipulated that out-of-pocket expenses for long-term care, including personal care, were deductible as medical expenses. The Alzheimer's Association offered the example of an AD patient who was still being cared for in the home by his wife, the primary caregiver. Their 1997 expenses for his care were about $15,200:

- $6,000 for adult day care.

- $2,500 for in-home care assistance.

- $5,000 for out-of-pocket health expenses, including Medicare copayments, deductibles, and prescription drugs.

- $1,200 for premiums for long-term care insurance.

The Alzheimer's Association estimated that, at an annual income of $42,000, approximately $12,000 of these expenses could be deducted under the new law's tax provisions. Previously, medical expenses were deductible only for medical services provided in skilled nursing facilities.

Alzheimer's disease has become a disease of particular concern because the nation's elderly population is growing rapidly. Approximately 10 percent of the population over age 65 is afflicted with AD. This percentage rises to more than 47 percent in those over age 85, the fastest-growing segment of our society. By 2050 the United States will have an estimated 78.9 million people over age 65. (See Figure 8.1.)

According to the U.S. Bureau of the Census, the numbers of cases of AD were expected to increase by more than 12 percent every five years through 2015. (See Table 8.1.) Prevalence (how many people have a disease at a given time) is partially determined by the length of time people with AD survive. Therefore, improvements in AD care, as well as increased length of life of the elderly population in general, will increase the numbers of AD patients.

In November 1994 former President Ronald Reagan, age 83, announced that he had developed Alzheimer's disease and wanted to make Americans more aware of the disease. Some experts believe that it is theoretically possible that AD had affected Reagan before he left the White House in January 1989.

Possible Causes of Alzheimer's Disease

Scientists are still looking for the cause of AD. While 90 percent of cases appear to have no genetic link, researchers have found some promising genetic clues to the disease. The first breakthrough was reported in the February 1991 issue of the British journal, *Nature.* Researchers reported that they had discovered that a mutation in a single gene could cause this progressive neurological illness.

Scientists found the defect (mutation) in the gene that directs cells to produce a substance called amyloid protein. Researchers at the Massachusetts Institute of Technology have found that low levels of the brain chemical acetylcholine contribute to the formation of hard deposits of amyloid protein that clog the brain tissue of Alzheimer patients. In normal people, the protein fragments are broken down and excreted by the body. Amyloid protein is found in cells throughout the body, and researchers do not know how it becomes a deadly substance in the brain cells of some people and not others.

In 1995 three more genes linked to AD were identified. One gene appears to be related to the most devastating form of AD, which can strike people in their thirties. When defective, the gene may prevent brain cells from correctly processing a substance called beta amyloid precursor protein. The second gene is linked to an early-onset form of Alzheimer's disease that strikes before age 65. This gene also appears to be involved in producing beta amyloid. Researchers believe that the discovery of these two genes will allow them to narrow their search for the proteins responsible for early-onset AD and give them clues to the causes of AD in older people.

The third gene, known as apolipoprotein E (apoE), was actually reported as associated with AD in 1993, but its role in the body was not known at that time. Researchers have since found that the gene plays several roles. Within the body, it regulates lipid metabolism within the organs and helps to redistribute cholesterol. In the brain, apoE participates in repairing nerve tissue that has been injured. There are three forms (alleles) of the gene: apoE-2, apoE-3, and apoE-4. Until recently, people with two copies of apoE-4, one from each parent, were thought to have a greatly increased risk of developing AD before age 70. From one-half to one-third of all Alzheimer's patients have at least one apoE-4 gene, while only 15 percent of the general population have an apoE-4 gene. In 1998, however, researchers discovered that the apoE-4 gene seems to affect *when* a person may get Alzheimer's, not *whether* the person will develop the disease.

Another newly discovered gene, A2M-2, seems to affect *whether* a person will develop Alzheimer's. Thirty percent of Americans may carry A2M-2, a genetic variant that more than triples a person's risk of developing late-onset Alzheimer's compared to siblings with the normal version of the A2M gene. The discovery of A2M-2 opens up the possibility of developing a drug that mimics the A2M gene's normal function. This has the potential to protect susceptible persons against brain damage or perhaps even reverse it.

Symptoms of Alzheimer's Disease

Alzheimer's begins slowly. The symptoms include difficulty with memory and a loss of intellectual abilities. The AD patient may also experience confusion; language problems, such as trouble finding words; impaired judgment; disorientation in place and time; and changes in mood, behavior, and personality. How fast these changes occur varies from person to person, but eventually, the disease leaves its victims unable to care for themselves. In their terminal stages, AD victims require care 24 hours a day. They no longer recognize family members or themselves, and they need help with such daily activities as eating, dressing, bathing, and using the toilet. Eventually, they may become incontinent, blind, and unable to communicate. Finally, their bodies may "forget" how to breathe or make the heart beat. The disease may kill its victims in only a few years, but patients have also been known to live with AD as long as 25 years. The average duration for the disease is eight years.

Testing for Alzheimer's Disease

A complete physical, psychiatric, and neurological evaluation can usually produce a diagnosis of AD that is about 90 percent accurate. For many years, the only sure way to diagnose the disease was to examine brain tissue under a microscope, which was not possible while the AD victim was still alive. An autopsy of someone who has died of AD shows the presence of tangles of fibers (neurofibrillary tangles) and clusters of degenerated nerve endings (neuritic plaques) in areas of the brain that are crucial for memory and intellect. Also, the cortex (thinking center) of the brain is shrunken.

In 1994 a Harvard Medical School group announced that they had possibly stumbled across a simple test for AD. The researchers found that the pupils of persons with AD dilated in response to an atropine solution (similar to the drops doctors use for eye examinations) that was one one-hundredth the strength needed for normal dilation, while people with other brain diseases responded normally. The scientists also reported that preliminary evidence suggested that future Alzheimer's patients would test positive several months before their symptoms became obvious. Several follow-up studies, however, were unable to repeat the findings of the 1994 test, and in 1997 the Mayo Clinic determined that the atropine test had no value.

In 1996 a San Francisco biotechnology firm also developed a new test for AD. The test, which involves analysis of blood and spinal fluid, gave conclusive results in 60 percent of older patients with dementia.

Experts have long been eager for a simple and accurate test. An accurate test would allow the detection of AD early enough for the use of experimental medications to slow the progression of the disease, as well as identifying persons at risk of developing AD. But the availability of tests raises other questions: Do patients really want to know their risks of developing AD? Will health insurers use test results to deny coverage?

Treatments for Alzheimer's Disease

There is no cure, treatment, or prevention for AD. Medication can lessen some of the symptoms, such as agitation, anxiety, unpredictable behavior, and depression. Physical exercise and good nutrition are important, as is a calm and highly structured environment. The object is to help the AD patient maintain as much comfort, normalcy, and dignity as possible.

Until 1997 tacrine (marketed as Cognex) was the nation's only Alzheimer's medication. But in early 1997, the FDA approved a new drug, donepezil, to be marketed under the trade name Aricept. Both drugs are cholinesterase inhibitors, which produce some improvement in memory and other cognitive skills. Both drugs offer only mild improvements at best, but at the moment, they are the only alternatives available to Alzheimer's patients.

In 1996 clinical (human testing) trials were underway on several other drugs. The drugs being tested included acetyl-L-carnitine, metrifonate, estrogen, nimodipine, and propentofylline. All of the drugs being tested are intended to improve the symptoms of AD and slow its progression, but none is expected to "cure" AD.

Second Victims

Unfortunately, the AD victim's suffering is only part of the devastating emotional, physical, and financial trauma of AD. People who care for loved ones with Alzheimer's are considered "second victims" of the disease. Caregivers often neglect their own needs, including their health and social lives, and the needs of other family members. As a result, they may develop more stress-related illnesses, such as heart attacks and strokes.

Many professionals recommend support groups for caregivers of AD patients, made up of family members, friends, and health care professionals. These groups encourage members to share information and ideas, give and receive mutual support, and exchange coping skills with each other. A study of 206 spouses of AD patients found that caregivers benefited greatly from support groups and counseling. Those who received this kind of support were able to care for the patients at home for almost one year longer than caregivers who lacked support.

CHAPTER 9
GENETIC DISEASES

Genetics, the study of biological inheritance, explains how and why certain traits such as hair color and blood types run in families. Each individual develops from a single fertilized egg, which contains all the information necessary for the development of innate mental and physical characteristics. This information is carried in 23 pairs of rod-shaped chromosomes (containing thousands of genes) that are responsible for determining and transmitting hereditary characteristics. Each pair of chromosomes includes one inherited from the mother and one from the father.

Genes determine specific physical features of a person, such as height and eye color. Genes also direct the production of cell proteins needed for health and development. There are two types of genes—dominant and recessive. When a dominant gene is passed on to offspring, the feature it determines will appear regardless of the characteristics of the corresponding gene on the chromosome inherited from the other parent. If the gene is recessive, the feature it determines will not show up in a child unless both the mother's and the father's chromosomes contain a recessive gene for that characteristic.

GENETIC TESTING

As scientists learn more about the genes responsible for a variety of illnesses, including Alzheimer's, mental health diseases, cancer, and heart disease, they can design tests to predict whether a person is at risk of developing the disease. In some cases, it is even possible to make a diagnosis on an unborn child. The issue of genetic testing, however, has turned out to be far more ethically complicated than scientists originally anticipated.

Initially, physicians believed that a test to determine in advance who would develop or escape a disease would be welcomed by at-risk families. They would be able to plan more realistically about having children, choosing jobs, getting insurance, and living their lives. Neverthe-

less, many people with family histories of a genetic disease—for example, Huntington's disease (see below)—have decided that not knowing is better than anticipating a grim future and an agonizing, slow death. Many prefer to live with the hope that they won't get the disease than with the certainty that they will.

People are also reluctant to be tested because they fear they will lose their health, life, and disability insurance. The tests are sometimes costly, and some insurers agree to reimburse the expenses only if they are informed of the results. The insurance companies feel they cannot risk selling policies to a person they know will become disabled or die prematurely.

The discovery of genetic links and the development of tests designed to predict the likelihood or certainty of developing a disease raise ethical questions for persons who carry a defective gene. Should women who are carriers of Huntington's disease or cystic fibrosis (see below) have children? Should a fetus with the defective gene be carried to term or aborted? One insurance company agreed to pay for prenatal cystic fibrosis testing for a mother who already had one affected child. But, the company insisted, if the baby was affected, the mother would have to terminate the pregnancy, or the insurance would not cover the child's future medical bills.

MUSCULAR DYSTROPHY

Muscular dystrophy is a term that applies to a group of hereditary muscle-destroying disorders. Some type of muscular dystrophy (MD) affects approximately 1 million Americans. Each variant of the disease is caused by defects in the genes that play important roles in the growth and development of muscles. In MD, the proteins produced by the defective genes are abnormal, causing the muscles to waste away. Unable to function properly, the muscle cells die and are replaced by fat and connective tissue. The symptoms of MD may not be noticed until as much as 50 percent of the muscle tissue has been affected.

All of the various disorders labeled muscular dystrophy cause progressive weakening and wasting of muscle tissues. They vary, however, as to the usual age at the onset of symptoms, rate of progression, and the initial group of muscles affected. The most common type, Duchenne MD, affects young boys, who show symptoms in early childhood and usually die from respiratory weakness or damage to the heart before adulthood. The gene is passed from the mother to her children. Females who inherit the defective gene generally do not manifest symptoms—they become carriers of the defective genes, and their children have a 50 percent chance of inheriting the disease. Other forms of muscular dystrophy manifest later in life and are usually not fatal.

In 1992 scientists discovered the defect in the gene that causes myotonic dystrophy. In persons with this disorder, a segment of the gene is enlarged and unstable. This finding helps doctors more accurately diagnose myotonic dystrophy, which affects at least 1 in 8,000 people. Researchers have since identified genes linked to other types of MD, including Duchenne MD, Becker MD, limb-girdle MD, and Emery-Dreifuss MD.

In addition to its commitment to MD research, the Muscular Dystrophy Association supports research into the causes and treatments of other groups of related neuromuscular illnesses, such as amyotrophic lateral sclerosis (also known as Lou Gehrig's disease), Charcot-Marie-Tooth disease, and myasthenia gravis. All of these are progressive, wasting, and weakening conditions that rob individuals of their ability to live, work, and function normally. Genes linked to these and other diseases were also identified in the 1990s.

Treatment—and Hope

There is no cure for muscular dystrophy, but patients can be made more comfortable and functional by a combination of physical therapy, exercise programs, and orthopedic devices (special shoes, braces, or powered wheelchairs) that help maintain mobility and independence as long as possible.

Genetic research gives hope of finding effective treatments, and even cures, for these diseases. Gene therapy experiments specifically aimed toward a cure or a treatment for one or more of these types of MD are currently underway. Research teams have identified the crucial proteins produced by these genes, such as dystrophin, beta sarcoglyan, gamma sarcoglyan, and adhalin.

When defective or absent, these proteins cause MD. Researchers hope that experimental treatments to inject normal muscle cells into wasting muscles will replace the diseased cells. Muscle cells, unlike other cells in the body,

fuse together to become giant cells. Scientists hope that if cells with healthy genes can be introduced into the muscles and accepted by the body's immune system, the muscle cells will then begin to make the missing proteins.

New delivery methods are also being tested, such as implanting a healthy gene into a virus that has been stripped of all of its harmful properties, and then injecting the modified virus into a patient. Researchers hope this will reduce the amount of rejection by the patient's immune system, allowing the healthy gene to do its work.

HUNTINGTON'S DISEASE

Huntington's disease (HD), or Huntington's chorea, is an inherited, progressive brain disorder. It causes the degeneration of cells in the basal ganglia, a pair of nerve clusters deep in the brain that affect both the body and the mind. HD is caused by a single dominant gene that affects both men and women of all races and ethnic groups. It does not usually strike until mid-adulthood, although there is a juvenile form that can affect children and adolescents. Early symptoms, such as forgetfulness, a lack of muscle coordination, or a loss of balance, are often ignored. The disease gradually takes its toll over a 10- to 25-year period.

Within a few years, characteristic involuntary jerking (chorea) of the body, limbs, and facial muscles appears. As HD progresses, speech becomes slurred and swallowing becomes difficult. The victim's thinking abilities decline, and there are distinct personality changes—depression and withdrawal, sometimes countered with euphoria. Eventually, nearly all patients must be institutionalized, and they usually die of choking or infections.

Prevalence of HD

HD, once considered rare, is now recognized as one of the more common hereditary diseases. HD is known to affect about 30,000 Americans; another 150,000 are at a 50 percent risk of inheriting it from an affected parent. Estimates of its prevalence are about 1 in every 10,000 persons.

Prediction Test

In 1983 researchers identified a DNA "marker" that made it possible to offer a test to determine, before symptoms appear, whether someone has inherited the HD gene. In some cases, it is even possible to make a prenatal diagnosis on the child. Many people, however, prefer not to know whether or not they carry the defective gene.

For those who have gone through with the testing, a positive result rarely brings shock and denial, according to those who conduct pre- and post-test counseling. Most people who learn that they will eventually get the disease are upset, but there is an acceptance of their fate. Among those whose tests come back negative, there is often a newfound freedom. They are more willing to set goals and enjoy life.

A testing center at Johns Hopkins Hospital reported that a high proportion of the people who come in for testing find out that they are not carrying the gene. Of the people who do not choose to be tested, the center's doctors think that many may already have very mild symptoms and suspect that they have the disease.

Gene behind Huntington's Disease Found

In 1993 an international team of scientists from the United States, England, and Wales announced that after 10 years of research, it had discovered the gene behind Huntington's disease. In the HD gene, the mutation involves a triplet of genetic subunits, or bases, known by the chemical initials CAG. In non-Huntington persons, the gene has 30 or fewer of these triplets, but HD patients have 40 or more. These increased multiples either destroy the gene's ability to make the necessary protein or cause it to produce a misshapen and malfunctioning protein. Either way, the defect results in the death of brain cells.

The researchers, who examined 75 families with a history of HD, found the abnormal expansion in each case of an afflicted patient. Currently, they are trying to determine if the exact number of excess triplets bears any indication of when in life a person will be affected by the disease. Some scientists fear that the ability to tell people that they are going to get an incurable disease and when they will get it will make genetic testing (see above), already a difficult decision, even more complicated.

CYSTIC FIBROSIS

Cystic fibrosis (CF) is the most common inherited fatal disease of children and young adults in the United States. It occurs in about 1 of every 2,000 births, and there are approximately 30,000 young people who currently have the disease; their median (half above and half below) life span is 30 years. An estimated 12 million Americans (1 in 20) are symptomless carriers of the CF gene. In order to inherit this disease, a child must receive the CF gene from both parents. Cystic fibrosis almost exclusively strikes whites.

At first, a child with CF does not appear to be suffering from a serious illness, but the diagnosis is usually made by the age of three. Often, the only signs are a persistent cough, a large appetite but poor weight gain, an extremely salty taste to the skin, and large, foul-smelling bowel movements. A simple "sweat test" is currently the standard diagnostic test for CF. The test measures the amount of salt in the sweat; abnormally high levels indicate cystic fibrosis.

Children with CF have great difficulty breathing. The CF gene causes the body to produce a thick, sticky mucus in the lungs and pancreas, causing difficulty in breathing and interference with digestion. This thick drainage must constantly be removed.

Cystic Fibrosis Gene-Screening Falters ←

In August 1989 researchers isolated the specific gene that causes CF. The mutation of this gene accounts for about 70 percent of the cases of the disease. In 1990 scientists managed to successfully correct the biochemical defect by inserting a healthy gene into diseased cells grown in the laboratory, a major step toward developing new therapies for the disease. In 1992 they injected healthy genes into laboratory rats by using a deactivated common cold virus as the delivery agent. The rats began to manufacture the missing protein, which regulates the chloride and sodium in the tissues, preventing the deadly buildup of mucus. Scientists were hopeful that within only a few years CF would be eliminated as a fatal disease, giving many children the chance for healthy, normal lives.

In 1993, however, optimism faded when the medical community discovered that the CF gene was more complicated than expected four years earlier. Biologists found that the gene can be mutated at more than 350 points, and more points are appearing at an alarming rate. At the same time, they discovered that many people who have inherited mutated genes from both parents do not have cystic fibrosis. With so many possible mutations, the potential combinations in a person who inherits one gene from each parent are immeasurable.

The combinations of different mutations create different effects. Some may result in crippling and fatal cystic fibrosis, while others may cause less serious disorders, such as infertility, asthma, or chronic bronchitis. To further complicate the picture, other genes can alter the way different mutations of the CF gene affect the body.

The Cystic Fibrosis Foundation is currently supporting nine research studies in human gene therapy. Several studies are using the adenovirus rather than the common cold virus as the vehicle for delivering healthy genes to lung or nasal tissue. Another study is using liposomes (fat cells) as a delivery vehicle.

Researchers are also finding that CF mutations may be much more common than previously thought. Five thousand healthy women receiving prenatal care at Kaiser Permanente in northern California were tested for the CF gene, thought to be present in less than 1 percent of the population. Of those screened, 11 percent had the mutation. This may show that many more common diseases, such as asthma, may be caused by mutations of the CF gene.

SICKLE-CELL DISEASE

Sickle-cell disease (SCD) is a group of hereditary diseases, including sickle-cell anemia and sickle B-thalassemia, in which the red blood cells contain an abnormal hemoglobin, termed hemoglobin S. Hemoglobin S is responsible for the premature destruction of red blood cells, or hemolysis. In addition, it causes the red cells to become deformed, actually taking on a sickle shape, particularly in parts of the body where the amount of oxygen is relatively low. These abnormally shaped cells cannot travel smoothly through the smaller blood vessels and capillaries. They tend to clog the vessels and prevent blood from reaching vital tissues. This blockage is called anoxia (lack of oxygen), and this blockage in turn causes more sickling and more damage.

Symptoms of Sickle-Cell Anemia

Persons with sickle-cell anemia have the symptoms of anemia, including fatigue, weakness, fainting, and palpitations or an increased awareness of their heartbeat. These palpitations result from the heart's trying to compensate for the anemia by pumping blood faster than normal.

In addition, they experience occasional sickle-cell crises—attacks of pain in the bones and stomach. Blood clots may also develop in the lungs, kidneys, brain, and other organs. A severe crisis or several acute crises can damage the organs of the body by impeding the flow of blood. This damage can lead to death from heart failure, kidney failure, or stroke. The frequency of these crises varies from patient to patient. A sickle-cell crisis, however, occurs more often during infections and after an accident or an injury.

Who Contracts Sickle-Cell Disease?

Both the sickle-cell trait and the disease exist almost exclusively in people of African, American Indian, and Hispanic descent and in persons from parts of Italy, Greece, Middle Eastern countries, and India. A sickle-cell trait, different from the actual disease, is inherited from one parent. Only if both the mother and the father have the trait can they produce a child with sickle-cell anemia. This trait is relatively common among blacks, and about 6 of every 1,000 black couples carry the risk of having a child with the disease. Persons of African descent are advised to seek genetic counseling and to be tested for the trait before marrying and starting a family. The sickle-cell trait is present in 8 percent of African Americans, about 2.54 million people. More than 50,000 Americans have sickle-cell anemia—one in every 375. One in every 3,000 American Indians and one in every 20,000 Hispanics has the disease. Numbers are much lower for other groups.

A CALL FOR UNIVERSAL SCREENING. In 1993 a federal panel of experts called for sickle-cell screening of all newborns. Because of intermarriage, it is becoming more difficult to be certain of a person's racial or ethnic background based on physical appearance, surname, or self-reporting. Many sickle-cell sufferers could possibly be missed by screening only a target population such as blacks.

By 1993, 34 states and jurisdictions had already instituted the universal screening of infants recommended by an earlier study group of the National Institutes of Health in 1988. Another 10 states had targeted screening aimed at groups traditionally considered at higher risk, and 8 states and jurisdictions had no sickle-cell screening program. The cost of universal screening has not been studied, but many experts feel that the investment would pay great dividends. A machine to run sickle-cell tests could cost between $5,000 and $30,000; material to conduct a single test costs $1 to $3. The American Academy of Pediatrics, the American Nurses Association, the National Medical Association (an organization of black physicians), and the Sickle Cell Disease Association of America endorsed the new guidelines for universal screening.

Early diagnosis (soon after birth) could save the lives of children born with SCD. Studies have found wide differences in the mortality rates of children with SCD. To improve survival rates for children with SCD living in high mortality areas, public health advocates recommend further study of the accessibility and quality of available screening and medical care, and the duplication of successful treatment programs. In addition, they emphasize the importance of educating parents about the disease and its treatments ("Mortality among Children with Sickle Cell Disease Identified by Newborn Screening during 1990–1994—California, Illinois, and New York," *Mortality and Morbidity Weekly Report,* vol. 46, no. 9, March 13, 1998; "Geographic Differences in Mortality of Young Children with Sickle Cell Disease in the United States," *Public Health Reports,* vol. 112, no. 1, January/February 1997).

Treatment of Sickle-Cell Disease

There is no universal cure for SCD, but the symptoms can be treated. Crises accompanied by extreme pain are the most common problems and can usually be treated with painkillers. Maintaining healthy eating and behavior habits and getting prompt treatment for any type of infection or injury is important. Special precautions are often necessary before any type of surgery. In early 1995 a medication that prevented the cells from clogging vessels and cutting off oxygen was approved.

The 1993 federal panel of experts on SCD (see above) recommended that all infants diagnosed with the disease receive daily doses of penicillin to prevent infections. The cost of preventive penicillin now being administered is estimated to be about $12 monthly for the liquid form and $10 for tablets. Parents are urged to make sure that these children receive the scheduled childhood immunizations and are vaccinated against influenza, pneumonia, and hepatitis B by age two. In the mid-1980s, 20 percent of children with SCD died before their first birthday; by 1993, primarily because of preventive antibiotics, that proportion had dropped to less than 3 percent.

BIOMEDICAL ADVANCES. Many adults with SCD now take hydroxyurea, a cancer drug that causes the body to produce red blood cells that resist sickling. In 1995 a multicenter study showed that among adults with three or more painful crises per year, hydroxyurea lowered the median number of crises requiring hospitalization by 58 percent. In 1996 an international study found that bone marrow transplants were successful in curing SCD in 16 of 22 patients—72.7 percent of the patients in the five-year study. All of the participants in the study were under age 14, had advanced symptoms, and had siblings who were compatible bone marrow donors. Four of the patients (18 percent) rejected the donor marrow, and their sickle-cell symptoms returned. Two of the patients (9 percent) died.

Because of the high risks of bone marrow transplants and the difficulties of matching donors, transplants are not appropriate for every patient. Further studies are needed to test the procedure with older patients and to reduce the proportion of tissue rejects. Blood harvested from umbilical cords and placentas has been found to be less likely to trigger rejection or graft-versus-host disease, in which the transplanted cells attack the cells of the bone marrow recipient, causing organ damage.

TAY-SACHS DISEASE

Tay-Sachs disease (TSD) is a fatal genetic disorder in children that causes the progressive destruction of the central nervous system. It is caused by the absence of an important enzyme called hexosaminidase A (hex-A). Without hex-A, a fatty substance builds up abnormally in the cells, particularly the brain's nerve cells. Eventually, these cells degenerate and die. This destructive process begins early in the development of a fetus, but the disease is not usually diagnosed until the baby is several months old. By the time a child with TSD is four or five years old, the nervous system is so badly damaged that the child dies.

Symptoms of Tay-Sachs

A baby with TSD seems normal at birth and tends to develop normally for about the first six months of life. But then development slows down. The child begins to regress and loses skills one by one—the ability to crawl, to sit, to reach out, and to turn over. The victim gradually becomes blind, deaf, and unable to swallow. The muscles begin to atrophy and paralysis sets in. Mental retardation occurs, and the child is unable to relate to the outside world. Death usually occurs between ages three and five. There is no cure or treatment for this disease.

How Is Tay-Sachs Inherited?

Tay-Sachs is transmitted from parent to child the same way eye or hair color is inherited. Both the mother and the father must be carriers of the TSD gene in order to give birth to a child with the disease.

Being a carrier does not affect the parents in any way. When both parents carry the recessive TSD gene, they have a one in four chance in every pregnancy of having a child with the disease. They also have a 50 percent chance of bearing a child who is also a carrier. If only one parent is a carrier, however, the couple will not have a child with TSD. Prenatal diagnosis early in pregnancy can predict if the unborn child has TSD. If the fetus has the disease, the couple may choose to terminate the pregnancy.

Who Is at Risk?

Some genetic diseases, such as Tay-Sachs, occur most frequently in a specific population. Individuals of Eastern European (Ashkenazi) Jewish descent have the highest risk of being carriers of TSD. According to the National Tay-Sachs and Allied Diseases Association, approximately 1 in every 27 Jews in the United States is a carrier of the TSD gene, and 85 percent of the children who are victims of this disease are Jewish. Italians also have a higher than average risk of being carriers. In the general population, the carrier rate is 1 in 250.

CHAPTER 10
INFECTIOUS DISEASES

Infectious (contagious) diseases are those caused by viruses or bacteria transmitted from one person to another through casual contact, such as influenza, or through bodily fluids, such as AIDS. Infectious diseases are the leading cause of death in the world. Not long ago, the federal government and medical experts believed that—due to the development of vaccines, antibiotics, and public health measures—infectious diseases were no longer a major public health problem. All over the world, however, new and rare diseases are emerging, and old diseases are making a comeback. Some of these infections reflect changes associated with increasing population, growing poverty, urban migration, drug-resistant germs, and expanding international travel.

The mistaken belief that infectious diseases were a thing of the past led many governments, including that of the United States, to neglect public health programs aimed at treating and preventing infectious disease. By 1994, however, enough troubling new diseases had arisen and old ones reoccurred that a federal commission recommended that the United States spend $125 million to implement a plan to respond to and contain infections.

As part of the U.S. Public Health Service (PHS), the U.S. Centers for Disease Control and Prevention (CDC) tracks certain infectious diseases ("notifiable diseases"). Physicians, clinics, and hospitals must report any occurrences of these diseases to the CDC each week. Table 10.1 shows the 52 infections tracked in 1998.

TABLE 10.1

The 52 infectious diseases designated as notifiable at the national level during 1998

Acquired immunodeficiency syndrome (AIDS)	Haemophilus influenzae (Invasive Disease)	Rabies, animal
Anthrax	Hansen disease (leprosy)	Rabies, human
Botulism	Hantavirus pulmonary syndrome	Rocky Mountain spotted fever
Brucellosis	Hemolytic uremic syndrome, post-diarrheal	Rubella
Chancroid	Hepatitis A	Salmonellosis
Chlamydia trachomatis, genital infection	Hepatitis B	Shigellosis
Cholera	Hepatitis, C/non-A, non-B	Streptococcal disease, invasive, group A
Coccidioidomycosis*	HIV infection, pediatric	Streptococcus pneumoniae, drug-resistant*
Congenital rubella syndrome	Legionellosis	Streptococcal toxic-shock syndrome
Cryptosporidiosis	Lyme disease	Syphilis
Diphtheria	Malaria	Syphilis, congenital
Encephalitis, California	Measles (Rubeola)	Tetanus
Encephalitis, eastern equine	Meningococcal disease	Toxic-shock syndrome
Encephalitis, St. Louis	Mumps	Trichinosis
Encephalitis, western equine	Pertussis	Tuberculosis
Escherichia coli O157:H7	Plague	Typhoid fever
Gonorrhea	Poliomyelitis, paralytic	Yellow fever
	Psittacosis	

Note: Although varicella is not a nationally notifiable disease, the Council of State and Territorial Epidemiologists recommends reporting of cases of this disease to CDC.
* Not published in the *MMWR* weekly tables as of 1998.

SOURCE: "Summary of Notifiable Diseases, United States, 1998," *Morbidity and Mortality Weekly Report*, vol. 47, no. 53, December 31, 1999

TABLE 10.2

Notifiable diseases--Summary of reported cases, by month, 1997

NAME	Total	Jan.	Feb.	Mar.	Apr.	May	June	July	Aug.	Sept.	Oct.	Nov.	Dec.	Unk.
AIDS*	58,492	4,682	5,066	5,364	4,586	5,072	5,234	4,281	4,803	4,964	4,636	4,016	5,788	–
Botulism, total	132	9	5	8	2	14	9	19	16	8	8	20	14	–
Brucellosis	98	20	1	6	4	7	6	10	13	8	3	9	11	–
Chancroid†	243		·····65·····			·····80·····			·····58·····			·····40·····		–
Chlamydia‡§	526,671		·····119,217·····			·····130,697·····			·····135,403·····			·····141,354·····		–
Cholera	6	–	–	–	–	–	1	–	2	–	2	–	–	–
Cryptosporidiosis	2,566	146	94	154	121	152	117	211	358	311	293	310	299	–
Diphtheria	4	–	–	2	1	–	1	–	–	–	–	–	–	–
Escherichia coli O157:H7	2,555	82	73	107	71	173	190	400	432	335	281	196	215	–
Gonorrhea†	324,907		·····74,417·····			·····76,126·····			·····87,378·····			·····86,986·····		–
Haemophilus influenzae, invasive	1,162	71	86	123	98	116	103	69	82	76	58	103	177	–
Hansen disease (leprosy)	122	6	4	12	11	12	5	4	7	11	2	19	29	–
Hepatitis A	30,021	1,716	2,184	2,885	2,033	3,124	2,163	2,091	2,628	2,517	2,526	2,524	3,630	–
Hepatitis B	10,416	696	637	947	736	1,022	774	731	955	809	735	923	1,451	–
Hepatitis, C/non-A non-B	3,816	273	257	322	246	384	291	304	370	319	242	312	496	–
Legionellosis	1,163	61	84	72	63	83	69	75	116	112	127	152	149	–
Lyme disease	12,801	512	254	390	293	612	724	1,638	3,197	1,944	1,057	988	1,192	–
Malaria	2,001	124	98	111	100	168	181	188	279	160	147	181	264	–
Measles (rubeola)	138	3	3	9	14	31	10	21	13	9	11	3	11	–
Meningococcal disease	3,308	138	348	469	282	360	248	175	184	171	168	230	535	–
Mumps	683	32	46	72	63	101	57	25	37	61	45	72	72	–
Pertussis (whooping cough)	6,564	607	403	512	537	475	404	393	543	475	397	740	1,078	–
Plague	4	–	–	–	–	1	1	–	–	1	–	1	–	–
Poliomyelitis, paralytic	3	1	–	–	–	1	–	–	–	1	–	–	–	–
Psittacosis	33	2	2	4	5	5	2	–	4	3	2	–	4	–
Rabies, animal	8,105	268	422	667	741	781	678	599	830	832	862	707	718	–
Rabies, human	2	–	–	1	–	–	–	–	–	–	–	–	1	–
Rocky Mountain spotted fever	409	20	7	14	11	24	58	54	87	48	45	25	16	–
Rubella (German measles)	181	10	4	7	10	30	34	36	7	10	17	1	15	–
Rubella, congenital syndrome	5	–	–	1	–	1	–	–	1	1	–	–	2	–
Salmonellosis	41,901	1,663	2,030	2,544	2,351	3,391	3,175	3,626	5,398	4,364	3,961	4,219	5,179	–
Shigellosis	23,117	1,572	1,200	1,301	1,064	1,615	1,522	1,694	2,717	2,166	2,100	2,792	3,374	–
Syphilis, total all stages†	46,540		·····11,872·····			·····13,007·····			·····11,371·····			·····10,290·····		–
Primary and secondary†	8,550		·····2,264·····			·····2,252·····			·····2,198·····			·····1,836·····		–
Congenital <1 year†	1,049		·····331·····			·····279·····			·····243·····			·····196·····		–
Tetanus	50	5	3	5	2	8	5	4	3	2	2	7	4	–
Toxic-shock syndrome	157	15	9	13	14	12	9	12	16	12	10	12	22	–
Trichinosis	13	5	–	–	–	1	–	–	4	–	–	–	4	–
Tuberculosis¶	19,851	794	1,285	1,630	1,790	1,813	1,553	1,697	1,644	1,583	1,601	1,442	3,019	–
Typhoid fever	365	9	20	28	17	33	25	23	43	44	35	36	52	–
Varicella (chickenpox)**	98,727	5,463	10,792	15,484	11,394	17,909	6,744	2,665	1,370	2,159	3,069	6,748	14,930	–

* The total number of acquired immunodeficiency syndrome (AIDS) cases includes all cases reported to the Division of HIV/AIDS Prevention - Surveillance and Epidemiology, National Center for HIV, STD, and TB Prevention (NCHSTP) as of December 31, 1997.

† Cases were updated through the Division of Sexually Transmitted Diseases Prevention, NCHSTP, as of July 13, 1998.

‡ Chlamydia refers to genital infections caused by C. trachomatis.

§ Cases were updated through the Division of Tuberculosis Elimination, NCHSTP, as of April 15, 1998.

** Not nationally notifiable.

SOURCE: "Summary of Notifiable Diseases, United States, 1997," supplement to *Morbidity and Mortality Weekly Report*, vol. 46, no. 54, November 20, 1998.

TABLE 10.3

Number of reported cases of nationally notifiable diseases preventable by routine childhood vaccination, April–June 1998 and January–June 1997 and 1998*

Disease	No. cases, April–June 1998	Total cases January–June		No. cases among children aged <5 years† January–June	
		1997	1998	1997	1998
Congenital rubella syndrome	2	3	3	3	3
Diphtheria	1	4	1	1	0
Haemophilus influenzae§	275	588	544	113	132
Hepatitis B¶	2122	4430	3809	39	37
Measles	28	77	37	28	17
Mumps	129	339	236	64	41
Pertussis	1130	2537	2075	1021	818
Poliomyelitis, paralytic**	0	2	1	1	1
Rubella	147	64	251	7	13
Tetanus	10	22	12	0	1

* Data for 1997 and 1998 are provisional.

† For 1997 and 1998, age data were available for ≥ 96% of cases.

§ Invasive disease; *H. influenzae* serotype is not routinely reported to the National Notifiable Diseases Surveillance System. Of 132 cases among children aged <5 years, serotype was reported for 74 cases, and of those, 32 were type b, the only serotype of *H. influenzae* preventable by vaccination.

¶ Because most hepatitis B virus infections among infants and children aged <5 years are asymptomatic (although likely to become chronic), acute disease surveillance does not reflect the incidence of this problem in this age group or the effectiveness of hepatitis B vaccination in infants.

** One case with onset in 1998 and three cases with onset in 1997 have been confirmed. All were associated with administration of oral poliovirus vaccine. One suspected case with onset in 1997 remains under investigation.

SOURCE: "Quarterly Immunization Table," *Morbidity and Mortality Weekly Report,* vol. 47, no. 29, July 23, 1998

MOST FREQUENTLY REPORTED DISEASES

In 1997 the top 4 most frequently reported infectious diseases in the United States were chlamydia, gonorrhea, AIDS, and syphilis, all sexually transmitted diseases. The remaining notifiable infectious diseases in the top 10 were:

- Salmonellosis (a food-borne disease causing fever and intestinal disorders, such as food poisoning).

- Hepatitis A (a food- and water-borne disease causing inflammation of the liver).

- Shigellosis (food- and water-borne dysentery).

- Tuberculosis (an airborne disease that usually affects the lungs but can also affect the bones and other organs).

- Lyme disease (a disease spread by ticks).

- Hepatitis B (a blood-borne and sexually transmitted disease that causes inflammation of the liver).

Table 10.2 summarizes the number of cases of these and other notifiable diseases reported to the CDC in 1997.

Resistant Strains of Bacteria

In many cases, widespread use and misuse of antibiotics, generally considered "miracle drugs" that control or cure many bacterial infectious diseases, has led to the development of resistant bacteria. Bacteria such as pneumococcus, which causes pneumonia and children's ear infections—diseases long considered common and treatable—are evolving into strains that are proving to be untreatable by all known medications. Pneumococcus

bacteria cause many hundreds of thousands of cases of pneumonia and almost half of the 24 million annual visits to American pediatricians for earaches. Since the 1980s, national rates of penicillin resistance have soared from less than 5 percent of patients treated to more than 30 percent of patients treated in 1996.

Between February and June 1997, 1,047 strains of pneumococcus obtained from 34 hospitals in the United States and Canada were tested for susceptibility to 19 antibiotics. Among the 845 U.S. samples, only 56 percent were fully susceptible to penicillin, another 28 percent were moderately susceptible, and 16 percent were fully resistant.

Prevention through Immunization

Many infectious diseases can be prevented by childhood immunizations. (See Table 10.3.) Until the 1960s, for example, poliomyelitis (polio) was a serious threat to children, adolescents, and even adults. After the discovery of vaccines to prevent this disease, massive worldwide immunization programs were carried out. In 1994 an international health commission declared that indigenous (in-country) transmission of wild (not contained in laboratories or vaccines) poliovirus had been stopped in the Western hemisphere. In 1997 only three cases of polio were reported in the United States.

The incidence of polio has also decreased greatly in other parts of the world. At one time, polio killed or crippled 500,000 people worldwide every year. By 1998 there were only 35,000 cases reported, and the World Health

Assembly, encouraged by the huge drop in new cases, established a goal of eradicating polio by 2000. At the end of 2000, due in large part to funding and infrastructure problems in the 30 remaining polio-infected countries, that goal had not been met. Only 6,000 new cases, however, were reported in 1999, and most governments had made great strides toward tracking new infections and vaccinating children against the disease.

INFLUENZA

Influenza (flu) is a contagious respiratory disease caused by a virus. When a person infected with the flu sneezes, coughs, or even talks, the virus is expelled into the air and may be inhaled by anyone nearby. It can also be transmitted by direct hand contact. The flu primarily affects the lungs, but the whole body suffers symptoms. The sufferer usually becomes acutely ill, with fever, chills, weakness, loss of appetite, and aching of the head, back, arms, and legs. The victim may also suffer from a sore throat, a dry cough, nausea, and burning eyes. The accompanying fever rises quickly—sometimes reaching 104 degrees—but usually subsides after two or three days. Influenza leaves the patient exhausted.

For healthy individuals, the flu is typically a moderately severe illness, with most adults and children back to work or school within a week. For the very young, the very old, and persons who are not in good general health, however, the flu can be very severe and even fatal. Complications such as bacterial infections may develop, taking advantage of the body's weakened condition and lowered resistance. The most common bacterial complication is pneumonia, but sinuses, bronchi (lung tubes), or inner ears can also become inflamed and painful. Less common but very serious complications include viral pneumonia, encephalitis (inflammation of the brain), acute kidney failure, and nervous system disorders. These complications can be fatal.

Who Gets the Flu?

Anyone can get the flu, especially if there is an epidemic in the community. In an epidemic year, 20 to 30 percent of the population may contract influenza. Not surprisingly, persons who are not healthy are considered at "high risk" for flu and its complications. The high-risk population includes those who have chronic lung conditions, such as asthma, emphysema, chronic bronchitis, tuberculosis, or cystic fibrosis; those with heart disease, chronic kidney disease, diabetes, or severe anemia; persons residing in a nursing home; those over age 65; and health care professionals.

Vaccines

Influenza can be prevented by inoculation with a current influenza vaccine, which is made annually so that it contains the influenza viruses expected to cause the flu the next year. The viruses are killed or inactivated to prevent those who are vaccinated from getting influenza from the vaccine. Instead, the person develops antibodies in his or her body. The antibodies are most effective after one or two months. High-risk persons should be vaccinated early in the fall since peak flu activity occurs around the beginning of the new calendar year.

Each year's flu vaccine protects against only the viruses that were included in making it. If another strain of flu appears, people can still catch that strain even though they were vaccinated for the primary expected strains.

Most people have little or no reaction to the vaccine; 25 percent may have a swollen, red, tender area where the vaccination is injected. Children may suffer a slight fever for 24 hours or have chills or a headache. Those who already suffer from a respiratory disease may find worsened symptoms. Usually, these reactions are temporary. Because the egg in which the virus is grown cannot be completely extracted, persons with an egg protein allergy should consult their physicians before receiving the vaccine and, if vaccinated, should remain under close medical observation.

TUBERCULOSIS

Tuberculosis (TB), a communicable disease caused by the bacterium *Mycobacterium tuberculosis,* is spread from person to person through the inhalation of airborne particles containing *M. tuberculosis*. The particles, called droplet nuclei, are produced when a person with infectious TB of the lungs or larynx forcefully exhales, such as when coughing, sneezing, speaking, or singing. These infectious particles can remain suspended in the air and be inhaled by someone sharing the same air.

Most TB (approximately 85 percent) occurs in the lungs (pulmonary TB). Risk of transmission is increased where ventilation is poor and when susceptible persons share air for prolonged periods with a person who has untreated pulmonary TB. The disease, however, may occur at any site of the body, such as the larynx, the lymph nodes, the brain, the kidneys, or the bones (extrapulmonary). With the exception of laryngeal TB, persons with extrapulmonary TB are usually not considered infectious to others.

TB does not develop in everyone infected with the bacteria. In the United States, about 90 percent of infected persons never show symptoms of TB. Nevertheless, 5 percent of persons infected develop the disease in the first or second year after infection. Another 5 percent show symptoms later in life. For those whose immune systems are compromised, the risk of developing TB is much higher. Eight percent of those infected with both TB and HIV (the virus that causes AIDS) develop full-blown TB symptoms within a year.

TABLE 10.4

Number of persons with reported cases of tuberculosis and percentage change in number of cases, by country of birth, age group, and year: 1992 and 1997

Age group (yrs)	United States			Other		
	No. reported cases		% Change from 1992 to 1997	No. reported cases		% Change from 1992 to 1997
	1992	1997		1992	1997	
0-14	1,285	961	-25%	411	291	-29%
15-24	908	565	-38%	1,047	1,094	4%
25-44	7,363	3,753	-49%	3,007	3,070	2%
45-64	4,888	3,376	-31%	1,557	1,851	19%
≥65	4,750	3,198	-33%	1,244	1,429	15%
Total*	19,194	11,853	-38%	7,266	7,735	6%

*Persons for whom age was not stated were excluded (seven in 1997, 35 in 1992).

SOURCE: "Tuberculosis Morbidity-United States, 1998," *Morbidity and Mortality Weekly Report*, vol. 47, no. 13, April 10, 1998

On the Rise Again?

Latent TB is believed to be present in about 30 to 50 percent of adults in most developing countries. In 1995 there were an estimated 7.5 million cases of tuberculosis worldwide, causing about 3 million deaths, more than any other single infectious disease. This figure increased dramatically since the AIDS epidemic swept through many countries. In 1992 the World Health Organization (WHO) estimated that at least 4 million adults worldwide, primarily in sub-Saharan Africa, Latin America, and Asia, had been infected with both AIDS and *M. tuberculosis*. According to WHO, by 1997 TB had become the leading cause of death in people infected with HIV worldwide.

After several decades of decline, TB also made a comeback in the United States in the late 1980s and early 1990s. From 1985 to 1993, more than 64,000 new TB cases were reported. In 1992 the CDC in Atlanta reported 26,460 cases of TB, up from 22,201 in 1985. By 1997, however, the number of reported cases had dropped to 19,588. (See Table 10.4.) This decline may be due to new public health programs that monitor the complicated drug-taking protocol in TB patients. The success of prevention and treatment programs varies depending on the location and population. Although overall case rates in the United States have been declining, the TB case rate either stayed the same or increased in 23 states and Washington, D.C., between 1995 and 1996.

Treatment has become increasingly difficult as new strains of multidrug-resistant (MDR) TB germs have developed. If the disease is not properly treated or if treatment is not completed, some TB germs can become resistant to drugs, making it much harder to cure. Between 1993 and 1996, MDR TB was detected in a record-high 42 states and Washington, D.C., compared to only 13 states in 1991.

Because of the increase in TB cases in the 1980s and the fact that new antibiotic-resistant strains of TB were emerging, Congress mandated that the National Institutes of Health (NIH) increase its budget for TB research. The National Institute of Allergy and Infectious Diseases (NIAID) is the main TB research institute of NIH. NIAID's research budget soared from $3.1 million in 1991 to $35 million in 1996.

AIDS

AIDS is a blood-borne and sexually transmitted disease that weakens the body's immune system, making it susceptible to opportunistic infections and diseases that, under ordinary circumstances, would not be life threatening. AIDS is caused by HIV, which attacks and destroys certain white blood cells.

Around the World

AIDS and HIV were virtually unknown before 1981. By the end of 2000, 36.1 million people worldwide were estimated to be living with HIV/AIDS, according to the NIH. Of those infected in 2000, 34.7 million were adults and 1.4 million were children under the age of 15. Forty-seven percent were female. More than 70 percent of people infected with HIV lived in sub-Saharan Africa; 16 percent resided in South or Southeast Asia. Worldwide, approximately 1 in every 100 adults aged 15 to 49 was HIV-infected.

Since the epidemic began, 21.8 million people have died of AIDS, and an estimated 3 million died in 2000 alone. Of those, approximately 500,000 were children under 15 years of age.

In the United States

By December 1998, AIDS had struck a reported 688,200 persons of all ages in the United States, resulting

TABLE 10.5

AIDS cases by sex, age at diagnosis, and race/ethnicity, reported through December 1998

Male Age at diagnosis (years)	White, not Hispanic		Black, not Hispanic		Hispanic		Asian/Pacific Islander		American Indian/ Alaska Native		Total[1]	
	No.	(%)	No.	(%)	No.	(%)	No.	(%)	No.	(%)	No.	(%)
Under 5	508	(0)	2,040	(1)	741	(1)	16	(0)	11	(1)	3,319	(1)
5-12	329	(0)	424	(0)	271	(0)	9	(0)	4	(0)	1,039	(0)
13-19	824	(0)	761	(0)	446	(0)	23	(1)	19	(1)	2,075	(0)
20-24	7,323	(3)	6,385	(3)	3,839	(4)	153	(3)	70	(4)	17,797	(3)
25-29	36,485	(13)	23,263	(12)	15,090	(15)	539	(12)	299	(19)	75,773	(13)
30-34	65,304	(23)	39,387	(21)	24,450	(24)	957	(22)	429	(27)	130,672	(23)
35-39	63,280	(23)	42,407	(23)	22,705	(22)	953	(22)	354	(22)	129,884	(23)
40-44	46,052	(17)	33,062	(18)	15,857	(16)	764	(17)	245	(15)	96,120	(17)
45-49	27,663	(10)	18,916	(10)	8,827	(9)	460	(10)	97	(6)	56,034	(10)
50-54	14,875	(5)	9,710	(5)	4,639	(5)	243	(6)	39	(2)	29,550	(5)
55-59	8,097	(3)	5,362	(3)	2,574	(3)	151	(3)	25	(2)	16,236	(3)
60-64	4,513	(2)	2,926	(2)	1,403	(1)	64	(1)	15	(1)	8,935	(2)
65 or older	3,735	(1)	2,420	(1)	1,120	(1)	57	(1)	9	(1)	7,349	(1)
Male subtotal	**278,988**	**(100)**	**187,063**	**(100)**	**101,962**	**(100)**	**4,389**	**(100)**	**1,616**	**(100)**	**574,783**	**(100)**

Female Age at diagnosis (years)												
Under 5	474	(2)	2,013	(3)	736	(3)	14	(2)	13	(4)	3,255	(3)
5-12	174	(1)	458	(1)	206	(1)	7	(1)	—	—	848	(1)
13-19	223	(1)	893	(1)	222	(1)	7	(1)	2	(1)	1,348	(1)
20-24	1,481	(6)	3,722	(6)	1,364	(6)	35	(6)	27	(8)	6,640	(6)
25-29	4,202	(17)	9,448	(15)	3,717	(16)	76	(13)	48	(15)	17,507	(15)
30-34	5,719	(23)	14,299	(22)	5,364	(23)	111	(19)	76	(24)	25,617	(23)
35-39	4,990	(20)	14,154	(22)	4,675	(20)	104	(18)	64	(20)	24,023	(21)
40-44	3,230	(13)	9,642	(15)	3,014	(13)	82	(14)	39	(12)	16,025	(14)
45-49	1,703	(7)	4,636	(7)	1,606	(7)	61	(10)	28	(9)	8,060	(7)
50-54	944	(4)	2,284	(4)	885	(4)	26	(4)	14	(4)	4,158	(4)
55-59	638	(3)	1,277	(2)	549	(2)	18	(3)	6	(2)	2,493	(2)
60-64	432	(2)	759	(1)	287	(1)	22	(4)	3	(1)	1,505	(1)
65 or older	894	(4)	760	(1)	254	(1)	22	(4)	3	(1)	1,935	(2)
Female subtotal	**25,104**	**(100)**	**64,345**	**(100)**	**22,879**	**(100)**	**585**	**(100)**	**323**	**(100)**	**113,414**	**(100)**
Total[2]	**304,094**		**251,408**		**124,841**		**4,974**		**1,940**		**688,200**	

[1] Includes 765 males and 178 females whose race/ethnicity is unknown.

[2] Includes 3 persons whose sex is unknown.

SOURCE: *HIV/AIDS Surveillance Report*, vol. 10, no. 2, 1998

in 390,692 deaths. (By the end of 2000, that number had risen to 753,907, and 438,795 Americans had died from the disease.) The NIH estimated that another 150,000 Americans might be unaware that they have the infection. From 1996 to 1999, the number of new AIDS cases decreased 29.6 percent, from 60,618 to 42,697 (National Institute of Allergy and Infectious Diseases, NIH, *HIV/AIDS Statistics, NIAID Fact Sheet*).

In 2000, 70 percent of all HIV-infected individuals in the United States were male, down from 83.9 percent in 1998. Worldwide, AIDS was more evenly divided between men and women (53 percent male and 47 percent female). Table 10.5 shows the number of AIDS cases reported in the United States as of December 1998, by age at time of diagnosis and by race/ethnicity. Figure 10.1 shows the rates of male and female adult/adolescent AIDS cases per 100,000 population reported in 1998 in the 50 states, the District of Columbia, Puerto Rico, and the U.S. Virgin Islands.

How Is AIDS Spread?

HIV/AIDS is not a disease that can be transmitted through casual contact with an infected person. The CDC has identified several behavioral risk factors that greatly increase the likelihood of a person's chances of being infected. Table 10.6 shows the numbers reported through December 1998 and the cumulative totals of infections through these contacts. The only known methods of transmission of HIV are by:

FIGURE 10.1

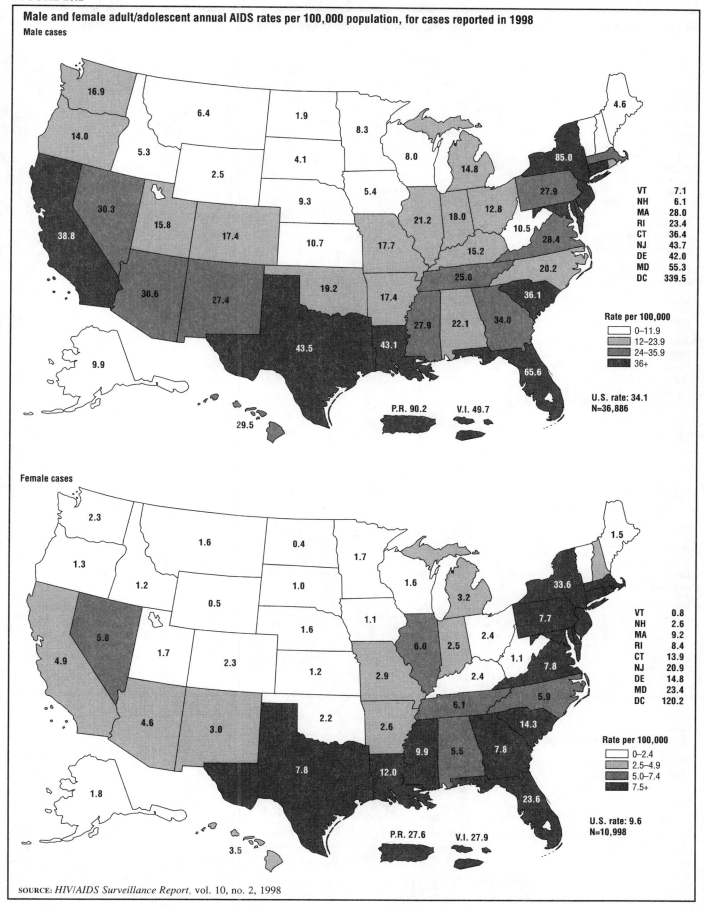

Male and female adult/adolescent annual AIDS rates per 100,000 population, for cases reported in 1998

Male cases

VT	7.1
NH	6.1
MA	28.0
RI	23.4
CT	36.4
NJ	43.7
DE	42.0
MD	55.3
DC	339.5

Rate per 100,000

- 0–11.9
- 12–23.9
- 24–35.9
- 36+

U.S. rate: 34.1
N=36,886

P.R. 90.2   V.I. 49.7

Female cases

VT	0.8
NH	2.6
MA	9.2
RI	8.4
CT	13.9
NJ	20.9
DE	14.8
MD	23.4
DC	120.2

Rate per 100,000

- 0–2.4
- 2.5–4.9
- 5.0–7.4
- 7.5+

U.S. rate: 9.6
N=10,998

P.R. 27.6   V.I. 27.9

SOURCE: *HIV/AIDS Surveillance Report*, vol. 10, no. 2, 1998

TABLE 10.6

AIDS cases by age group, exposure category, and sex, reported through December 1998

Adult/adolescent exposure category	Males				Females				Totals[1]			
	1998		Cumulative total		1998		Cumulative total		1998		Cumulative total[2]	
	No.	(%)	No.	(%)	No.	(%)	No.	(%)	No.	(%)	No.	(%)
Men who have sex with men	16,642	(45)	326,051	(57)	—	—	—	—	16,642	(35)	326,051	(48)
Injecting drug use	7,869	(21)	126,889	(22)	3,201	(29)	46,804	(43)	11,070	(23)	173,693	(26)
Men who have sex with men and inject drugs	1,984	(5)	43,640	(8)	—	—	—	—	1,984	(4)	43,640	(6)
Hemophilia/coagulation disorder	145	(0)	4,663	(1)	17	(0)	248	(0)	162	(0)	4,911	(1)
Heterosexual contact:	2,610	(7)	23,361	(4)	4,125	(38)	43,128	(39)	6,736	(14)	66,490	(10)
Sex with injecting drug user	631		8,015		1,212		18,231		1,843		26,246	
Sex with bisexual male	—		—		190		3,132		190		3,132	
Sex with person with hemophilia	4		47		28		382		32		429	
Sex with transfusion recipient with HIV infection	23		373		24		562		47		935	
Sex with HIV-infected person, risk not specified	1,952		14,926		2,671		20,821		4,624		35,748	
Receipt of blood transfusion, blood components, or tissue[3]	156	(0)	4,784	(1)	137	(1)	3,598	(3)	293	(1)	8,382	(1)
Other/risk not reported or identified[4]	7,480	(20)	41,037	(7)	3,518	(32)	15,533	(14)	11,000	(23)	56,572	(8)
Adult/adolescent subtotal	36,886	(100)	570,425	(100)	10,998	(100)	109,311	(100)	47,887	(100)	679,739	(100)

Pediatric (<13 years old) exposure category	Males				Females				Totals[1]			
	No.	(%)	No.	(%)	No.	(%)	No.	(%)	No.	(%)	No.	(%)
Hemophilia/coagulation disorder	—	—	227	(5)	—	—	7	(0)	—	—	234	(3)
Mother with/at risk for HIV infection:[4]	172	(91)	3,818	(88)	169	(88)	3,869	(94)	341	(89)	7,687	(91)
Injecting drug use	42		1,525		41		1,507		83		3,032	
Sex with injecting drug user	26		715		18		685		44		1,400	
Sex with bisexual male	2		82		2		83		4		165	
Sex with person with hemophilia	1		17		—		12		1		29	
Sex with transfusion recipient with HIV infection	—		11		1		14		1		25	
Sex with HIV-infected person, risk not specified	48		555		38		582		86		1,137	
Receipt of blood transfusion, blood components, or tissue	1		73		2		81		3		154	
Has HIV infection, risk not specified	52		840		67		905		119		1,745	
Receipt of blood transfusion, blood components, or tissue[3]	1	(1)	238	(5)	—	—	140	(3)	1	(0)	378	(4)
Risk not reported or identified[4]	17	(9)	75	(2)	23	(12)	87	(2)	40	(10)	162	(2)
Pediatric subtotal	190	(100)	4,358	(100)	192	(100)	4,103	(100)	382	(100)	8,461	(100)
Total	**37,076**		**574,783**		**11,190**		**113,414**		**48,269**		**688,200**	

[1] Includes 3 persons whose sex is unknown.

[2] Includes 12 persons known to be infected with human immunodeficiency virus type 2 (HIV-2).

[3] Thirty-seven adults/adolescents and 2 children developed AIDS after receiving blood screened negative for HIV antibody. Thirteen additional adults developed AIDS after receiving tissue, organs, or artificial insemination from HIV-infected donors. Four of the 13 received tissue, organs, or artificial insemination from a donor who was negative for HIV antibody at the time of donation.

[4] "Other" also includes 113 persons who acquired HIV infection perinatally but were diagnosed with AIDS after age 13. These 113 persons are tabulated under the adult/adolescent, not pediatric, exposure category.

SOURCE: *HIV/AIDS Surveillance Report*, vol. 10, no. 2, 1998

- Having oral, anal, or vaginal sex with an infected person.

- Sharing drug needles or syringes with an infected person.

- Passing from an infected mother to her baby perinatally (around the time of birth) and possibly through breast milk.

- Receiving a transplanted organ or a body fluid, such as blood or blood products, from an infected person.

By avoiding these methods of transmission, a person can virtually eliminate the possibility of becoming infected with HIV.

Opportunistic Infections

Because of the advancing damage to the body's immune system, so-called opportunistic infections (those that the body could ordinarily fight off) are very common among HIV/AIDS sufferers. Two of the most common opportunistic infections are Pneumocystis carinii pneumonia, a lung infection caused by a fungus, and Kaposi's sarcoma, a once-rare cancer of the blood vessel walls that causes conspicuous purple lesions on the skin. Some of the other infections to which AIDS patients are susceptible are toxoplasmosis (a contagious disease caused by a protozoan), oral candidiasis (thrush)—as well as esophageal or bronchial candidiasis—extrapulmonary cryptococcosis, HIV wasting syndrome, pulmonary TB, extrapulmonary TB, and severe herpes simplex.

Treatment of AIDS

Several drugs have recently been developed that help to control the effects of HIV, delay the progression of the disease, and fight opportunistic infections. The latest treatment programs use combinations of several drugs, and seem to give better results than any single drug discovered so far. Some of the newest antiviral drugs used against AIDS and its related opportunistic infections include the protease inhibitors, such as Viracept and Crixivan. Combined with azidothymidine (AZT), the first U.S. Food and Drug Administration (FDA) approved drug for the treatment of AIDS, these drugs can often diminish a patient's viral "load" of HIV to undetectable levels, and allow patients to live normal lives for many years. The drugs, however, do produce severe side effects in a number of patients. The cost of protease inhibitors ranges from $4,800 to $8,000 for a year's supply. When used in combination with AZT, the cost of AIDS drugs is approximately $18,000 per year. The total per-patient cost of AIDS drugs falls between $12,000 and $70,000, depending on the severity of the patient's condition.

The development of these new protease inhibitor drugs, often called the AIDS drug "cocktail," has increased patient life spans and dramatically diminished the number of deaths from AIDS in the United States in recent years. While the NIH reported 50,610 deaths from AIDS in 1995, only 16,273 Americans died from AIDS in 1999. Many patients taking the AIDS drugs can now live with the HIV virus for years, even decades, without developing symptoms. Few of these expensive drugs are available to patients in developing countries, however, where 95 percent of new AIDS cases are reported.

AIDS and TB

TB occurs with increasing frequency among persons infected with HIV. In fact, HIV infection is one of the strongest-known risk factors for the progression of TB from infection to disease. The PHS reported that approximately 5 percent of all AIDS patients also have TB, and it is very likely that the HIV epidemic has contributed substantially to the increased number of TB cases. In some geographic areas, as many as 58 percent of persons with TB are HIV-positive. Of the many diseases associated with HIV infection, however, TB is one of the few that are treatable and preventable.

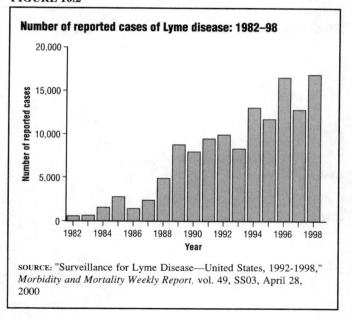

FIGURE 10.2

Number of reported cases of Lyme disease: 1982–98

SOURCE: "Surveillance for Lyme Disease—United States, 1992-1998," *Morbidity and Mortality Weekly Report*, vol. 49, SS03, April 28, 2000

LYME DISEASE

Spread by the bites of infected deer ticks, Lyme disease is the most commonly reported vector-borne (spread by a "carrier" animal or insect) disease in the United States. The disease is caused by the *Borrelia burgdorferi* organism and produces early symptoms such as skin rashes, headache, fever, and general illness; if untreated, the disease can cause arthritis and heart damage.

The CDC began to track Lyme disease in 1982, and the disease was added to the list of nationally notifiable diseases in 1990. Figure 10.2 shows the dramatic increase in the number of reported cases from 1982 to 1998. In 1997 the CDC received reports of 12,801 cases of Lyme disease from 46 states and the District of Columbia, with the majority of cases occurring in the northeastern and north central states. Ten states—Connecticut, Rhode Island, New Jersey, New York, Pennsylvania, Delaware, Massachusetts, Wisconsin, Minnesota, and Maryland— accounted for 92 percent of the total cases reported. (See Figure 10.3.)

In December 1998 the FDA announced approval for the world's first vaccine against Lyme disease. Doctors warned, however, that while the vaccine, LYMErix, developed by SmithKline Beecham, would help prevent Lyme disease, it would not eliminate the threat entirely. In order to build the best immunity, a person must have three shots over a full year.

As LYMErix is not 100 percent protective, the FDA warned that people still must take precautions against ticks. Wearing long-sleeved shirts and long pants, tucking pants legs into socks, and spraying the skin and/or clothing with tick repellents can keep ticks away from the skin.

FIGURE 10.3

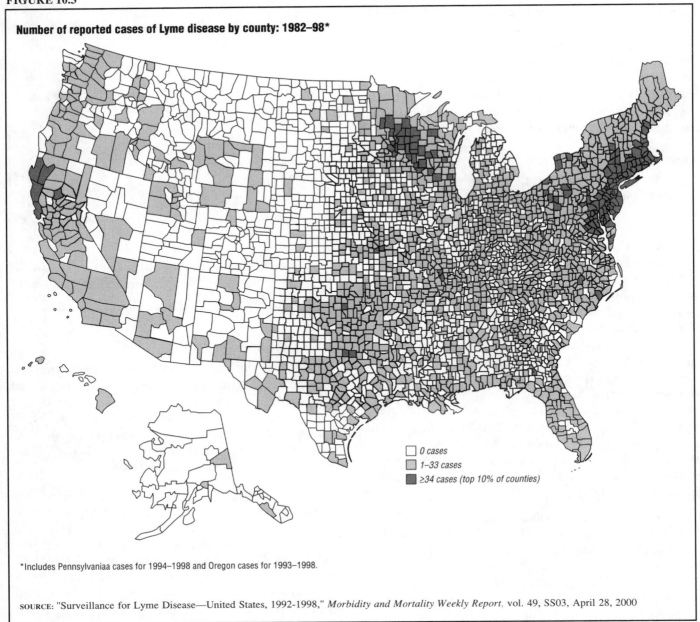

Number of reported cases of Lyme disease by county: 1982–98*

0 cases

1–33 cases

≥34 cases (top 10% of counties)

*Includes Pennsylvaniaa cases for 1994–1998 and Oregon cases for 1993–1998.

SOURCE: "Surveillance for Lyme Disease—United States, 1992-1998," *Morbidity and Mortality Weekly Report,* vol. 49, SS03, April 28, 2000

If a tick is found on the body, one should remove it promptly and be alert for any of the early symptoms of the disease. Immediate medical care is imperative to prevent long-term health damage from Lyme disease.

CHAPTER 11
MENTAL HEALTH

Mental illness is difficult to classify into clearly defined diseases. While the symptoms of mental illness may distinguish one type of problem from another, the symptoms vary far more widely in both type and intensity than do the symptoms of a physical illness. In general, people are usually considered mentally healthy if they are able to keep their mental and emotional balance in times of crisis and stress and cope effectively with the problems of daily life. If that coping ability is lost, then there is some degree of mental dysfunction. The goal is to recognize and understand the problems, alleviate the underlying causes, and work toward regaining mental and emotional equilibrium.

HOW MANY PEOPLE ARE MENTALLY ILL?

It is difficult to determine how many people suffer from mental illness. There are social stigmas attached to being labeled "crazy," keeping some sufferers of mental disease from seeking help. Many of those seeking help do not reveal it on surveys. Some patients do not realize that the source of their symptoms is a mental disorder, and the experts themselves often have a hard time defining mental illness.

Types of Disorders

Psychiatrists have identified a wide range of mental disorders, from phobias (irrational fears) to depression and chronic problems such as schizophrenia. Some disorders are relatively mild and affect a victim's life in only a minor way. Others can be overwhelming and completely debilitating.

Phobias are the most common mental disorder, with 20 million Americans reporting at least one phobia serious enough to affect their daily routines. Depressions are the next most common disorder: about 17 million people suffer each year from manic-depressive (bipolar) disorder, major (unipolar) depression, or minor chronic depression (dysthymia). The medical community also classifies substance abuse as a mental disorder. Alcoholism, which affects close to 14 million people a year, is very common. Many people suffer from more than one disorder at a time (comorbidity); as many as 6 million Americans suffer from drug abuse combined with one or more other mental disorders. (See Table 11.1.)

NATIONAL INSTITUTE OF MENTAL HEALTH STUDY

In 1993 the Division of Epidemiology and Services Research at the National Institute of Mental Health (NIMH), released the results of the most comprehensive study of the nation's mental health ever conducted ("The de Facto U.S. Mental and Addictive Disorders Service System," *Archives of General Psychiatry,* vol. 50, February 1993). The study was based on intensive interviews of 20,000 men and women in 1980 and follow-up interviews of 16,000 people between 1981 and 1985 from randomly selected households representative of the entire population.

The study found that approximately 52 million adults in the United States—more than one in four—experience a mental disorder at some point during a year, but only 28 percent of those affected seek help. In a given year, about 9 million Americans develop a mental disorder for the first time, another 8 million suffer a relapse, and 35 million are plagued by continuing symptoms. The NIMH study pointed out that the new cases (9 million) are balanced by the same number of persons whose disorders clear up, causing the general proportion of persons with mental disorders to remain relatively constant at about 28 percent of the total population.

Some Undercounting

The totals reported in the study may represent a small undercount of persons with mental disorders since not everyone met all the official criteria for a disorder. For example, if someone suffered a panic attack three times a month, rather than the four times that were required to

TABLE 11.1

Prevalence of disorders in five ECA site combined community and institutionalized population: per 100 persons, 18 years and older*

(Standard Error in Parentheses)

Disorders	One month at wave 1		One year new at wave 2		One year prevalence		Number of persons[+] (000's omitted)
Any DIS ADM Disorder	15.7	(0.4)	12.3	(0.4)	28.1	(0.5)	51,311
Any DIS Disorder							
except Alcohol or Drug	13.0	(0.4)	9.0	(0.3)	22.1	(0.4)	40,355
Any Mental Disorder							
with Comorbid Substance Use	1.0	(0.1)	2.3	(0.1)	3.3	(0.2)	6,067
Any Substance Use Disorder	3.8	(0.2)	5.6	(0.3)	9.5	(0.3)	17,288
Any Alcohol Disorder	2.8	(0.2)	4.6	(0.2)	7.4	(0.3)	13,512
Any Drug Disorder	1.3	(0.1)	1.8	(0.1)	3.1	(0.2)	5,661
Schizophrenic/							
Schizophrenifom Disorders	0.7	(0.1)	0.3	(0.1)	1.1	(0.1)	2,009
Affective Disorders	5.2	(0.2)	4.3	(0.2)	9.5	(0.3)	17,391
Any Bipolar	0.6	(0.1)	0.5	(0.1)	1.2	(0.1)	2,191
Unipolar Major Depression	1.8	(0.1)	3.2	(0.1)	5.0	(0.2)	9,130
Dysthymia	3.3	(0.2)	2.1	(0.1)	5.4	(0.2)	9,860
Anxiety Disorders	7.3	(0.3)	5.3	(0.2)	12.6	(0.3)	23,008
Phobia	6.3	(0.2)	4.7	(0.2)	10.9	(0.3)	19,903
Panic Disorder	0.5	(0.1)	0.7	(0.1)	1.3	(0.1)	2,374
Obsessive-Campulsive Disorder	1.3	(0.1)	0.8	(0.1)	2.1	(0.1)	3,835
Somatization Disorder	0.1	(0.0)	0.1	(0.0)	0.2	(0.0)	419
Antisocial Personality Disorder	0.5	(0.1)	1.0	(0.1)	1.5	(0.1)	2,739
Cognitive Impairment (Severe)	1.7	(0.1)	1.0	(0.1)	2.7	(0.1)	4,930

* DIS indicates Diagnostic Interview Schedule; ECA, Epidemiologic Catchment Area, and ADM, alcohol, drug or mental. Rates are standardized to the age, sex and race distribution of the 1980 institutionalized and noninstitutionalized population of the United States aged 18 years and older.

+ Based on 1990 population estimates. The combined household and institutionalized, civilian adult population was 182.6 million in 1990.

SOURCE: R.W. Manderscheid and M.A. Somenschein, *Mental Health, United States, 1994*, Center for Mental Health Services, Washington D.C., 1994

meet the specified criteria, he or she would not be included in the count of those with panic disorders.

Another factor in undercounting is that interviewers asked respondents only about symptoms of eight of the most common mental disorders: drug and alcohol abuse, schizophrenia, depression, anxiety problems, "antisocial" personality, severe cognitive impairment, and somatization (chronic complaints of multiple physical symptoms without medical cause). The study did not concern itself with what are often considered "problems in living," such as marital difficulties. While not counted among major mental disorders, relationship problems cause a great many people to seek psychotherapy.

Treatment

The NIMH study noted that not all mental disorders require treatment and that many people with mental disorders have relatively brief, self-limiting illnesses that are not disabling enough to warrant treatment. The study found that 70 percent of mental illness cases go untreated. Among those who seek help, 43 percent see their general physicians. About 40 percent visit psychiatrists, clinical psychologists, clinical social workers, or other trained mental health professionals.

The majority of those with the most serious problems sought help from mental health specialists and saw them more frequently than those who sought help from a general doctor. Of those who went to specialists for treatment, each visited his or her doctor an average of 14 visits per year, while those who went to their family physicians averaged only three or four visits per year. NIMH encourages general practitioners, who often lack special training to recognize mental disorders, to send patients who seek help to mental health professionals for screening to ensure that mental disorders are properly diagnosed and treated.

In addition, NIMH recommends that general physicians receive more training to recognize and treat psychiatric disorders. For instance, many angiograms (medical procedures to study the heart and blood vessels) are unnecessary because they are really cases of undiagnosed panic attacks. People suffering panic attacks often mistakenly believe they are having heart attacks and rush to hospital emergency rooms.

A significant proportion of those seeking help sought out nonprofessionals. About 18 percent reported going to such self-help groups as Alcoholics Anonymous or to family members or friends. About one in five went to clergy, family service agencies, welfare workers, or lay healers. About 18 percent of those seeking help went to more than one source.

A probable explanation for the relatively small number of persons seeking help from psychiatrists, clini-

TABLE 11.2

Lifetime and 12-month prevalence of UM/CIDI DSM-III-R disorders

Disorders	Male				Female				Total			
	Lifetime		12-Month		Lifetime		12-Month		Lifetime		12-Month	
	%	(se*)	%	(se)	%	(se)	%	(se)	%	(se)	%	(se)
A. Affective Disorders												
Major Depressive Episode	12.7	(0.9)	7.7	(0.8)	21.3	(0.9)	12.9	(0.8)	17.1	(0.7)	10.3	(0.6)
Manic Episode	1.6	(0.3)	1.4	(0.3)	1.7	(0.3)	1.3	(0.3)	1.6	(0.3)	1.3	(0.2)
Dysthymia	4.8	(0.4)	2.1	(0.3)	8.0	(0.6)	3.0	(0.4)	6.4	(0.4)	2.5	(0.2)
Any Affective disorder	14.7	(0.8)	8.5	(0.8)	23.9	(0.9)	14.1	(0.9)	19.3	(0.7)	11.3	(0.7)
B. Anxiety Disorders												
Panic Disorder	2.0	(0.3)	1.3	(0.3)	5.0	(1.40	3.2	(0.4)	3.5	(0.3)	2.3	(0.3)
Agoraphobia without Panic	3.5	(0.4)	1.7	(0.3)	7.0	(0.60	3.8	(0.4)	5.3	(0.4)	2.8	(0.3)
Social Phobia	11.1	(0.8)	6.6	(0.4)	15.5	(1.0)	9.1	(0.7)	13.3	(0.7)	7.9	(0.4)
Simple Phobia	6.7	(0.5)	4.4	(0.5)	15.7	(1.1)	13.2	(0.9)	11.3	(0.6)	8.8	(0.5)
Generalized Anxiety Disorder	3.6	(0.5)	2.0	(0.3)	6.6	(0.5)	4.3	(0.4)	5.1	(0.3)	3.1	(0.3)
Any Anxiety Disorder	19.2	(0.9)	11.8	(0.6)	30.5	(1.2)	22.6	(0.1)	24.9	(0.8)	17.2	(0.7)
C. Substmce Use Disorders												
Alcohol Abuse	12.5	(0.8)	3.4	(0.4)	6.4	(0.6)	1.6	(0.2)	9.4	(0.5)	2.5	(0.2)
Alcohol Dependence	20.1	(1.0)	10.7	(0.9)	8.2	(0.7)	3.7	(0.4)	14.1	(0.7)	7.2	(0.5)
Drug Abuse	5.4	(0.5)	1.3	(0.2)	3.5	(0.4)	0.3	(0.1)	4.4	(0.3)	0.8	(0.1)
Drug Dependence	9.2	(0.7)	3.8	(0.4)	5.9	(0.5)	1.9	(0.3)	7.5	(0.4)	2.8	(0.3)
Any Substance												
Abuse/Dependence	35.4	(1.2)	16.1	(0.7)	17.9	(1.1)	6.6	(0.4)	26.6	(1.0)	11.3	(0.5)
D. Other Disorders												
Antisocial Personality	5.8	(0.5)	–	–	1.2	(0.3)	–	–	3.5	(0.3)	–	–
Non-Affective Psychosis+	0.6	(0.1)	0.5	(0.1)	0.6	(0.2)	0.6	(0.2)	0.7	(0.1)	0.5	(0.1)
E. Any NCS Disorder	48.7	(0.2)	27.7	(0.9)	47.3	(1.5)	31.2	(1.3)	48.0	(1.1)	29.5	(1.0)

* se = standard error.
+ Non-Affective Psychosis = schizophrenia, schizophreniform disorder, schizoaffective disorder, delusional disorder, and atypical psychosis.

SOURCE: Ronald C. Kessler et al., *Lifetime and 12-Month Prevalence of DSM-III-R Psychiatric Disorders in the United States,* University of Michigan Institute for Social Research, Ann Arbor, MI, 1994

psychologists, or other specifically trained professionals is the higher cost of those services, and the reluctance of insurance companies to cover mental health problems. Many private insurance policies offer only limited coverage for mental health services. In addition, mental health practitioners covered by insurance and mental health care facilities are often unevenly distributed throughout the country. In January 1998, however, Congress made significant progress toward more equitable mental health when the Mental Health Parity Act of 1996 (PL 104-204) took effect. The act requires that mental health benefits have the same standing as medical/surgical benefits in health plans with 50 or more employees. Thirteen states have also enacted statewide mental illness parity laws. (Three more states have enacted parity laws applicable to state employees only.)

UNIVERSITY OF MICHIGAN STUDY

In 1994 Ronald C. Kessler of the University of Michigan (UM) Institute for Social Research reported the results of a national survey of 8,000 civilian, noninstitutionalized persons. The survey found that nearly half of all Americans between the ages of 15 and 54 had suffered from an episode of psychiatric disorder at some time in their lives. Nearly 30 percent of those interviewed had had

such an episode in the year preceding the survey. The interviews, conducted between September 1990 and February 1992, were designed to identify disorders described in the third edition of the *Diagnostic and Statistical Manual of Mental Disorders of the American Psychiatric Association (DSM III),* the standard classification system used in this country. (In 1994, the updated DSM IV was released with some new classifications and clarifications.)

Many of the UM findings differed from those reported in the NIMH survey. While the NIMH study found phobia the most common disorder, the UM study concluded that major depression was the most common disorder, with 17.1 percent of the population suffering an episode at some time in their lives and over 10.3 percent in the year prior to the study. The second-most common disorder was alcohol dependence, with 14.1 percent experiencing a problem during their lives and 7.2 percent in the past year. The UM study found that some of the most common disorders were social phobias (13.3 percent), such as fear of speaking in public or meeting new people, and simple phobias (11.3 percent), such as fear of flying or enclosed spaces (claustrophobia). Table 11.2 from the UM study shows that 7.9 percent of the population had experienced social phobias in the previous year, and 8.8 percent had suffered a simple phobia.

The study found that comorbidity increased the severity of the disorders. Roughly one-fourth of persons who had a lifetime history of several different simultaneously occurring disorders, such as depression combined with alcohol dependence, accounted for almost 90 percent of the severe recent disorders in the total population.

Demographic Characteristics

The UM study found that the rates for almost all disorders declined with increasing income and education; in other words, the poor and those with the least education were more profoundly affected by mental disorders than the nonpoor and those with more education. The exception to this generalization was the middle education group, which had a significantly higher incidence of lifetime substance abuse disorders.

Persons between the ages of 25 and 34 had the highest overall rates of mental illness; after age 34, the rates declined. Men had much higher rates for substance abuse and antisocial personality disorders, while women had much higher rates for affective (depression) and anxiety disorders. Table 11.2 shows that women were much more likely than men to suffer from an affective disorder or an anxiety disorder during their lifetimes. On the other hand, men were about twice as likely as women to experience a substance use disorder (primarily alcohol use or dependence). Men also experienced antisocial personality nearly five times as frequently as women did.

Persons who lived in the West experienced the highest rates of lifetime substance use disorders and antisocial personality disorder. People who lived in the Northeast, which is known for its fast-paced way of life, experienced the highest incidence of lifetime anxiety disorders. The South, on the other hand, which is known for a slower, more relaxed pace, had the lowest rates of all lifetime disorders. Rural living, however, may not be as idyllic as often portrayed, since the UM study noted that rural residents were no less likely than were urban residents to suffer from a lifetime or one-year psychiatric disorder.

Conclusions of the UM Study

The UM survey noted that only about 40 percent of those with a lifetime disorder ever received professional treatment. Fewer than 20 percent of those with a recent occurrence had received treatment in the previous year. Like the 1993 NIMH survey (see above), however, the UM study cautioned that not everyone who has had a psychiatric disorder at some time in his or her life needs psychiatric treatment. Many problems are minor and are resolved without treatment. Nonetheless, the study argued that some psychiatric disorders can cause tremendous pain and suffering, and people who suffer from these disorders should have access to help.

The UM study concluded that while psychiatric disorders affect many people, the most severe are concentrated among a small number of people (less than 15 percent of the population) who have a lifetime history of comorbidity. Within a given year, an estimated 3 to 5 percent of the total population suffers from disorders severe enough to need treatment. If the overwhelming majority of people with severe disorders have a lifetime history of comorbidity, early intervention to stop or slow the progression of these interrelated disorders could reduce the number of severe psychiatric episodes in the future.

SCHIZOPHRENIA

The "crazy person" who hears voices, becomes violent, and sometimes ends up as a street person, muttering and shouting incomprehensibly, frequently suffers from schizophrenia. This disease generally attacks in adolescence, causing hallucinations, paranoia, delusions, and social isolation. The effects begin slowly and, initially, are often considered the normal behavioral changes of adolescence. Gradually, voices take over in the schizophrenic's mind, obliterating reality and directing the person into all kinds of erratic behavior. Suicide attempts and violent attacks are common in the lives of schizophrenics. Many schizophrenics turn to drugs in an attempt to escape the torment inflicted by their brains. NIMH estimated that as many as half of all schizophrenics are also drug abusers.

In 1994 the Center for Mental Health Services (CMHS) reported that 2 million Americans suffered from schizophrenia and similar disorders. (See Table 11.1.) Doctors are not sure what causes schizophrenia or even whether it is a single disease or a variety of conditions with similar symptoms but different causes. It might be caused by a virus, brain damage, or a biochemical disorder, or it may be genetic. Stress can aggravate the symptoms but is not the cause of the disease.

Some studies suggest that the brain of a schizophrenic manufactures too much dopamine, a chemical vital to normal nerve activity. Drug treatments focus on suppressing the dopamine, but not all schizophrenics respond to the available treatments. The most effective medication, clozapine, has a potentially fatal side effect—it can hamper the body's ability to make white blood cells, which fight infection. Patients who take it must be closely monitored.

DEPRESSION

According to the CMHS, an estimated 17.4 million Americans, the majority of whom are women, suffer from depressive (affective) disorders. (See Table 11.1.) Depression occurs most often in adults between the ages of 25 and 44 years of age and can interfere with normal functioning and cause pain and suffering not only to the victims, but also to their families and others who care about them. Unfortunately, many people with these disorders do not seek help, although about 80 percent, including those with the most severe symptoms, can be helped with medications and therapy.

What Is a Depressive Disorder?

Depression is a "whole body" illness, involving physical, mental, and emotional problems. A depressive disorder is not a temporary sad mood, and it is not a sign of personal weakness or a condition that can be willed away. People with depressive illness cannot just "pull themselves together" and get well. Without treatment, the symptoms can go on for months or even years. (See Table 11.3 for a list of symptoms that characterize depression.) Not everyone who is depressed experiences all of the symptoms. Some people have very few symptoms; some have many. In addition, the severity and duration of the symptoms may vary.

There are several types of depressive disorders. The most common form, according to the 1994 CMHS report, was dysthymia, a less severe but chronic form of depression. Dysthymia may not disable its victims as severely as other forms of depression, but it can rob a life of its joy, energy, and productivity. In 1994 an estimated 10 million persons suffered from dysthymia. (See Table 11.1.)

Unipolar major depression is a more severe and disabling form; over 9 million persons were diagnosed with major depression in 1994. The victims may lose the ability to work, eat, sleep, and enjoy the activities that once gave them pleasure. Manic depression (now called bipolar disorder) is characterized by wide mood swings from excessive elation and hyperactivity to the more common symptoms of depression.

Causes of Depression

Usually, combinations of genetic, psychological, and environmental factors are involved in depressive disorders. Some types of depression run in families, indicating that it may be genetic. Major depression seems to recur in generation after generation of some families, but it can also occur in people without a family history of depression.

Whether a genetic factor exists or not, studies of the brain show that depression is a biological disease based on a chemical disorder. Researchers suggest that the problem may be caused by the complex neurotransmission (chemical messaging) system of the brain and that the person suffering from the disorder has either too much or too little of certain neurochemicals in the brain. Most of the antidepressant drugs now used to treat the disorder try to correct these chemical imbalances.

A person's psychological makeup is another factor in depressive disorders. People who are easily overwhelmed by stress or who suffer from low self-esteem or a pes-

TABLE 11.3

The symptoms of depression and mania

Depression
- Persistent sad, anxious, or "empty" mood
- Loss of interest or pleasure in activities, including sex
- Feelings of hopelessness, pessimism
- Feelings of guilt, worthlessness, helplessness
- Sleeping too much or too little, early-morning awakening
- Appetite and/or weight loss or overeating and weight gain
- Decreased energy, fatigue, feeling "slowed down"
- Thoughts of death or suicide, or suicide attempts
- Restlessness, irritability
- Difficulty concentrating, remembering, or making decisions
- Persistent physical symptoms that do not respond to treatment, such as headaches, digestive disorders, and chronic pain

Mania
- Abnormally elevated mood
- Irritability
- Severe insomnia
- Grandiose notions
- Increased talking
- Racing thoughts
- Increased activity, including sexual activity
- Markedly increased energy
- Poor judgement that leads to risk-taking behavior
- Inappropriate social behavior

A thorough diagnostic evaluation is needed if five or more of these symptoms persist for more than two weeks, or if they interfere with work or family life. An evaluation involves a complete physical checkup and information-gathering on family health history.

SOURCE: *Depression: What Every Woman Should Know,* National Institute of Mental Health, Washington, D.C., 1995

simistic view of life, themselves, and the world, tend to be prone to depression. Events outside the person's control can also trigger a depressive episode. A major change in the patterns of daily living, such as a serious loss, a chronic illness, a difficult relationship, or financial problems, can cause the onset of depression.

Treatment of Depression

Psychotherapy and a variety of antidepressant medications that alter brain chemistry are used to treat depressive disorders. Some people respond well to psychotherapy and others to antidepressants. Many do best with a combination of treatment—drugs for relatively quick relief of symptoms and therapy to learn how to cope with life's problems more effectively. Antidepressant drugs are not addictive, but the patient must be carefully watched by a physician to check for effectiveness. In some cases of chronic depression, medication may need to be taken on a continuous basis to avoid the symptoms of the disease.

ANXIETY DISORDERS

Everyone experiences anxiety almost every day. In today's world, a certain amount of anxiety is unavoidable and, in some cases, may even be beneficial. For example, anxiety before an exam or a job interview can actually improve performance. Anxiety prior to a surgical operation, giving a speech, or driving in bad weather is normal.

Nevertheless, when anxiety becomes extreme or when an attack of anxiety strikes suddenly, without an apparent external cause, it can be both debilitating and destructive. Its symptoms may include nervousness, fear, a "knot" in the stomach, a rapid heartbeat, or increased blood pressure. If the anxiety is severe and long lasting, more serious problems may develop. People suffering from anxiety over an extended period may have headaches, ulcers, irritable bowel syndrome, insomnia, and depression. Because anxiety tends to create various other emotional and physical symptoms, a "snowball" effect can occur in which these problems produce even more anxiety.

Chronic anxiety can interfere with one's ability to lead a normal life. People who suffer from prolonged anxiety are considered to have anxiety disorders by mental health specialists. The CMHS reported an estimated 23 million Americans suffered from anxiety disorders in 1994. (See Table 11.1.)

Panic Disorder

If anxiety reaches high levels, panic attacks that are both unexpected and seemingly without cause may occur. One characteristic of a panic attack is that the victim can never predict when he or she will be suddenly overcome. These unpredictable panic episodes are marked by an overwhelming sense of impending doom while the person's heart races and breathing quickens to the point of gasping for air. Sweating, weakness, dizziness, terror, and feelings of unreality are also typical. Individuals undergoing a panic attack fear they are going to die, go crazy, or, at the very least, lose control.

Repeated panic attacks can lead to a panic disorder. Panic disorder, which can run in families, has a lifetime prevalence (according to the UM survey) in about 3.5 percent of the population. (See Table 11.2.) For most victims, the attacks start between the ages of 15 and 19.

Many of those affected are convinced they are suffering heart attacks and end up in hospital emergency rooms. When they are found to be free of heart disease, they may turn to neurologists and other specialists to seek an answer to their problems. Research has found that of the patients who make the most visits to doctors, spend the most time in the hospital, and use the most prescription medications, approximately 12 percent suffer from undiagnosed panic disorder.

The usual treatment for panic disorder is behavior therapy combined with antianxiety drugs to treat the fear of the attacks. Sometimes, antidepressant medications are used, even though the victim is not clinically depressed. Relaxation therapy has also proved beneficial.

Phobias

Phobias are defined as unreasonable fears associated with a particular situation or object. The most common of the many varieties of phobias is simple phobia. Bees, germs, heights, odors, and storms are examples of things commonly feared in simple phobias. Simple phobias, especially animal phobias, are common in children, but they can occur at any age. About 20 million American adults suffered from phobias in 1994. (See Table 11.1.) Most phobics understand that their fears are unreasonable, but that awareness does not make them feel any less anxious.

Simple phobias, such as a fear of heights, usually do not interfere with daily life or cause as much distress as more severe forms, such as agoraphobia (see below). Persons suffering from severe phobias may rearrange their lives drastically to avoid the situations they fear will trigger panic attacks.

SOCIAL PHOBIAS. Social phobias can be more serious than simple phobias. The person with a social phobia is intensely afraid of being judged by others. At social gatherings, the social phobic expects to be singled out, scrutinized, and found lacking. People with social phobias are usually very anxious about feeling humiliated or embarrassed. They are often so crippled by their own fears that they may have a hard time thinking clearly, remembering facts, or carrying on a normal conversation. Thus, the social phobic tries to avoid public situations and gatherings of people. Social phobias tend to start between the ages of 15 and 20 and, if not treated, can continue throughout life.

AGORAPHOBIA. Many people who experience panic attacks go on to develop agoraphobia, the fear of crowds and open spaces. The term comes from the Greek word *agora,* which means marketplace. This type of phobia is a severely disabling disorder that often keeps its victims virtual prisoners in their own homes, unable to go out for work, shopping, or social activities.

Agoraphobia normally develops slowly, following an initial unexpected panic attack. For example, on an ordinary day, while shopping, driving to work, or doing errands, the individual is suddenly struck by a wave of terror. He or she experiences symptoms such as trembling, a pounding heart, profuse sweating, and difficulty in breathing normally. The person desperately seeks safety, reassurance from friends and family, or a physician. All is well—until another panic attack occurs.

The agoraphobic begins to avoid all places and situations where an attack occurred and then begins to avoid places where an attack could possibly occur or where it might be difficult to escape and get help. Gradually, the victim becomes more and more limited in the choice of places that are "safe." Eventually, the agoraphobic cannot venture outside the immediate neighborhood or leave the house. The fear ultimately expands to touch every aspect of life.

Agoraphobia usually begins during the late teens or twenties. The UM survey reported that 5.3 percent of the adult population suffers from agoraphobia. Women tend to be affected two to four times more often than are men. (See Table 11.2.)

PHOBIA TREATMENT PROGRAMS. Phobia treatment centers now exist throughout the United States. The programs use a wide variety of behavioral therapy techniques to help patients face and overcome their fears. In addition, drugs may be used to ease the symptoms of anxiety, fear, and depression and to help the person return to a normal life more quickly. Antidepressants have been shown to help people who suffer from panic attacks and agoraphobia. In addition, antianxiety drugs are useful in treating the generalized anxiety that accompanies phobias.

EATING DISORDERS

American society is preoccupied with body image. Americans are constantly bombarded with images of very thin, beautiful young women in magazines, on television, on billboards, and in the movies. The advertisers of many products suggest that to be thin and beautiful is to be happy. Many prominent weight-loss programs reinforce this suggestion. A well-balanced, low-fat food plan, combined with exercise can help most people achieve a healthier weight and lifestyle without dieting to become "model" thin, which may be harmful to many people.

According to NIMH, dieting plays a role in the onset of two serious eating disorders—anorexia nervosa and bulimia. Teenage and college-age women are at special risk. In fact, more than 90 percent of those who develop an eating disorder are young women, although experts are beginning to study the rising rates of anorexia and bulimia among men. No one knows how many men and teenage boys are afflicted. Until recently, there has been a lack of awareness that eating disorders can be a problem for males, perhaps because men are more likely to hide their illness behind such excuses as avoiding heart disease or diabetes or trying to build a more muscular physique. Studies suggest that for every 10 women with an eating disorder, 1 male is afflicted.

Anorexia Nervosa

Anorexia nervosa involves severe weight loss—a minimum of 15 percent below normal body weight. Anorexic people literally starve themselves, even though they may be very hungry. For reasons that researchers do not yet fully understand, anorexics become terrified of gaining weight. Both food and weight become obsessions. They often develop strange eating habits, refuse to eat with other people, and exercise strenuously to keep off extra pounds. Anorexic individuals continue to believe they are overweight even when they are bone-thin.

The medical complications of anorexia are similar to starvation. When the body attempts to protect its most vital organs, the heart and the brain, it goes into "slow gear." Monthly menstrual periods stop, and breathing, pulse, blood pressure, and thyroid function slow down. The nails and hair become brittle, and the skin dries. Water imbalance causes constipation, and the lack of body fat causes an inability to withstand cold temperatures. Depression, weakness, and a constant obsession with food are also symptoms of the disease. In addition, personality changes may occur. The victim may have outbursts of anger and hostility or may withdraw socially. In the most serious cases, death can result.

Bulimia

The person who is bulimic eats compulsively and then purges (gets rid of the food) through self-induced vomiting, use of laxatives, diuretics, strict diets, fasts, exercise, or a combination of the above. Bulimia often begins when a young person is disgusted with the amount of "bad" food he or she has just eaten and vomits to rid the body of the calories. NIMH estimated that half of those with anorexia will turn to binge eating and purging.

Many bulimics are at a normal body weight or above due to their frequent binge-purge behavior, which can occur from once or twice a week to several times a day. In fact, a bulimic who maintains a normal weight can manage to keep his or her eating disorder a secret for years. As with anorexia, bulimia usually begins during the teen years, but many bulimics do not seek help until they are in their thirties or forties.

Binge eating and purging is dangerous. In rare cases, bingeing can cause stomach ruptures, or purging can result in heart failure because the body loses vital minerals. The acid in vomit wears down the teeth and the stomach lining and can cause scarring on the hands when fingers are pushed down the throat to induce vomiting. The esophagus becomes inflamed, and glands in the neck become swollen.

Bulimics often talk of being "hooked" on certain foods and needing to feed their "habit." This addictive behavior carries over into other areas of their lives, including alcohol and drug abuse. Many bulimic people suffer from severe depression, which increases their risk for suicide.

Causes of Eating Disorders

Bulimics and anorexics seem to have different personalities. Bulimics are likely to be impulsive (acting without thought of the consequences) and are more likely to abuse alcohol and drugs. Anorexics tend to be perfectionists, good students, and good athletes. They usually keep their feelings to themselves and rarely disobey their parents. Bulimics and anorexics share certain traits: they lack self-esteem, have feelings of helplessness, and fear gaining weight. In both disorders, the eating problems appear to develop as a way of handling stress and anxiety.

The bulimic consumes huge amounts of food (often junk food) in a search for comfort and stress relief. The bingeing, however, brings only guilt and depression. On the other hand, the anorexic restricts food to gain a sense of control in some part of her life. Controlling her weight seems to offer two advantages—she can take control of her body, and she can gain approval from others.

Demographics of Eating Disorders

Individuals with eating disorders usually come from white middle- or upper-class families. NIMH noted that while eating disorders have increased substantially in industrialized countries during the past 20 years, they are almost unheard of in Third World countries. Thinness is not necessarily admired among all people throughout the world, especially in those places where hunger is not a matter of choice.

Treatment of Eating Disorders

Many anorexics tend to deny their illness, and getting and keeping the anorexic patient in treatment can be difficult. Treating bulimia is also not easy. Many bulimics are easily frustrated and want to leave treatment if their symptoms are not quickly relieved.

A physician treats the medical complications of the disease, while a nutritionist advises on specific diet and eating plans. To help the patient face his or her underlying problems and emotional issues, psychotherapy is usually necessary. Group therapy has been found helpful for bulimics, who are relieved to find that they are not alone or unique in their binge-eating behavior. A combination of behavioral therapy and family therapy is often the most effective with anorexics. If the patient also suffers from depression, antidepressants are often prescribed.

A long-term study (approximately 11.5 years) of 173 young women diagnosed with bulimia reiterated the strong hold eating disorders have on their victims (P. K. Keel, et al., "Long-Term Outcome of Bulimia Nervosa," *Archives of General Psychiatry,* vol. 56, January 1999). At the final follow-up, 30 percent of the patients still showed symptoms of eating disorders. Eighteen percent were diagnosed with "eating disorder not otherwise specified," 11 percent with bulimia nervosa, and 1 percent with anorexia nervosa.

Of the 70 percent who were in remission, one-third had achieved only partial remission. Patients who had longer periods of symptoms before beginning treatment and those who had a history of substance abuse were less likely to be successful.

SUICIDE

Suicide can be the ultimate consequence of depression. Not all victims of depression, however, contemplate suicide, nor do all those who attempt suicide suffer from depressive illnesses. In 1998 suicide ranked as the eighth-leading cause of death in the United States—the 29,264 suicides reported that year accounted for 1.2 percent of total deaths. The death rate for suicide for all ages and races was 10.4 per 100,000 population. (See Table 11.4 and Table 1.10 in Chapter 1.)

Who Commits Suicide?

Suicide occurs among all age, sex, racial, occupational, religious, and social groups. Table 11.4 lists the suicide death rates by age, sex, and race/ethnicity from 1950 to 1998. While the overall rate of suicide has remained fairly stable, the rate nearly tripled from 1950 to 1998 among adolescents and young adults. In 1998, among children aged 5 to 14, suicide was the fifth-most-common cause of death; for those between 15 and 24 years of age, it was the third-leading cause of death.

Usually, suicide attempts outnumber completed suicides by about eight to one. Among teens, however, the ratio is 25 to 30 attempts for every successful suicide. According to NIMH, approximately 1 million teens go through "suicide crises" each year.

While four times as many women as men attempt suicide, the overwhelming majority of completed suicides are male. Men make up about three-fourths of total suicides, and white males account for about 70 percent of that number. Men use more deadly weapons than women—over half shoot themselves, and the use of guns is increasing rapidly. In the younger age brackets for women (ages 15 to 24), however, over half who completed a suicide used a gun.

In 1998 the suicide rate for white males (18.3 per 100,000 population) was almost double that for black males (10.5 per 100,000). The highest level was among American Indian/Alaska Native males, who committed suicide at a rate of 21.4 per 100,000. Between 1950 and 1998, suicide rates among young (15 to 24 years old) white and black men increased dramatically—from 6.6 to 19.3 per 100,000 population for whites, and from 4.9 to 15 per 100,000 population for blacks. The highest rate in that age group, again, was among American Indian and Alaska Native males, who committed suicide at a rate of 41.8 per 100,000. (See Table 11.4.)

In 1998, among older white males, the suicide rate was far higher than for any other racial groups. White males aged 65 and older had death rates (36.6 per 100,000) from suicide three times higher than the rates for black males (11.6 per 100,000). For those aged 85 and over, white men committed suicide at a rate of 62.7 per 100,000 population, while among black men of the same age, the rate was statistically indeterminate (fewer than 20 deaths). For white males, suicide rates increased dramatically from age 65 on. The rates for black men, on the

TABLE 11.4

Death rates for suicide, according to sex, detailed race, Hispanic origin, and age: selected years 1950–98

[Data are based on the National Vital Statistics System]

Sex, race, Hispanic origin, and age	1950[1]	1960[1]	1970	1980	1985	1990	1995	1996	1997	1998	1996–98[2]
All persons					Deaths per 100,000 resident population						
All ages, age adjusted	11.0	10.6	11.8	11.4	11.5	11.5	11.2	10.8	10.6	10.4	10.6
All ages, crude	11.4	10.6	11.6	11.9	12.4	12.4	11.9	11.6	11.4	11.3	11.5
Under 1 year	...	...	...	...	...	...	...	...	...	...	...
1–4 years	...	...	...	...	...	...	...	...	...	...	...
5–14 years	0.2	0.3	0.3	0.4	0.8	0.8	0.9	0.8	0.8	0.8	0.8
15–24 years	4.5	5.2	8.8	12.3	12.8	13.2	13.3	12.0	11.4	11.1	11.5
25–44 years	11.6	12.2	15.4	15.6	15.0	15.2	15.3	15.0	14.8	14.6	14.8
25–34 years	9.1	10.0	14.1	16.0	15.3	15.2	15.4	14.5	14.3	13.8	14.2
35–44 years	14.3	14.2	16.9	15.4	14.6	15.3	15.2	15.5	15.3	15.4	15.4
45–64 years	23.5	22.0	20.6	15.9	16.3	15.3	14.1	14.4	14.2	14.1	14.3
45–54 years	20.9	20.7	20.0	15.9	15.7	14.8	14.6	14.9	14.7	14.8	14.8
55–64 years	27.0	23.7	21.4	15.9	16.8	16.0	13.3	13.7	13.5	13.1	13.4
65 years and over	30.0	24.5	20.8	17.6	20.4	20.5	18.1	17.3	16.8	16.9	17.0
65–74 years	29.3	23.0	20.8	16.9	18.7	17.9	15.8	15.0	14.4	14.1	14.5
75–84 years	31.1	27.9	21.2	19.1	23.9	24.9	20.7	20.0	19.3	19.7	19.7
85 years and over	28.8	26.0	19.0	19.2	19.4	22.2	21.6	20.2	20.8	21.0	20.7
Male											
All ages, age adjusted	17.3	16.6	17.3	18.0	18.8	19.0	18.6	18.0	17.4	17.2	17.5
All ages, crude	17.8	16.5	16.8	18.6	20.0	20.4	19.8	19.3	18.7	18.6	18.8
Under 1 year	...	...	...	...	...	...	...	...	...	...	...
1–4 years	...	...	...	...	...	...	...	...	...	...	...
5–14 years	0.3	0.4	0.5	0.6	1.2	1.1	1.3	1.1	1.2	1.2	1.2
15–24 years	6.5	8.2	13.5	20.2	21.0	22.0	22.5	20.0	18.9	18.5	19.2
25–44 years	17.2	17.9	20.9	24.0	23.7	24.4	24.9	24.3	23.8	23.5	23.8
25–34 years	13.4	14.7	19.8	25.0	24.7	24.8	25.6	24.0	23.6	22.9	23.5
35–44 years	21.3	21.0	22.1	22.5	22.3	23.9	24.1	24.6	23.9	24.0	24.1
45–64 years	37.1	34.4	30.0	23.7	25.3	24.3	22.5	23.0	22.5	22.4	22.6
45–54 years	32.0	31.6	27.9	22.9	23.6	23.2	22.8	23.3	22.5	23.1	22.9
55–64 years	43.6	38.1	32.7	24.5	27.1	25.7	22.0	22.7	22.4	21.3	22.1
65 years and over	52.8	44.0	38.4	35.0	40.9	41.6	36.3	35.2	33.9	34.1	34.4
65–74 years	50.5	39.6	36.0	30.4	33.9	32.2	28.7	27.7	26.4	26.2	26.8
75–84 years	58.3	52.5	42.8	42.3	53.1	56.1	44.8	43.4	40.9	42.0	42.1
85 years and over	58.3	57.4	42.4	50.6	56.2	65.9	63.1	59.9	60.3	57.8	59.3
Female											
All ages, age adjusted	4.9	5.0	6.8	5.4	4.9	4.5	4.1	4.0	4.1	4.0	4.1
All ages, crude	5.1	4.9	6.6	5.5	5.2	4.8	4.4	4.4	4.4	4.4	4.4
Under 1 year	...	...	...	...	...	...	...	...	...	...	...
1–4 years	...	...	...	...	...	...	...	...	...	...	...
5–14 years	0.1	0.1	0.2	0.2	0.4	0.4	0.4	0.4	0.4	0.4	0.4
15–24 years	2.6	2.2	4.2	4.3	4.3	3.9	3.7	3.6	3.5	3.3	3.5
25–44 years	6.2	6.6	10.2	7.7	6.5	6.2	5.8	5.8	6.0	6.0	5.9
25–34 years	4.9	5.5	8.6	7.1	5.9	5.6	5.2	5.0	5.0	4.9	5.0
35–44 years	7.5	7.7	11.9	8.5	7.1	6.8	6.5	6.6	6.8	6.9	6.8
45–64 years	9.9	10.2	12.0	8.9	8.0	7.1	6.1	6.4	6.5	6.4	6.4
45–54 years	9.9	10.2	12.6	9.4	8.3	6.9	6.7	7.0	7.3	7.0	7.1
55–64 years	9.9	10.2	11.4	8.4	7.8	7.3	5.3	5.5	5.4	5.5	5.5
65 years and over	9.4	8.4	8.1	6.1	6.6	6.4	5.5	4.8	4.9	4.7	4.8
65–74 years	10.1	8.4	9.0	6.5	6.9	6.7	5.4	4.8	4.7	4.3	4.6
75–84 years	8.1	8.9	7.0	5.5	6.7	6.3	5.5	5.0	5.2	4.9	5.0
85 years and over	8.2	6.0	5.9	5.5	4.7	5.4	5.5	4.4	4.9	5.8	5.0
White male											
All ages, age adjusted	18.1	17.5	18.2	18.9	19.9	20.1	19.7	19.1	18.4	18.3	18.6
All ages, crude	19.0	17.6	18.0	19.9	21.6	22.0	21.4	20.9	20.2	20.3	20.5
15–24 years	6.6	8.6	13.9	21.4	22.3	23.2	23.5	20.9	19.5	19.3	19.9
25–44 years	17.9	18.5	21.5	24.6	24.8	25.4	26.3	25.7	25.3	25.2	25.4
45–64 years	39.3	36.5	31.9	25.0	27.0	26.0	24.2	24.9	24.2	24.2	24.4
65 years and over	55.8	46.7	41.1	37.2	43.7	44.2	38.7	37.8	36.1	36.6	36.8
65–74 years	53.2	42.0	38.7	32.5	35.8	34.2	30.3	29.6	28.0	27.9	28.5
75–84 years	61.9	55.7	45.5	45.5	57.0	60.2	47.5	46.1	43.4	44.7	44.7
85 years and over	61.9	61.3	45.8	52.8	60.9	70.3	68.2	65.4	65.0	62.7	64.3

other hand, showed virtually no increase in their later years. (See Table 11.4.)

For white and black women, the suicide rates were far lower than those for men in all age groups. The death rate from suicide for white women was 4.4 per 100,000 in 1998, and for black women the rate was less than half that at 1.8 per 100,000. Young white women aged 15 to 24 had a suicide rate (3.5 per 100,000) about one-sixth the rate for white men (19.3 per 100,000) in the same age group. For black women of all

TABLE 11.4

Death rates for suicide, according to sex, detailed race, Hispanic origin, and age: selected years 1950–98 [CONTINUED]

[Data are based on the National Vital Statistics System]

Sex, race, Hispanic origin, and age	1950[1]	1960[1]	1970	1980	1985	1990	1995	1996	1997	1998	1996–98[2]
					Deaths per 100,000 resident population						
Black male											
All ages, age adjusted	7.0	7.8	9.9	11.1	11.5	12.4	12.4	11.8	11.2	10.5	11.2
All ages, crude	6.3	6.4	8.0	10.3	11.0	12.0	11.9	11.4	10.9	10.2	10.8
15–24 years	4.9	4.1	10.5	12.3	13.3	15.1	18.0	16.7	16.0	15.0	15.9
25–44 years	9.8	12.6	16.1	19.2	17.8	19.6	18.6	17.8	17.0	15.2	16.7
45–64 years	12.7	13.0	12.4	11.8	12.9	13.1	11.8	11.8	10.5	11.1	11.1
65 years and over	9.0	9.9	8.7	11.4	15.8	14.9	14.3	12.6	13.6	11.6	12.6
65–74 years	10.0	11.3	8.7	11.1	16.7	14.7	13.5	12.7	12.9	11.4	12.4
75–84 years	---	6.6	8.9	10.5	15.6	14.4	16.6	12.5	14.1	12.5	13.0
85 years and over	---	6.9	*	*	*	*	*	*	*	*	13.1
American Indian or Alaska Native male[3]											
All ages, age adjusted	---	---	---	20.8	19.9	21.0	20.1	20.0	21.3	21.4	20.9
All ages, crude	---	---	---	20.9	20.3	20.9	19.6	19.9	20.9	21.1	20.6
15–24 years	---	---	---	45.3	42.0	49.1	34.2	32.1	38.4	41.8	37.5
25–44 years	---	---	---	31.2	30.2	27.8	31.8	34.8	32.6	33.3	33.5
45–64 years	---	---	---	*	*	*	15.0	11.5	15.5	11.3	12.8
65 years and over	---	---	---	*	*	*	*	*	*	*	14.0
Asian or Pacific Islander male[4]											
All ages, age adjusted	---	---	---	9.0	8.5	8.8	9.7	8.6	9.4	9.1	9.1
All ages, crude	---	---	---	8.8	8.4	8.7	9.4	8.6	9.2	9.1	9.0
15–24 years	---	---	---	10.8	14.2	13.5	16.0	11.9	12.2	10.9	11.7
25–44 years	---	---	---	11.0	9.3	10.6	11.5	11.5	10.6	11.9	11.3
45–64 years	---	---	---	13.0	10.4	9.7	9.1	8.6	12.3	10.2	10.4
65 years and over	---	---	---	18.6	16.7	16.8	20.3	16.0	21.0	21.0	19.4
Hispanic male[5]											
All ages, age adjusted	---	---	---	---	10.4	12.4	12.3	11.1	10.4	10.1	10.5
All ages, crude	---	---	---	---	9.8	11.4	11.5	10.6	9.8	9.4	9.9
15–24 years	---	---	---	---	13.8	14.7	18.3	15.5	14.4	13.4	14.4
25–44 years	---	---	---	---	14.8	16.2	15.5	14.6	13.9	13.0	13.8
45–64 years	---	---	---	---	12.3	16.1	14.2	13.3	11.6	11.5	12.1
65 years and over	---	---	---	---	14.7	23.4	19.9	17.7	17.7	20.0	18.5
White, non-Hispanic male[5]											
All ages, age adjusted	---	---	---	---	20.3	20.8	20.2	19.7	19.3	19.2	19.4
All ages, crude	---	---	---	---	22.3	23.1	22.3	22.0	21.5	21.6	21.7
15–24 years	---	---	---	---	22.6	24.4	23.8	21.4	20.2	20.2	20.6
25–44 years	---	---	---	---	25.1	26.4	27.3	27.1	26.8	26.7	26.9
45–64 years	---	---	---	---	27.3	26.8	24.8	25.6	25.1	25.1	25.2
65 years and over	---	---	---	---	46.4	45.4	39.2	38.6	36.8	37.3	37.5
White female											
All ages, age adjusted	5.3	5.3	7.2	5.7	5.3	4.8	4.4	4.4	4.4	4.4	4.4
All ages, crude	5.5	5.3	7.1	5.9	5.6	5.3	4.8	4.8	4.9	4.8	4.8
15–24 years	2.7	2.3	4.2	4.6	4.7	4.2	3.9	3.8	3.7	3.5	3.6
25–44 years	6.6	7.0	11.0	8.1	7.0	6.6	6.3	6.4	6.6	6.6	6.5
45–64 years	10.6	10.9	13.0	9.6	8.7	7.7	6.7	7.0	7.2	7.1	7.1
65 years and over	9.9	8.8	8.5	6.4	6.9	6.8	5.7	5.0	5.1	5.0	5.0

ages, the rate (1.8 per 100,000) was about one-sixth the black male rate (10.5 per 100,000). (See Table 11.4.)

In contrast to men, female suicide rates change very little as women age. Black women 65 years and older had a suicide rate of 1.2 per 100,000, compared to 11.6 per 100,000 black men. For white women age 65 and older, the rate was 5 per 100,000 in 1998, compared to the white male rate of 36.6 per 100,000. (See Table 11.4.) One generally held theory about the very high rates among white men over age 75 is that these men, who have traditionally been in positions of power, have great difficulty adjusting to a life they may consider useless or diminished.

Other minority groups showed similar disparities between the suicide rates of women and men in 1998.

American Indian/Alaska Native males (21.4 per 100,000) had a suicide rate almost four times that of American Indian/Alaska Native females (5.6 per 100,000). The suicide rate for Asian/Pacific Islander men was 9.1 per 100,000, while the rate for Asian/Pacific Islander women was 3.1 per 100,000. While Hispanic males had a rate of 10.1 per 100,000, Hispanic females (1.9 per 100,000), along with black females (1.8 per 100,000), had the lowest suicide rates. (See Table 11.4.)

Why Do People Commit Suicide?

There are many reasons for committing suicide. Notes left by people who have killed themselves usually tell of unbearable life crises. Many describe what it is like to endure chronic pain, to lose loved ones, to be unable to

TABLE 11.4

Death rates for suicide, according to sex, detailed race, Hispanic origin, and age: selected years 1950–98 [CONTINUED]

[Data are based on the National Vital Statistics System]

Sex, race, Hispanic origin, and age	1950[1]	1960[1]	1970	1980	1985	1990	1995	1996	1997	1998	1996–98[2]
Black female					Deaths per 100,000 resident population						
All ages, age adjusted	1.7	1.9	2.9	2.4	2.1	2.4	2.0	2.0	1.9	1.8	1.9
All ages, crude	1.5	1.6	2.6	2.2	2.1	2.3	2.0	2.0	1.9	1.8	1.9
15–24 years	1.8	*	3.8	2.3	2.0	2.3	2.2	2.3	2.4	2.2	2.3
25–44 years	2.3	3.0	4.8	4.3	3.2	3.8	3.4	2.9	2.7	2.7	2.8
45–64 years	2.7	3.1	2.9	2.5	2.8	2.9	2.0	2.3	2.4	2.2	2.3
65 years and over	2.0	1.9	2.6	*	2.7	1.9	2.2	2.1	1.6	1.2	1.6
American Indian or Alaska Native female[3]											
All ages, age adjusted	- - -	- - -	- - -	5.0	4.4	3.8	4.4	5.9	4.4	5.6	5.3
All ages, crude	- - -	- - -	- - -	4.7	4.4	3.7	4.2	5.6	4.2	5.4	5.1
15–24 years	- - -	- - -	- - -	*	*	*	*	10.2	*	*	8.3
25–44 years	- - -	- - -	- - -	10.7	*	*	7.1	9.0	6.4	8.0	7.8
45–64 years	- - -	- - -	- - -	*	*	*	*	*	*	*	5.6
65 years and over	- - -	- - -	- - -	*	*	*	*	*	*	*	*
Asian or Pacific Islander female[4]											
All ages, age adjusted	- - -	- - -	- - -	4.7	4.4	3.4	3.7	3.6	3.4	3.1	3.3
All ages, crude	- - -	- - -	- - -	4.7	4.3	3.4	3.8	3.7	3.6	3.3	3.5
15–24 years	- - -	- - -	- - -	*	5.8	3.9	5.2	3.0	4.7	2.7	3.5
25–44 years	- - -	- - -	- - -	5.4	4.2	3.8	3.8	4.5	3.7	4.0	4.1
45–64 years	- - -	- - -	- - -	7.9	5.4	5.0	4.9	5.2	4.4	4.3	4.6
65 years and over	- - -	- - -	- - -	*	13.6	8.5	9.0	8.4	8.9	7.2	8.1
Hispanic female[5]											
All ages, age adjusted	- - -	- - -	- - -	- - -	1.8	2.3	2.0	2.2	1.7	1.9	1.9
All ages, crude	- - -	- - -	- - -	- - -	1.6	2.2	1.9	2.1	1.6	1.8	1.8
15–24 years	- - -	- - -	- - -	- - -	2.1	3.1	2.6	3.3	2.4	2.8	2.8
25–44 years	- - -	- - -	- - -	- - -	2.1	3.1	2.7	2.8	2.2	2.2	2.4
45–64 years	- - -	- - -	- - -	- - -	3.2	2.5	2.7	2.6	2.3	2.7	2.5
65 years and over	- - -	- - -	- - -	- - -	*	*	*	2.5	*	2.5	2.3
White, non-Hispanic female[5]											
All ages, age adjusted	- - -	- - -	- - -	- - -	5.7	5.0	4.6	4.5	4.7	4.6	4.7
All ages, crude	- - -	- - -	- - -	- - -	6.2	5.6	5.1	5.0	5.3	5.2	5.2
15–24 years	- - -	- - -	- - -	- - -	4.7	4.3	4.0	3.8	3.9	3.6	3.8
25–44 years	- - -	- - -	- - -	- - -	7.7	7.0	6.7	6.7	7.2	7.2	7.0
45–64 years	- - -	- - -	- - -	- - -	9.2	8.0	7.0	7.3	7.6	7.4	7.4
65 years and over	- - -	- - -	- - -	- - -	7.5	7.0	5.8	5.1	5.2	5.2	5.2

. . . Category not applicable.
- - - Data not available.
* Based on fewer than 20 deaths.
[1] Includes deaths of persons who were not residents of the 50 States and the District of Columbia.
[2] Average annual death rate.
[3] Interpretation of trends should take into account that population estimates for American Indians increased by 45 percent between 1980 and 1990, partly due to better enumeration techniques in the 1990 decennial census and to the increased tendency for people to identify themselves as American Indian in 1990.
[4] Interpretation of trends should take into account that the Asian population in the United States more than doubled between 1980 and 1990, primarily due to immigration.
[5] Excludes data from States lacking an Hispanic-origin item on their death certificates.

Notes: Rates are age adjusted to the 1940 U.S. standard million population. Age groups chosen to show data for American Indians, Asians, Hispanics, and non-Hispanic whites were selected to minimize the presentation of unstable age-specific death rates based on small numbers of deaths and for consistency among comparison groups. The race groups, white, black, Asian or Pacific Islander, and American Indian or Alaska Native, include persons of Hispanic and non-Hispanic origin. Conversely, persons of Hispanic origin may be of any race. Bias in death rates results from inconsistent race identification between the death certificate (source of data for numerator of death rates) and data from the Census Bureau (denominator); and from undercounts of some population groups in the census. The net effects of misclassification and under coverage result in death rates estimated to be overstated by 1 percent for the white population and 5 percent for the black population; and death rates estimated to be understated by 21 percent for American Indians, 11 percent for Asians, and 2 percent for Hispanics (Rosenberg HM, Maurer JD, Sorlie PD, Johnson NJ, et al. Quality of death rates by race and Hispanic origin: A summary of current research, 1999. National Center for Health Statistics. Vital Health Stat 2(128). 1999).

SOURCE: *Health, United States, 2000*, National Center for Health Statistics, Hyattsville, MD, 2000

pay bills, or to be incapable of living independently. Other commonly cited reasons are:

- To punish loved ones.
- To gain attention.
- To join a deceased loved one.
- To avoid punishment.
- To express love.

Some suicides are committed on an irrational, impulsive whim. Suicide researchers note that even among those most determined to end their lives, the desire is not as much to die as it is to escape the lives they are leading and the pain they are suffering. Whatever the cause of their despair, many are desperately crying for help.

Follow-up studies on suicide survivors reveal their intense ambivalence about actually dying. Not all the survivors are glad to be alive, but for most, the attempted suicide marked a definite turning point. It was an urgent and dramatic signal that their problems demanded serious and quick attention. Most of the survivors said that what they really wanted was to change their lives.

Suicide among the Terminally Ill

Not all suicides are categorized as the acts of mentally ill persons. Some people consider suicides committed by terminally ill people as rational acts. Many people believe that a terminally ill person has a right to choose his or her own death. Until a few years ago, persons with cancer and AIDS were, of the terminally ill, the most likely to commit suicide. Patients with terminal disease often worry that they will suffer long and painful deaths, and that they stand a good chance of losing everything—health, independence, jobs, insurance, homes, contact with loved ones and friends.

Researchers have found that factors that have an impact on the quality of life include security, family, love, pleasurable activity, and freedom from pain and suffering. Sufferers of debilitating disease may lose all of these. For some, suicide is an apparently attractive alternative that relieves pain and suffering, insecurity, self-pity, dependence, and hopelessness.

Suicide's Warning Signs

Researchers believe that most suicidal people convey their intentions to someone among their friends and family—either openly or indirectly. The people they signal are those who know them well and are in the best position to recognize the signs and give help. Comments such as "You'd be better off without me," "No one will have to worry about me much longer," or a casual "I've had it" can be signals of upcoming attempts. Some suicidal persons put their affairs in order. They draw up wills, give away prized possessions, or act as if they are preparing for a long trip. They may even talk about going away.

Often the indicator is a distinct change in personality or behavior. A normally happy person may become increasingly depressed. A regular churchgoer may stop attending services, or an avid runner may quit exercising. These types of changes, if added to expressions of worthlessness or hopelessness, can indicate not only that the person is seriously depressed but also that he or she may have decided on a suicide attempt. While the vast majority of depressed people are not suicidal, most of the suicide-prone are depressed.

People who have a record of previous suicide attempts are at the highest risk of actually killing themselves—over six hundred times higher than the rate for the general population. Between 20 to 50 percent of those who complete suicide have tried it before.

CHAPTER 12
HEALTH PROMOTION AND DISEASE PREVENTION

This chapter contains a number of surveys concerning personal nutrition and health care. Surveys on these topics are generally considered less accurate than surveys dealing with impersonal matters, since respondents in personal surveys often give the answer that they believe is expected of them or that reflects what they *should* be doing. Therefore, it is best to use these surveys as indicators rather than as statistical truth.

SELF-CARE

While Americans have traditionally cared for themselves with treatments ranging from cod-liver oil to vitamin E to chicken soup, many Americans are taking an even greater responsibility for their own health and wellness. They are trying to contribute to their own disease prevention through diet and lifestyle changes. In addition, more people are trying to treat themselves for minor health problems before calling a doctor.

Various demographic changes are promoting this focus on health and wellness, including an aging population. In 1998 baby boomers (ages 34–52) accounted for nearly 80 million adults—approximately 40 percent of the adult U.S. population. Baby boomers will be the most educated older generation in American history, and the most interested in the aging process. Simultaneously, the nation's health care system is changing, and there is more health care information available to the public than ever before.

Today, Americans are better informed about the relationship between good health and proper diet. In 1998 *Prevention Magazine,* well known for its recommendations for healthful living, along with the Food Marketing Institute, published *A Look at the Self-Care Movement: A Shopping for Health Report* (Rodale Press, Emmaus, PA, 1998), which looked at the ways Americans try to maintain good health on their own. The survey, conducted in March 1998, was based upon telephone interviews with 1,008 adults who had primary or shared responsibility for

the household's food shopping and had shopped in the two-week period prior to the survey. Table 12.1 gives the demographics of the survey participants.

TABLE 12.1

Demographics of survey participants

	Total Shoppers
Base size:	1,000
Gender	
Female	68%
Male	32%
Age	
18-24	7 %
25-39	32%
40-49	24%
50-64	24%
65+	13%
Working women	43%
Household composition	
1 Adult in household	26%
2+ Adults in household	74%
Marital Status	
Married	62%
Single, never married	14%
All others	24%
Education	
H.S. graduate or less	44%
Any college	22%
College graduate+	33%
Race	
White	83%
Black	9%
Other	8%
Household income	
Less than $35,000	47%
$35,000-$49,999	21%
$50,000+	32%
Region	
Northeast	20%
North Central	24%
South	35%
West	21%

SOURCE: *A Look at the Self-Care Movement: A Shopping for Health Report, 1998,* Food Marketing Insititute and PREVENTION Magazine, Rodale Press, Inc., Emmaus, PA, 1998

FIGURE 12.1

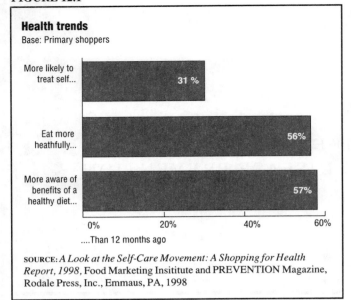

Health trends
Base: Primary shoppers

SOURCE: *A Look at the Self-Care Movement: A Shopping for Health Report, 1998,* Food Marketing Insititute and PREVENTION Magazine, Rodale Press, Inc., Emmaus, PA, 1998

FIGURE 12.2

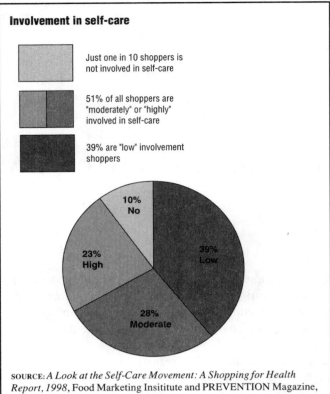

Involvement in self-care

Just one in 10 shoppers is not involved in self-care

51% of all shoppers are "moderately" or "highly" involved in self-care

39% are "low" involvement shoppers

SOURCE: *A Look at the Self-Care Movement: A Shopping for Health Report, 1998,* Food Marketing Insititute and PREVENTION Magazine, Rodale Press, Inc., Emmaus, PA, 1998

More than half (57 percent) of those surveyed claimed that they were more aware of the benefits of a good diet than they were the year before. About the same proportion of respondents (56 percent) also said they were eating more healthily. Nearly one in three survey participants (31 percent) was more likely to attempt to self-treat before consulting a doctor for minor health problems than he or she was 12 months before. (See Figure 12.1.)

Just over half (51 percent) of survey respondents claimed they were moderately or highly involved in self-care by making educated purchases, while just less than half (49 percent) had little or no involvement in self-care. (See Figure 12.2.) In addition, half of all respondents reported they actively sought information about diet, nutrition, and disease prevention. Most of those consumers said that health care professionals and magazines were their favorite sources for health information.

Health Awareness

Nearly 90 percent of survey respondents believed that eating healthily can greatly reduce the risk of contracting some diseases, and most of them reported eating more healthily than they did the year before. Awareness of the benefits of a good diet, however, differed by generation. Two-thirds (66 percent) of Generation Xers (those between the ages of 18 and 33) and 57 percent of baby boomers, but only 49 percent of those over the age of 53, said they were more aware of the benefits of a good diet.

Nutrition

Well-balanced meals are essential to every person's health. The food guide pyramid (Figure 12.3) is the U.S. Department of Agriculture's guide to the recommended portions of different types of food in American diets. A healthful diet is especially important for children. Growing children

need good nourishment to develop properly. Furthermore, lifetime eating habits are determined, in many cases, by diets developed in childhood. According to the Centers for Disease Control and Prevention (CDC), the typical diet of American children and adolescents is too high in fat, saturated fat, and sodium, and too low in fruits, vegetables, and calcium ("Guidelines for School Health Programs to Promote Lifelong Healthy Eating," supplement to *Morbidity and Mortality Weekly Report,* Vol. 45, No. RR-9, June 14, 1996).

Children and adolescents, on average, obtain 33–35 percent of their calories from fat and 12–13 percent from saturated fat (somewhat above the recommended levels of 30 percent and 10 percent, respectively). In the 1997 CDC *Youth Risk Behavior Surveillance—United States,* high school students were asked what they had eaten the day before the survey. Their responses showed that only 29.3 percent had eaten the recommended five servings of fruits and vegetables the day before the survey. Another study, reported in "Adolescents' Views on Food and Nutrition" (M. Story and M. D. Resnick, *Journal of Nutritional Education,* Vol. 18, No. 4, 1986), indicated that teenagers were well informed about nutrition but did not use their knowledge to make healthful food choices.

KEYS TO PREVENTION—DIET AND EXERCISE

The CDC stated that a combination of poor diet and inadequate physical exercise accounts for a minimum of

300,000 deaths in the United States each year ("Guidelines for School Health Programs to Promote Lifelong Healthy Eating"; see above). The diet- and exercise-related risk factors for coronary heart disease, the nation's number-one killer, are high cholesterol, high blood pressure, and obesity (although a person can exercise and still be obese). The CDC estimated that deaths from cancer, the number-two killer, could be reduced by 35 percent by changing dietary habits. Stroke, the third-leading cause of death, and diabetes, the seventh-leading cause, also have strong diet-related risk factors.

The CDC, in its *Third National Health and Nutrition Examination Survey,* conducted between 1988 and 1994, found that 13.7 percent of children, 11.5 percent of adolescents, and 34.9 percent of adults were overweight. ("Overweight" means about 124 percent of desirable weight for men, and 120 percent for women.) Diet modification alone is not enough for an effective weight-control strategy. Regular physical activity must be part of one's daily lifestyle.

In a survey of American adults attempting to lose weight, 33.3 percent of overweight men and 37.8 percent of overweight women reported that they did not participate in any leisure-time physical activity as part of their weight-loss program. Only 22.2 percent of men and 19 percent of women exercised the recommended 30 minutes or more, five or more times a week. The older and more overweight survey participants reported less physical activity than did the younger and less overweight participants. The less educated reported less physical activity during leisure time than those with more education. Those who lived in the southern United States were less likely to engage in physical activity than were those from other regions. Hispanics were also less likely than whites or blacks to report physical activity. (See Table 12.2.)

TAKING CONTROL

Approximately 80 percent of consumers surveyed for *Prevention Magazine*'s 1998 *Shopping for Health* report said their purchasing decisions were at least partially influenced by a desire to prevent or manage a specific health condition on their own, or to follow a doctor's advice. In particular, they wanted to control high cholesterol, hypertension, obesity, heart disease, and diabetes. Over half (52 percent) said they were trying to prevent the risk of developing one or more specific health conditions. The three conditions cited most often were heart disease, high cholesterol, and high blood pressure. (See Table 12.3.)

Most Americans rely on their own best judgment when it comes to dealing with everyday health problems. In a 1997 joint survey conducted by *Prevention Magazine* and the American Pharmaceutical Association, respondents were asked what they would do first if they had each

FIGURE 12.3

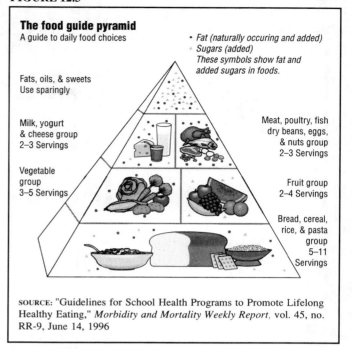

The food guide pyramid
A guide to daily food choices

• *Fat (naturally occuring and added)*
▲ *Sugars (added)*
These symbols show fat and added sugars in foods.

Fats, oils, & sweets
Use sparingly

Milk, yogurt & cheese group
2–3 Servings

Vegetable group
3–5 Servings

Meat, poultry, fish dry beans, eggs, & nuts group
2–3 Servings

Fruit group
2–4 Servings

Bread, cereal, rice, & pasta group
5–11 Servings

SOURCE: "Guidelines for School Health Programs to Promote Lifelong Healthy Eating," *Morbidity and Mortality Weekly Report,* vol. 45, no. RR-9, June 14, 1996

of 12 different symptoms and/or conditions. Most respondents said they would self-treat first for headaches (80 percent), stomach upset (76 percent), diarrhea (75 percent), cold or cough (73 percent), fever (71 percent), menstrual cramps (69 percent), and muscle or joint pain (59 percent). Survey participants said that for more serious conditions, such as chest pain (78 percent), toothaches (63 percent), and yeast infections (48 percent), they would talk to a doctor first. (See Table 12.4.)

Products Used to Maintain Health

Consumers use many products to maintain their health. A large majority of survey respondents (85 percent) said they used over-the-counter medicines, prescription medication (71 percent), and vitamin and mineral supplements (67 percent). Better than one in four respondents (28 percent) said they used herbal remedies. College graduates were more likely than high school graduates to use alternative care products (vitamins and minerals, herbal remedies, and homeopathic remedies). Those earning over $50,000 were more likely to use alternative care products than those who earned less than $50,000, and baby boomers (ages 34–52) were more likely to use alternative care products than either Generation Xers (ages 18–33) or "Matures" (53 and older). Generation Xers were more apt to turn to aromatherapies, and Matures used more in-home diagnostic tests. (See Table 12.5.)

RISK FACTORS

Smoking and Tobacco Use

The proportion of adults who smoked cigarettes declined from 42 percent in a 1965 survey to 24 percent in

TABLE 12.2

Leisure-time physical activity patterns among overweight adults trying to lose weight, by selected characteristics, 1998

Characteristic	Men					Women				
	Sample size	% using physical activity to lose weight	(95% CI*)	% meeting physical activity guidelines†	(95% CI)	Sample size	% using physical activity to lose weight	(95% CI)	% meeting physical activity guidelines	(95% CI)
Age (yrs)										
18–24	903	83.8	(80.3–87.3)	25.7	(21.6–29.8)	1,294	77.5	(73.4–81.6)	20.3	(16.8–23.8)
25–34	2,570	76.7	(74.4–79.1)	22.5	(20.0–25.1)	3,790	72.0	(69.8–74.2)	20.4	(18.4–22.4)
35–44	3,685	68.2	(65.7–70.8)	18.8	(16.8–20.8)	5,173	65.5	(63.3–67.7)	18.6	(16.8–20.4)
45–54	3,499	63.0	(60.5–65.6)	21.0	(18.8–23.2)	4,391	62.1	(59.8–64.5)	18.4	(16.6–20.2)
55–64	2,256	57.2	(54.1–60.3)	23.8	(21.1–26.5)	3,183	55.4	(52.7–58.1)	18.3	(16.1–20.5)
≥65	2,120	55.1	(51.8–58.4)	25.5	(22.6–28.4)	3,734	46.7	(44.2–49.3)	18.7	(16.5–20.9)
Race/Ethnicity§										
White	12,426	66.5	(65.3–67.7)	22.8	(21.6–24.0)	16,622	63.5	(62.3–64.7)	20.1	(19.1–21.1)
Black	1,049	70.1	(66.2–74.0)	22.6	(18.9–26.3)	2,687	62.8	(60.1–65.5)	16.9	(14.6–19.3)
Hispanic	1,017	63.8	(59.1–68.5)	17.1	(13.6–20.6)	1,614	52.7	(48.8–56.6)	14.3	(11.8–16.9)
Other	541	68.4	(60.6–76.2)	23.0	(15.6–30.5)	642	63.5	(55.7–71.3)	20.6	(14.7–26.5)
Education level										
Less than high school	1,575	47.4	(43.3–51.5)	17.7	(14.4–21.0)	2,921	44.6	(41.7–47.5)	12.7	(10.7–14.7)
High school graduate	4,327	65.7	(63.5–67.9)	19.9	(18.1–21.7)	7,811	60.6	(58.8–62.4)	17.4	(16.0–18.8)
Some college	4,018	68.5	(66.3–70.7)	22.5	(20.5–24.5)	6,234	66.2	(64.2–68.2)	21.0	(19.4–22.6)
College graduate	5,113	72.7	(70.7–74.7)	25.5	(23.5–27.5)	4,599	71.9	(69.9–73.9)	23.5	(21.5–25.5)
Region¶										
Northeast	2,939	68.9	(66.2–71.6)	23.0	(20.5–25.6)	3,777	62.0	(59.5–64.6)	18.4	(16.2–20.6)
Midwest	2,365	69.7	(67.2–72.3)	24.6	(22.3–27.0)	3,593	64.1	(61.9–66.3)	18.3	(16.7–19.9)
South	4,060	62.0	(60.0–64.0)	20.1	(18.5–21.7)	6,518	59.2	(57.6–60.8)	17.8	(16.4–19.2)
West	5,669	67.1	(64.8–69.5)	21.9	(19.9–23.9)	7,677	63.6	(61.4–65.8)	20.8	(19.2–22.4)
BMI status**										
Overweight	8,729	69.7	(68.1–71.3)	24.5	(23.1–25.9)	12,042	66.2	(64.8–67.6)	21.3	(20.1–22.5)
Obese	6,304	62.3	(60.5–64.1)	18.8	(17.2–20.4)	9,523	57.1	(55.5–58.7)	16.1	(14.9–17.3)
Total	**15,033**	**66.6**	**(65.4–67.8)**	**22.2**	**(21.2–23.2)**	**21,565**	**62.2**	**(61.2–63.2)**	**19.0**	**(18.2–19.8)**

* Confidence interval.

† Five or more times per week and ≥30 minutes per session.

§ Racial groups other than white, black, and Hispanic were combined because, when analyzed separately, data were too small for meaningful analysis.

¶ *Northeast*=Connecticut, Maine, Massachusetts, New Hampshire, New Jersey, New York, Pennsylvania, Rhode Island, and Vermont; *Midwest*=Illinois, Indiana, Iowa, Kansas, Michigan, Minnesota, Missouri, Nebraska, North Dakota, Ohio, South Dakota, and Wisconsin; *South*=Alabama, Arkansas, Delaware, District of Columbia, Florida, Georgia, Kentucky, Louisiana, Maryland, Mississippi, North Carolina, Oklahoma, South Carolina, Tennessee, Texas, Virginia, and West Virginia; and *West*=Arizona, California, Colorado, Hawaii, Idaho, Montana, Nevada, New Mexico, Oregon, Utah, Washington, and Wyoming.

** Body mass index (BMI) of 25.0–29.9 for overweight persons and ≥30.0 for obese persons.

SOURCE: "Prevalence of Leisure-Time Physical Activity Among Overweight Adults—United States, 1998," *Morbidity and Mortality Weekly Report*, vol. 49, no. 15, April 21, 2000

TABLE 12.3

Managing health conditions

	Shoppers attempting to manage* condition through purchases		Shoppers attempting to prevent** condition through purchases	
		Number of shopper households		Number of shopper households
Total shoppers	100%	78,940,000	100%	64,800,000
NET Heart disease/high chol./hypert.	30%	23,682,000	52%	33,696,000
High cholesterol/watch cholesterol	12%	9,472,800	14%	9,007,200
High blood pressure/hypertension	12%	9,472,800	12%	7,581,600
Obesity	12%	9,157,040	6%	3,758,400
Nothing/none	11%	8,525,520	3%	2,138,400
Heart disease	9%	7,262,480	31%	19,828,800
Health maintenance	9%	6,946,720	4%	2,462,400
Diabetes	9%	6,788,840	10%	6,220,800
Weight management/fat intake	6%	4,815,340	4%	2,721,600
Colds/flu/sinus condition	4%	3,394,420	3%	1,749,600
Allergies	3%	2,526,080	4%	2,786,400
Cancer	1%	947,280	9%	5,961,600
All Others	12%	9,630,680	1%	583,200

*Base = Respondents who said that "trying to manage condition" on their own and/or "follow doctor's advice" affects their grocery shopping purchases
**Base = Respondents who said that "reducing risk of specific condition" affects their grocery shopping purchases
Note: Projections are based on number of U.S. phone households per 1996 census estimates assuming one primary shopper per household.

SOURCE: *A Look at the Self-Care Movement: A Shopping for Health Report, 1998,* Food Marketing Insititute and PREVENTION Magazine, Rodale Press, Inc., Emmaus, PA, 1998

TABLE 12.4

What consumers do first when treating common health conditions

	Talk to a pharmacist	Call a doctor	Treat yourself in some way	Do nothing	Don't know	Sample size
A fever	7	16	71	5	1	(1202)
Headache pain	6	7	80	7	–	(1202)
Muscle or joint pain	6	23	59	11	1	(1202)
Chest pain	5	78	10	6	1	(1202)
Stomach upset or heartburn	7	9	76	7	1	(1202)
Diarrhea	7	8	75	9	1	(1202)
A cold or cough	8	11	73	8	–	(1202)
A yeast infection (women only)	8	48	38	3	3	(654)
Menstrual Cramps (women only)	4	6	69	18	3	(654)
Allergies, asthma, or sinus congestion	8	37	46	7	2	(1202)
A toothache	6	63	25	5	1	(1202)
And what about if you wanted to quit smoking (38% volunteered they do not smoke)	12	25	51	9	3	(745)

SOURCE: *Navigating the Medication Marketplace: How Consumers Choose,* PREVENTION Magazine and the American Pharmaceutical Association, Rodale Press, Inc., Emmaus, PA, 1998

1998. In 1998 men (25.9 percent, down from 51.2 percent in 1965) were still more likely than women (22.1 percent, down from 33.7 percent in 1965) to smoke. White men and women aged 18–24 were far more likely to smoke than black men and women in the same age group. (See Table 12.6.) About 57 percent of current or former smokers reported starting to smoke before the age of 18, while 42 percent were 18 or older.

Alcohol Use

In 1995 almost two in five adults (37 percent) reported that they never drank—a small change from 1983 (34 percent). The proportion of reported nondrinkers had risen as high as 44 percent, in 1993. (See Table 12.7.) Among those who drink, the frequency of drinking and the quantity drunk have remained fairly stable.

TABLE 12.5

Health-care product usage by demographics

	Total Shoppers	Education				Household income		Age		
		< H.S. grad	H.S. grad	Some college	College grad +	<$50,000	$50,000+	Xers	Boomers	Matures
Base size:	1,000	96	362	211	327	607	278	238	459	293
OTC medications	85%	79%	88%	87%	84%	85%	88%	88%	89%	77%
Rx drugs	71%	70%	71%	74%	69%	68%	76%	62%	70%	79%
Vitamins & minerals	67%	56%	62%	74%	72%	65%	72%	65%	69%	68%
Herbal remedies	28%	27%	22%	30%	33%	25%	35%	26%	31%	23%
Homeopathic remedies	15%	9%	11%	16%	21%	13%	20%	10%	19%	13%
Aromatherapy products	13%	6%	13%	17%	14%	12%	18%	19%	15%	6%
In-home diagnostic tests	9%	4%	8%	11%	11%	8%	10%	6%	10%	12%

SOURCE: *A Look at the Self-Care Movement: A Shopping for Health Report, 1998,* Food Marketing Insititute and PREVENTION Magazine, Rodale Press, Inc., Emmaus, PA, 1998

IMMUNIZATIONS

Diseases that used to kill or cripple many thousands of children—such as mumps, measles, diphtheria, and poliomyelitis—are now controlled through immunizations. Polio and diphtheria, two diseases that once struck terror in the hearts of parents, have been virtually eliminated. The Childhood Immunization Initiative is a national strategy to achieve high vaccination levels among children during their first two years of life. (See Figure 12.4 for the recommended schedule for immunizations.) The very success of the nation's immunization efforts since the 1960s, however, has given some parents a false sense of security and made them feel that having their children vaccinated is not a critical priority.

Although the incidence rates for these diseases have dropped dramatically, they have not disappeared. In 1998 there were 666 cases of mumps, 7,405 cases of whooping cough (pertussis), and 100 cases of measles (rubeola) reported to the CDC. (See Table 12.8.) If immunization rates decline, however, these diseases could become active again.

All children should be vaccinated during their first 18 months of life. Nonetheless, adolescents (ages 11–21, as defined by the American Medical Association and the American Academy of Pediatrics) and young adults (ages 22–39) can still be at risk for these diseases. The CDC recommends that adolescents ages 11–12 be vaccinated according to the guidelines shown in Table 12.9.

TABLE 12.6

Current cigarette smoking by persons 18 years of age and over according to sex, race, and age: selected years 1965–98

[Data are based on household interviews of a sample of the civilian noninstitutionalized population]

Sex, race, and age	1965	1974	1979	1983	1985	1990	1992	1993	1994	1995	1997	1998
18 years and over, age adjusted						Percent of persons						
All persons	41.9	37.0	33.3	31.9	29.9	25.3	26.3	24.8	25.3	24.6	24.6	24.0
Male	51.2	42.8	37.0	34.8	32.2	28.0	28.1	27.3	27.6	26.5	27.1	25.9
Female	33.7	32.2	30.1	29.4	27.9	22.9	24.6	22.6	23.1	22.7	22.2	22.1
White male	50.4	41.7	36.4	34.2	31.3	27.6	27.7	26.6	27.1	26.2	26.8	26.0
Black male	58.8	53.6	43.9	41.7	40.2	32.8	33.3	33.7	34.3	29.4	32.4	29.0
White female	33.9	32.0	30.3	29.6	27.9	23.5	25.3	23.4	24.0	23.4	22.8	23.0
Black female	31.8	35.6	30.5	31.3	30.9	20.8	24.5	20.6	21.6	23.5	22.5	21.1
18 years and over, crude												
All persons	42.4	37.1	33.5	32.1	30.1	25.5	26.5	25.0	25.5	24.7	24.7	24.1
Male	51.9	43.1	37.5	35.1	32.6	28.4	28.6	27.7	28.2	27.0	27.6	26.4
Female	33.9	32.1	29.9	29.5	27.9	22.8	24.6	22.5	23.1	22.6	22.1	21.9
White male	51.1	41.9	36.8	34.5	31.7	28.0	28.2	27.0	27.7	26.6	27.2	26.3
Black male	60.4	54.3	44.1	40.6	39.9	32.5	32.2	32.7	33.7	28.5	32.2	29.0
White female	34.0	31.7	30.1	29.4	27.7	23.4	25.1	23.1	23.7	23.1	22.5	22.6
Black female	33.7	36.4	31.1	32.2	31.0	21.2	24.2	20.8	21.7	23.5	22.5	21.0
All males												
18–24 years	54.1	42.1	35.0	32.9	28.0	26.6	28.0	28.8	29.8	27.8	31.7	31.3
25–34 years	60.7	50.5	43.9	38.8	38.2	31.6	32.8	30.2	31.4	29.5	30.3	28.6
35–44 years	58.2	51.0	41.8	41.0	37.6	34.5	32.9	32.0	33.2	31.5	32.1	30.2
45–64 years	51.9	42.6	39.3	35.9	33.4	29.3	28.6	29.2	28.3	27.1	27.6	27.7
65 years and over	28.5	24.8	20.9	22.0	19.6	14.6	16.1	13.5	13.2	14.9	12.8	10.4
White male												
18–24 years	53.0	40.8	34.3	32.5	28.4	27.4	30.0	30.4	31.8	28.4	34.0	34.1
25–34 years	60.1	49.5	43.6	38.6	37.3	31.6	33.5	29.9	32.5	29.9	30.4	29.2
35–44 years	57.3	50.1	41.3	40.8	36.6	33.5	30.9	31.2	32.0	31.2	32.1	29.6
45–64 years	51.3	41.2	38.3	35.0	32.1	28.7	28.1	27.8	26.9	26.3	26.5	27.0
65 years and over	27.7	24.3	20.5	20.6	18.9	13.7	14.9	12.5	11.9	14.1	11.5	10.0
Black male												
18–24 years	62.8	54.9	40.2	34.2	27.2	21.3	*16.2	*19.9	*18.7	*14.6	23.5	19.7
25–34 years	68.4	58.5	47.5	39.9	45.6	33.8	29.5	30.7	29.8	25.1	31.6	25.2
35–44 years	67.3	61.5	48.6	45.5	45.0	42.0	47.5	36.9	44.5	36.3	33.9	36.2
45–64 years	57.9	57.8	50.0	44.8	46.1	36.7	35.4	42.4	41.2	33.9	39.4	37.3
65 years and over	36.4	29.7	26.2	38.9	27.7	21.5	28.3	*27.9	25.6	28.5	26.0	16.3
All females												
18–24 years	38.1	34.1	33.8	35.5	30.4	22.5	24.9	22.9	25.2	21.8	25.7	24.5
25–34 years	43.7	38.8	33.7	32.6	32.0	28.2	30.1	27.3	28.8	26.4	24.8	24.6
35–44 years	43.7	39.8	37.0	33.8	31.5	24.8	27.3	27.4	26.8	27.1	27.2	26.4
45–64 years	32.0	33.4	30.7	31.0	29.9	24.8	26.1	23.0	22.8	24.0	21.5	22.5
65 years and over	9.6	12.0	13.2	13.1	13.5	11.5	12.4	10.5	11.1	11.5	11.5	11.2
White female												
18–24 years	38.4	34.0	34.5	36.5	31.8	25.4	28.5	26.8	28.5	24.9	29.4	28.0
25–34 years	43.4	38.6	34.1	32.2	32.0	28.5	31.5	28.4	30.2	27.3	26.1	26.9
35–44 years	43.9	39.3	37.2	34.8	31.0	25.0	27.6	27.3	27.1	27.0	27.5	26.7
45–64 years	32.7	33.0	30.6	30.6	29.7	25.4	25.8	23.4	23.2	24.3	20.9	22.5
65 years and over	9.8	12.3	13.8	13.2	13.3	11.5	12.6	10.5	11.1	11.7	11.7	11.2
Black female												
18–24 years	37.1	35.6	31.8	32.0	23.7	10.0	10.3	*8.2	11.8	*8.8	11.5	8.3
25–34 years	47.8	42.2	35.2	38.0	36.2	29.1	26.9	24.7	24.8	26.7	22.5	21.5
35–44 years	42.8	46.4	37.7	32.7	40.2	25.5	32.4	31.5	28.2	31.9	30.1	30.0
45–64 years	25.7	38.9	34.2	36.3	33.4	22.6	30.9	21.3	23.5	27.5	28.4	25.3
65 years and over	7.1	*8.9	*8.5	*13.1	14.5	11.1	*11.1	*10.2	13.6	13.3	10.7	11.5

* Data preceded by an asterisk have a relative standard error of 20–30 percent.

SOURCE: *Health, United States, 2000*, National Center for Health Statistics, Hyattsville, MD, 2000

TABLE 12.7

Trends in alcohol use

Questions: In general, how often do you consume alcoholic beverages—that is, beer, wine, or liquor—never, less than one day a month, one to three days a month, one to two days a week, three to four days a week, five to six days a week or daily?

On a day when you drink alcoholic beverages, on average, how many drinks do you have?

By a "drink" I mean a shot of hard liquor, a can or bottle of beer, or a glass of wine.

	1995 %	1994 %	1993 %	1991 %	1989 %	1987 %	1985 %	1983 %
Frequency of alcohol consumption								
Total who drink	63	60	56	61	61	64	67	66
Less than once a month	17	16	17	16	16	13	15	16
1 - 3 days per month	21	18	14	20	16	19	20	16
1 - 2 days per week	15	14	14	15	18	21	19	19
3 - 4 days per week	5	5	5	5	5	5	6	9
5 - 7 days per week	5	7	6	5	7	6	6	6
Never drink	37	40	44	39	39	36	33	34
Quantity of alcohol consumption								
Heavy (4 or more drinks)	11	12	10	11	9	14	11	11
Moderate (1 - 3 drinks)	50	47	43	50	50	50	55	53
Never drink	37	40	44	39	39	36	33	34
Undesignated	2	0	3	0	2	0	1	2
Number of interviews	(1257)	(1262)	(1250)	(1256)	(1250)	(1250)	(1256)	(1252)

SOURCE: *The Prevention Index: A Report Card on the Nation's Health,* Rodale Press, Inc., Emmaus, PA, 1998

FIGURE 12.4

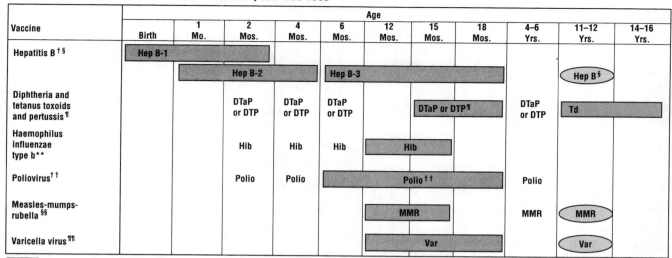

Recommended childhood immunization schedule*, Jan–Dec 1998

Vaccine	Age										
	Birth	1 Mo.	2 Mos.	4 Mos.	6 Mos.	12 Mos.	15 Mos.	18 Mos.	4–6 Yrs.	11–12 Yrs.	14–16 Yrs.
Hepatitis B † §	Hep B-1		Hep B-2		Hep B-3					Hep B §	
Diphtheria and tetanus toxoids and pertussis ¶			DTaP or DTP	DTaP or DTP	DTaP or DTP	DTaP or DTP¶			DTaP or DTP	Td	
Haemophilus influenzae type b**			Hib	Hib	Hib	Hib					
Poliovirus††			Polio	Polio	Polio††				Polio		
Measles-mumps-rubella §§						MMR			MMR	MMR	
Varicella virus ¶¶¶						Var				Var	

▨ Range of acceptable ages for vaccination

⬭ Vaccines to be assessed and administered if necessary

* This schedule indicates the recommended age for routine administration of currently licensed childhood vaccines; vaccines are listed under the ages for which they are routinely recommended. Catch-up immunization should be done during any visit when feasible. Some combination vaccines are available and may be used whenever administration of all components of the vaccine is indicated. Providers should consult the manufacturers' package inserts for detailed recommendations.

† **Infants born to hepatitis B surface antigen (HBsAg)-negative mothers** should receive 2.5 μg of Merck vaccine (Recombivax HB ®) or 10 μg of SmithKline Beecham (SB) vaccine (Engerix- B ®). The second dose should be administered at least 1 month after the first dose. The third dose should be administered at least 2 months after the second but not before 6 months of age. **Infants born to HBsAg-positive mothers** should receive 0.5 mL hepatitis B immune globulin (HBIG) within 12 hours of birth, and either 5 μg of Merck vaccine (Recombivax HB ®) or 10 μg of SB vaccine (Engerix- B ®) at a separate site. The second dose is recommended at age 1– 2 months and the third dose at age 6 months. **Infants born to mothers whose HBsAg status is unknown** should receive either 5 m g of Merck vaccine (Recombivax HB ®) or 10 μg of SB vaccine (Engerix- B ®) within 12 hours of birth. The second dose of vaccine is recommended at age 1 month and the third dose at age 6 months. Blood should be drawn at the time of delivery to determine the mother's HBsAg status; if it is positive, the infant should receive HBIG as soon as possible (no later than age 1 week). The dosage and timing of subsequent vaccine doses should be based on the mother's HBsAg status.

§ Children and adolescents who have not been vaccinated against hepatitis B in infancy may begin the series during any visit. Those who have not previously received three doses of hepatitis B vaccine should initiate or complete the series during the routine visit to a health-care provider at age 11– 12 years, and unvaccinated older adolescents should be vaccinated whenever possible. The second dose should be administered at least 1 month after the first dose, and the third dose should be administered at least 4 months after the first dose and at least 2 months after the second dose.

¶ Diphtheria and tetanus toxoids and acellular pertussis vaccine (DTaP) is the preferred vaccine for all doses in the vaccination series, including completion of the series in children who have received one or more doses of whole-cell diphtheria and tetanus toxoids and pertussis vaccine (DTP). Whole-cell DTP is an acceptable alternative to DTaP. The fourth dose (DTP or DTaP) may be administered as early as age 12 months, provided 6 months have elapsed since the third dose and if the child is unlikely to return at age 15–18 months. Tetanus and diphtheria toxoids, adsorbed, for adult use (Td), is recommended at age 11–12 years if at least 5 years have elapsed since the last dose of DTP, DTaP, or diphtheria and tetanus toxoids, adsorbed, for pediatric use (DT). Subsequent routine Td boosters are recommended every 10 years.

** Three type b (Hib) conjugate vaccines are licensed for infant use. If *Haemophilus* b conjugate vaccine (meningococcal protein conjugate) (PRP- OMP) (PedvaxHIB ® [Merck]) is administered at ages 2 and 4 months, a dose at age 6 months is not required.

†† Two poliovirus vaccines are currently licensed and distributed in the United States: inactivated poliovirus vaccine (IPV) and oral poliovirus vaccine (OPV). The following schedules are all acceptable to the ACIP, AAP, and AAFP. Parents and providers may choose among these options: 1) two doses of IPV followed by two doses of OPV; 2) four doses of IPV; or 3) four doses of OPV. ACIP recommends two doses of IPV at ages 2 and 4 months followed by a dose of OPV at age 12– 18 months and at age 4– 6 years. IPV is the only poliovirus vaccine recommended for immunocompromised persons and their household contacts.

§§ The second dose of measles-mumps-rubella vaccine (MMR) is recommended routinely at age 4–6 years but may be administered during any visit, provided at least 1 month has elapsed since receipt of the first dose and that both doses are administered beginning at or after age 12 months. Those who have not previously received the second dose should complete the schedule no later than the routine visit to a health-care provider at age 11–12 years.

¶¶¶ Susceptible children may receive varicella vaccine (Var) at any visit after the first birthday, and those who lack a reliable history of chickenpox should be vaccinated during the routine visit to a health-care provider at age 11–12 years. Susceptible children aged ≥ 13 years should receive two doses at least 1 month apart.

SOURCE: "Recommended childhood Immunization Schedule—United States, 1998," *Morbidity and Mortality Weekly Report*, vol. 47, no. 1, January 16, 1998

TABLE 12.8

Selected notifiable disease rates, according to disease: selected years 1950–98

[Data are based on reporting by State health departments]

Disease	1950	1960	1970	1980	1985	1990	1995	1996	1997	1998
					Cases per 100,000 population					
Diphtheria	3.83	0.51	0.21	0.00	0.00	0.00	–	0.01	0.01	0.00
Haemophilus influenzae, invasive	- - -	- - -	- - -	- - -	- - -	- - -	0.45	0.45	0.44	0.44
Hepatitis A	- - -	- - -	27.87	12.84	10.03	12.64	12.13	11.70	11.22	8.59
Hepatitis B	- - -	- - -	4.08	8.39	11.50	8.48	4.19	4.01	3.90	3.80
Lyme disease	- - -	- - -	- - -	- - -	- - -	- - -	4.49	6.21	4.79	6.39
Meningococcal disease	- - -	- - -	1.23	1.25	1.04	0.99	1.25	1.30	1.24	1.01
Mumps	- - -	- - -	55.55	3.86	1.30	2.17	0.35	0.29	0.27	0.25
Pertussis (whooping cough)	79.82	8.23	2.08	0.76	1.50	1.84	1.97	2.94	2.46	2.74
Poliomyelitis, total	22.02	1.77	0.02	0.00	0.00	0.00	0.00	0.01	0.01	0.00
Paralytic[1]	- - -	1.40	0.02	0.00	0.00	0.00	0.00	0.01	0.01	0.00
Rocky Mountain spotted fever	- - -	- - -	0.19	0.52	0.30	0.26	0.23	0.32	0.16	0.14
Rubella (German measles)	- - -	- - -	27.75	1.72	0.26	0.45	0.05	0.10	0.07	0.13
Rubeola (measles)	211.01	245.42	23.23	5.96	1.18	11.17	0.12	0.20	0.06	0.04
Salmonellosis, excluding typhoid fever	- - -	3.85	10.84	14.88	27.37	19.54	17.66	17.15	15.66	16.17
Shigellosis	15.45	6.94	6.79	8.41	7.14	10.89	12.32	9.80	8.64	8.74
Tuberculosis[2]	- - -	30.83	18.28	12.25	9.30	10.33	8.70	8.04	7.42	6.79
Sexually transmitted diseases:[3]										
Syphilis[4]	146.02	68.78	45.26	30.51	28.39	54.52	26.39	20.07	17.43	14.19
Primary and secondary	16.73	9.06	10.89	12.06	11.40	20.34	6.30	4.29	3.20	2.61
Early latent	39.71	10.11	8.08	9.00	9.11	22.27	10.15	7.61	6.21	4.71
Late and late latent[5]	70.22	45.91	24.94	9.30	7.74	10.35	9.25	7.68	7.62	6.56
Congenital[6]	8.97	2.48	0.97	0.12	0.11	1.53	0.70	0.49	0.40	0.30
Chlamydia[7]	- - -	- - -	- - -	- - -	17.42	160.83	190.42	192.87	206.95	236.57
Gonorrhea[8]	192.50	145.40	297.22	445.10	382.98	277.45	149.44	123.24	122.02	132.88
Chancroid	3.34	0.94	0.70	0.30	0.87	1.69	0.23	0.15	0.09	0.07
					Number of cases					
Diphtheria	5,796	918	435	3	3	4	–	2	4	1
Haemophilus influenzae, invasive	- - -	- - -	- - -	- - -	- - -	- - -	1,180	1,170	1,162	1,194
Hepatitis A	- - -	- - -	56,797	29,087	23,210	31,441	31,582	31,032	30,021	23,229
Hepatitis B	- - -	- - -	8,310	19,015	26,611	21,102	10,805	10,637	10,416	10,258
Lyme disease	- - -	- - -	- - -	- - -	- - -	- - -	11,700	16,455	12,801	16,801
Meningococcal disease	- - -	- - -	2,505	2,840	2,479	2,451	3,243	3,437	3,308	2,725
Mumps	- - -	- - -	104,953	8,576	2,982	5,292	906	751	683	666
Pertussis (whooping cough)	120,718	14,809	4,249	1,730	3,589	4,570	5,137	7,796	6,564	7,405
Poliomyelitis, total	33,300	3,190	33	9	8	6	7	5	5	1
Paralytic[1]	- - -	2,525	31	9	8	6	7	5	5	1
Rocky Mountain spotted fever	- - -	- - -	380	1,163	714	651	590	831	409	365
Rubella (German measles)	- - -	- - -	56,552	3,904	630	1,125	128	238	181	364
Rubeola (measles)	319,124	441,703	47,351	13,506	2,822	27,786	309	508	138	100
Salmonellosis, excluding typhoid fever	- - -	6,929	22,096	33,715	65,347	48,603	45,970	45,471	41,901	43,694
Shigellosis	23,367	12,487	13,845	19,041	17,057	27,077	32,080	25,978	23,117	23,626
Tuberculosis[2]	- - -	55,494	37,137	27,749	22,201	25,701	22,860	21,337	19,851	18,361
Sexually transmitted diseases:[3]										
Syphilis[4]	217,558	122,538	91,382	68,832	67,563	135,043	69,345	53,226	46,642	37,977
Primary and secondary	23,939	16,145	21,982	27,204	27,131	50,578	16,543	11,388	8,556	6,993
Early latent	59,256	18,017	16,311	20,297	21,689	55,397	26,657	20,187	16,631	12,613
Late and late latent[5]	113,569	81,798	50,348	20,979	18,414	25,750	24,295	20,356	20,385	17,570
Congenital[6]	13,377	4,416	1,953	277	329	3,865	1,850	1,295	1,070	801
Chlamydia[7]	- - -	- - -	- - -	- - -	25,848	323,663	478,577	490,615	531,529	607,602
Gonorrhea[8]	286,746	258,933	600,072	1,004,029	911,419	690,042	392,651	326,805	326,564	355,642
Chancroid	4,977	1,680	1,416	788	2,067	4,212	607	386	246	189

0.00 Rate greater than zero but less than 0.005.

– Quantity zero.

- - - Data not available.

[1] Data beginning in 1986 may be updated due to retrospective case evaluations or late reports.

[2] Case reporting for tuberculosis began in 1953. Data prior to 1975 are not comparable with subsequent years' data because of changes in reporting criteria effective in 1975.

[3] Newly reported civilian cases prior to 1991; includes military cases beginning in 1991 and adjustments to the number of cases through June 15, 1999, for states submitting hardcopy reports and through July 19, 1999, for states reporting electronically. For 1950, data for Alaska and Hawaii not included.

[4] Includes stage of syphilis not stated.

[5] Includes cases of unknown duration.

[6] Data reported for 1989 and later years reflect change in case definition introduced in 1988. Through 1994, all cases of congenitally acquired syphilis; as of 1995, congenital syphilis less than 1 year of age.

[7] Chlamydia was non-notifiable in 1994 and earlier years. For 1998, cases for New York based exclusively on those reported by New York City.

[8] Data for 1994 do not include cases from Georgia.

Notes: The total resident population was used to calculate all rates except sexually transmitted diseases, for which the civilian resident population was used prior to 1991. For sexually transmitted diseases, 1997 population estimates were used to calculate 1998 rates. Population data from those states where diseases were not notifiable or not available were excluded from rate calculation.

SOURCE: *Health, United States, 2000,* National Center for Health Statistics, Hyattsville, MD, 2000

TABLE 12.9

Recommended schedule of vaccinations for adolescents ages 11-12 years

Immunobiologic	Indications	Name	Dose	Frequency	Route
Hepatitis A vaccine	Adolescents who are at increased risk of hepatitis A infection or its complications	HAVRIX®*	720 EL.U.[†]/0.5 mL[§]	A total of two doses at 0,[¶] 6-12 mos	IM**
		VAQTA®*	25 U/0.5 mL	A total of two doses at 0, 6-18 mos	IM
Hepatitis B vaccine	Adolescents not vaccinated previously for hepatitis B	Recombivax HB®*	5 µg/0.5 mL	A total of three doses at 0, 1-2, 4-6 mos	IM
		Engerix-B®*	10 µg/0.5 mL	A total of three doses at 0, 1-2, 4-6 mos	IM
Influenza vaccine	Adolsecents who are at increased risk for complications caused by influenza or who have contact with persons at increased risk for these complications	Influenza virus vaccine[††]	0.5 mL	Annually (September-December)	IM
Measles, mumps, and rubella vaccine (MMR)	Adolescents not vaccinated previously with two doses of measles vaccine at ≥ 12 mos of age	MMR II®*	0.5 mL	One dose	SC[§§]
Pneumococcal polysaccharide vaccine	Adolescents who are at increased risk for pneumococcal disease or its complications	Pneumococcal vaccine polyvalent[††]	0.5 mL	One dose	IM or SC
Tetanus and diphtheria toxoids (Td)	Adolescents not vaccinated within the previous 5 yrs	Tetanus and diphtheria toxoids, adsorbed (for adult use)[††]	0.5 mL	Every 10 yrs	IM
Varicella virus vaccine	Adolescents not vaccinated previously and who have no reliable history of chickenpox	VARIVAX®*	0.5 mL	One dose[¶¶]	SC

* Manufacturer's product name.
[†] Enzyme-linked immunosorbent assay (ELISA) unit.
[§] Alternative dosage and schedule of 360 EL.U./0.5 mL and a total of three doses administered at 0, 1, and 6-12 months.
[¶] 0 months represents timing of the initial dose, and subsequent numbers represent months after the initial dose.
** Intramuscular injection.
[††] Generic name.
[§§] Subcutaneous injection.
[¶¶] Adolescents ≥13 years of age should be administered a total of two doses (0.5 mL/dose) subcutaneously at 0 and 4-8 weeks.

SOURCE: "Immunization of Adolescents," *Morbidity and Mortality Weekly Report,* vol. 45, no. RR-13, November 22, 1996

CHAPTER 13

PUBLIC OPINION ABOUT HEALTH CARE

In October 2000, when the Gallup Organization asked respondents to name the most important noneconomic problem facing the country today, 11 percent named health care. More people believed health care to be a bigger problem than crime, the government, drugs, taxes, and a long list of other American issues. Only education and a decline in moral values were considered to be more pressing than health care. (See Figure 13.1.)

HEALTH CARE COSTS—PERCEPTION VERSUS REALITY

Every year since 1998, the Employee Benefit Research Institute (EBRI), a public policy research and education organization that studies economic security and employee benefits, has conducted its *Annual Health Confidence Survey (HCS).* A number of the questions on the survey deal with health care costs. Questions vary from year to year.

All survey participants were concerned with the costs of health care. The perceptions, however, that respondents had about rising costs and the amount they were paying differed sharply from the facts. Eight of 10 Americans (81 percent) surveyed in 1998 believed that health care costs had increased over the past five years, 12 percent thought health care costs had stayed about the same, and 5 percent said costs were lower. (See Figure 13.2.) Nearly all persons (93 percent) in fee-for-service plans said their health care costs were higher, compared with 85 percent of preferred provider organization (PPO) plan members and 78 percent of health maintenance organization (HMO) plan members.

In fact, while health care costs have increased over the long term, they did not rise dramatically from 1993 to 1998. In 1960 out-of-pocket spending accounted for 31 percent of all private health care expenditures. By 1992 out-of-pocket spending accounted for 37 percent of all private health care spending, which now accounted for a far larger portion of the nation's gross domestic product.

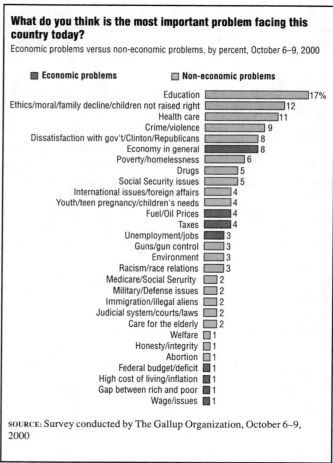

FIGURE 13.1

What do you think is the most important problem facing this country today?

Economic problems versus non-economic problems, by percent, October 6–9, 2000

■ Economic problems   ■ Non-economic problems

Education	17%
Ethics/moral/family decline/children not raised right	12
Health care	11
Crime/violence	9
Dissatisfaction with gov't/Clinton/Republicans	8
Economy in general	8
Poverty/homelessness	6
Drugs	5
Social Security issues	5
International issues/foreign affairs	4
Youth/teen pregnancy/children's needs	4
Fuel/Oil Prices	4
Taxes	4
Unemployment/jobs	3
Guns/gun control	3
Environment	3
Racism/race relations	3
Medicare/Social Serurity	2
Military/Defense issues	2
Immigration/illegal aliens	2
Judicial system/courts/laws	2
Care for the elderly	2
Welfare	1
Honesty/integrity	1
Abortion	1
Federal budget/deficit	1
High cost of living/inflation	1
Gap between rich and poor	1
Wage/issues	1

SOURCE: Survey conducted by The Gallup Organization, October 6–9, 2000

In the 1990s, however, most health care costs increased only modestly. According to *Health Care Financing Review,* published by the U.S. Department of Health and Human Services, out-of-pocket spending was still 37 percent in 1996.

Health insurance costs did not increase significantly for employers with 10 or more employees in the 1990s.

FIGURE 13.2

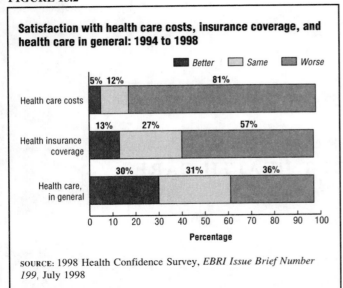

Satisfaction with health care costs, insurance coverage, and health care in general: 1994 to 1998

SOURCE: 1998 Health Confidence Survey, *EBRI Issue Brief Number 199*, July 1998

FIGURE 13.3

Americans' views of the health care system

- Does not need to be changed at all 3%
- Don't know 2%
- Needs some minor changes 36%
- Needs major changes 59%

SOURCE: 1998 Health Confidence Survey, *EBRI Issue Brief Number 199*, July 1998

Between 1993 and 1994, average health insurance costs decreased 1.1 percent. Health insurance costs increased 2.1 percent between 1994 and 1995, and 2.5 percent between 1995 and 1996. Between 1996 and 1997, health insurance costs increased less than 0.5 percent.

Dissatisfaction with health care costs increased at the end of the twentieth century. When asked in the 2000 *HCS* about satisfaction with health care costs over the past two years, 39 percent said they were "not too satisfied" or "not at all satisfied" with the cost of their health insurance, while 55 percent were "somewhat" to "extremely satisfied" with their costs. In 1998 only 32 percent of Americans said they were unsatisfied with health care costs, while 63 percent were somewhat or extremely satisfied. When asked about out-of-pocket costs—those not covered by their health plans—43 percent were unsatisfied in 2000. Levels of satisfaction were higher for quality of care received, and choice of physician.

HEALTH CARE CONCERNS

Nearly all Americans believe that the health care system needs some changes. Almost three in five (59 percent) respondents thought that the system required major change, and 36 percent said minor changes were needed. Only 3 percent said the system needed no changes. (See Figure 13.3.)

By Age

Not surprisingly, middle-aged Americans (ages 35–54) and those nearing retirement age (ages 55–64) were more concerned with the current health care situation than survey respondents between the ages of 20 and 34 or Americans over the age of 65, who are covered by Medicare. According to the 1998 *HCS*, one-fourth (25 percent) of Americans

ages 55–64 considered health care to be a critical issue, while only 9 percent of respondents between the ages of 20 and 34 considered health care to be a critical issue. Middle-aged respondents were more apt to say that health care had gotten worse during the previous five years. Most respondents (70 percent) between the ages of 45 and 54 said the health care system needed major changes, while only 44 percent of respondents aged 20–34 agreed.

By Gender

Women (64 percent) were somewhat more likely than men (53 percent) to feel that the health care system needed major changes in 1998. More women (83 percent) than men (71 percent) supported requiring employers to offer health insurance to their employees as a means of covering the uninsured. Half of women were extremely or very satisfied with almost all the elements of health care they had received in the preceding two years, compared with 42 percent of men.

By Income and Education

Survey participants with higher incomes were more satisfied with treatments and care received during the prior two years. Over half (52 percent) of those with annual household incomes of $50,000 were satisfied, compared with 39 percent of those with less than $30,000. Both college graduates and those earning $30,000 or more were more likely to be insured, to receive coverage from an employer, and to report that they had a choice of plans.

Minorities

The 1998 *HCS* found important differences in opinions between minority and white Americans. Just over half (52 percent) of the white survey respondents gave health care in the United States high ratings, but more

TABLE 13.1

Satisfaction with quality of care and choice of doctor

	White	Minority
Satisfied with quality of care during past 2 years	56%	43%
Pleased with choice of doctor	52%	42%

SOURCE: *Annual Health Confidence Survey,* Employee Benefit Research Institute, Washington D.C., 1998

TABLE 13.2

Percent enrolled in health care plans, by race

	White	Minority
Enrolled in HMO plans	30%	43%
Have traditional health insurance	34%	21%
Have coverage of any kind	89%	82%

SOURCE: *Annual Health Confidence Survey,* Employee Benefit Research Institute, Washington, D.C., 1998

TABLE 13.3

Support of health care reform issues, by race

	White	Minority
All Americans should have health care	76%	85%
Allow uninsured to purchase Medicare	66%	76%
Increase payroll tax 1%	52%	61%
Increase income tax 1%	40%	52%

SOURCE: *Annual Health Confidence Survey,* Employee Benefit Research Institute, Washington, D.C., 1998

than half (57 percent) of minorities rated it as fair or poor. While 56 percent of whites were satisfied with the quality of care they had received during the preceding two years, only 43 percent of minorities were satisfied. More than half (52 percent) of white survey participants were pleased with their choice of doctor, but only 42 percent of minorities were pleased. (See Table 13.1.)

More minorities (43 percent) than whites (30 percent) said they were enrolled in HMO plans, while more whites (34 percent) than minorities (21 percent) reported that they had traditional health insurance. About 82 percent of minorities said they had health coverage of any kind, compared with 89 percent of whites. (See Table 13.2.) Among minorities who were insured, however, 67 percent reported that they had a choice of two or more plans, while only 55 percent of whites had a choice.

When it came to the issue of government reform of health care, minorities were more supportive than whites. More minorities (85 percent) than whites (76 percent) favored proposals to give all Americans access to health care. Three-fourths (76 percent) of minorities, compared with 66 percent of whites, favored a proposal to allow the uninsured to purchase Medicare. Six of 10 (61 percent) minority survey participants supported a 1 percent increase in payroll tax, and 52 percent supported a 1 percent increase in income tax, while 52 percent of whites supported a payroll tax hike and 40 percent supported an income tax increase. (See Table 13.3.)

CONFIDENCE IN THE FUTURE OF HEALTH CARE

Only about a quarter of 1999 *HCS* participants were "extremely" or "very" confident about the future of health care over the next 10 years. Thirty-eight percent were unsure whether or not they would be able to afford that care, and 34 percent feared they would not be able to select their own medical providers. Nearly one-quarter (24 percent) of respondents were also not confident they would be able to get the treatments they needed.

Confidence by Age

Middle-aged (35–54 years old) survey participants were less confident than younger (20–34 years old) partic-

ipants about the quality of health care over the next 10 years. Twice as many middle-aged participants (30 percent) as younger participants (15 percent) were not confident they would have access to quality health care in the next 10 years. One-fourth of middle-aged survey respondents were not confident they would be able to get the treatments needed over the next 10 years, while only 16 percent of younger respondents were not confident.

Nearly half (47 percent) of middle-aged respondents were not confident they would be able to afford health care or that they would be able to select their own doctors (44 percent) over the next 10 years. Among the younger respondents, 34 percent were concerned about affordability and 30 percent about freedom to choose their own doctor.

Confidence by Income

Low-income survey respondents (those earning less than $30,000) were less confident in the future of health care than those with higher incomes ($50,000 or more). Almost half (49 percent) of respondents with lower incomes were not confident that they would be able to afford health care without facing financial hardship. Only 31 percent of high-income respondents shared this concern. One-fourth (26 percent) of lower-income respondents were not confident that they would be able to get the treatments they would need in the next 10 years, while 19 percent of high-income respondents felt that way. Three of 10 lower-income respondents (29 percent) were not confident that they would have access to quality health care in the next 10 years, compared with 21 percent of higher-income survey respondents.

FIGURE 13.4

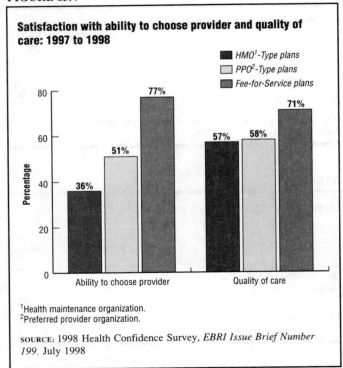

Satisfaction with ability to choose provider and quality of care: 1997 to 1998

Legend:
- HMO[1]-Type plans
- PPO[2]-Type plans
- Fee-for-Service plans

Ability to choose provider: HMO 36%, PPO 51%, Fee-for-Service 77%
Quality of care: HMO 57%, PPO 58%, Fee-for-Service 71%

[1]Health maintenance organization.
[2]Preferred provider organization.

SOURCE: 1998 Health Confidence Survey, *EBRI Issue Brief Number 199*, July 1998

THE MANAGED CARE PUZZLE

The EBRI found in its 2000 *HCS* that Americans were confused about the nation's health care system, beginning with the phrase, "managed care." Many people do not realize what kind of coverage they have. The vast majority of workers who participate in a health care plan are enrolled in some form of managed care (85 percent in 1998). According to the 2000 survey, however, well over half (61 percent) of people in managed care plans said they had never been in a managed care program at all. People in PPO-type plans were more likely to report that they had never been in managed care (66 percent) than those enrolled in HMO-type plans (52 percent).

What Americans Think of Managed Care

More people (49 percent) were extremely or very satisfied with their health plan, than were somewhat satisfied (37 percent), or dissatisfied (14 percent). The majority (62 percent) of those enrolled in fee-for-service plans were generally satisfied, compared with 47 percent of those in managed care plans.

Levels of Satisfaction

Those enrolled in fee-for-service plans in 1998 were most likely (77 percent) to be satisfied with their ability to select their own doctors. Slightly over half (51 percent) of those enrolled in PPO-type managed care plans were satisfied with their ability to select their own physician, compared with only one-third (36 percent) of persons enrolled in HMO-type managed care. More than half (59 percent)

of all survey participants were satisfied with the quality of care they received. Somewhat higher proportions of fee-for-service enrollees (71 percent) were satisfied with the quality of care than were managed care enrollees (57.5 percent). (See Figure 13.4.) There were no significant differences in satisfaction between fee-for-service members and managed care enrollees in the areas of general care received, cost of health insurance, health costs not covered by insurance, hospitals used, and benefits covered by health plans.

THE FUTURE OF MEDICARE

In 2000 most Americans were very concerned about the survival of Medicare. The Balanced Budget Act of 1997 (PL 105-33) reduced projected Medicare spending by $386 billion between 1998 and 2007, and the Medicare Trust Fund was expected to be depleted by 2010. Medicare reform was a major issue in the 2000 presidential election, and President George W. Bush was expected to introduce some sort of reform legislation during his term in office.

A joint survey released in October 1998 by the Kaiser Family Foundation and the Harvard School of Public Health illustrated the need for public debate about Medicare reform. Forty percent thought the problems facing Medicare were major; 26 percent considered them minor. Most survey participants (77 percent) felt that it was very important to them personally that the program be preserved.

In 1998, 68 percent of Americans surveyed believed that fraud and abuse in Medicare were the major reasons that the program was in trouble, yet only 20 percent believed that better management alone would save the program.

According to additional findings from the 2000 *HCS*, 75 percent of Americans favored using the federal budget surplus to pay some of the costs of Medicare and shore up the popular program for the future. Seventy-four percent also favored allowing defined contribution plans (where Medicare beneficiaries are permitted to choose from many private health plans and the government contributes a fixed amount to the cost of the plan). This figure varied significantly from the Kaiser/Harvard survey in 1998, which said that a vast majority opposed the idea of fixed payments.

According to the *HCS*, support has fallen among Americans for other proposed reforms:

- While 61 percent of Americans surveyed in 1999 supported requiring higher-income seniors to pay higher premiums, only 54 percent favored that option in 2000.

- Sixty-one percent of Americans in 1999 favored reducing Medicare payments to doctors and hospitals; only 53 percent supported that option in 2000.

TABLE 13.4

Rating Medicare 1998
The generation gap

	Over the age of 65	Under the age of 65
Medicare is doing a good job	74%	44%
Pleased with own health plan	41%	29%
Trust Medicare to provide health insurance	60%	38%
Trust private health plans to provide health insurance	14%	46%

SOURCE: *Annual Health Confidence Survey*, Employee Benefit Research Institute, Washington D.C., 1998

- The proposal to increase out-of-pocket payments for Medicare recipients remained unpopular—36 percent favored the idea in 1999, 31 percent in 2000.

- A large majority of Americans were also opposed to increasing payroll taxes for current workers—only 33 percent supported the idea in 1999, only 29 percent in 2000.

- In both years, almost three-quarters of Americans opposed the idea of increasing the Medicare eligibility age to 67 (27 percent supported the idea in 1999, 26 percent in 2000).

Despite questions concerning the solvency of Medicare, 72 percent favored expanding Medicare to cover prescription drugs in 1999, and two-thirds (69 percent) supported covering long-term care in 1998. Three-fifths (60 percent) favored expanding Medicare by allowing people close to the eligible age of 65 (62–64 years old) to buy into the program a few years early.

Rating Medicare—the Generation Gap

In 1998 most persons 65 years of age and older (74 percent) thought that Medicare was doing a "good job," compared with 44 percent of those under age 65. (See Table 13.4.) All ages, however, gave Medicare (49 percent) a higher rating of doing a "good job" than health insurance companies (36 percent) and HMOs and other managed care plans (30 percent).

Four in 10 seniors (41 percent) were likely to be pleased with their own health plan. Only 29 percent of those under age 65 were pleased with their private insurance. The survey also found that 60 percent of those 65 years and older trusted the current Medicare program to provide health insurance to seniors, compared with 38 percent of those under the age of 65. Younger persons (46 percent) were far more apt to trust privately run health plans to provide insurance than were older persons (14 percent). (See Table 13.4.)

TABLE 13.5

Percentage of survey respondents who reported that selected public health services were "very important" or "somewhat important", 1996*

Public health service	% Respondents	
	Very important	Somewhat important
Preventing the spread of infectious diseases (e.g., tuberculosis, measles, influenza, and AIDS)	93	7
Vaccinating to prevent diseases	90	9
Delivering medical care to ill patients by doctors and hospitals	85	13
Improving the quality of education and employment	83	14
Ensuring persons are not exposed to unsafe water supply, dangerous air pollution, or toxic waste	82	15
Conducting medical research on the causes and prevention of disease	82	15
Encouraging persons to live healthier lifestyles (e.g., eat well, exercise, and not to smoke)	72	24
Helping persons cope with stress from the problems of daily living and work	56	34

*Results of a random-digit-dialed telephone survey of U.S. residents aged ≥18 years (n=1004 respondents) conducted by Louis Harris and Associates, Inc., for the Harris Poll column, which is syndicated to the media but is not commissioned by any one client. The standard error was ±3% at the 95% confidence level.

SOURCE: "Public Opinion About Public Health-California and the United States, 1996," *Morbidity and Mortality Weekly Report*, vol. 47, no. 4, February 6, 1998

PUBLIC HEALTH

In December 1996, Louis Harris and Associates surveyed 1,004 U.S. residents aged 18 and over and asked respondents to rank the importance of eight services "to improve the health of the public." The rankings were "very important," "somewhat important," "not very important," "not at all important," or "did not know." The percentage of respondents who rated specific public health services as very important ranged from a high of 93 percent for preventing the spread of infectious diseases to a low of 56 percent for helping persons cope with stress. (See Table 13.5.)

Respondents also were asked who they thought should be mainly responsible for the performance of prevention rather than the treatment of disease. More than half (57 percent) thought the government should be responsible, while 40 percent said that "someone else" should be responsible. Of those respondents who named the government, 53 percent said the federal government should be responsible, 32 percent named state governments, and 13 percent chose city and local governments.

THE MOST URGENT HEALTH PROBLEMS FACING AMERICANS

Trends

In September 2000, a Gallup poll asked Americans to rate the nation's most urgent health problems. The largest

FIGURE 13.5

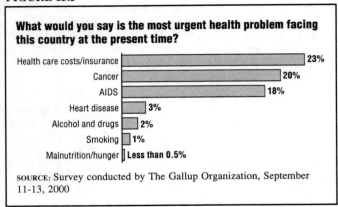

What would you say is the most urgent health problem facing this country at the present time?

Health care costs/insurance	23%
Cancer	20%
AIDS	18%
Heart disease	3%
Alcohol and drugs	2%
Smoking	1%
Malnutrition/hunger	Less than 0.5%

SOURCE: Survey conducted by The Gallup Organization, September 11-13, 2000

group, 23 percent, felt that health care costs and insurance posed the most pressing problem. Twenty percent of respondents felt that cancer was the most urgent health problem facing the United States. The biggest change at the close of the twentieth century was in the perception of the AIDS threat. In 1987, 68 percent of respondents felt that AIDS was the nation's most pressing problem. In 1997 only 29 percent felt AIDS was the country's biggest health threat. By 2000 that number had dropped to 18 percent, as AIDS death rates fell dramatically following the development of effective new medications. (See Figure 13.5.)

IMPORTANT NAMES AND ADDRESSES

Alzheimer's Association
919 N. Michigan Ave., #1100
Chicago, IL 60611-1676
(312) 335-8700
FAX: (312) 335-1110
Toll-free: (800) 272-3900
E-mail: info@alz.org
URL: http://www.alz.org

American Cancer Society
1599 Clifton Rd. NE
Atlanta, GA 30329-4251
(404) 320-3333
Toll-free: (800) ACS-2345
URL: http://www.cancer.org

American Dental Association
211 E. Chicago Ave.
Chicago, IL 60611
(312) 440-2500
FAX: (312) 440-2800
URL: http://www.ada.org

American Diabetes Association
1701 N. Beauregard St.
Alexandria, VA 22311
(703) 549-1500
FAX: (703) 836-7439
Toll-free: (800) DIABETES
URL: http://www.diabetes.org

American Heart Association
7272 Greenville Ave.
Dallas, TX 75231
(214) 373-6300
FAX: (214) 706-1341
Toll-free: (800) AHA-USA1
URL: http://www.americanheart.org

American Hospital Association
1 N. Franklin, #2700
Chicago, IL 60606
(312) 422-3000
FAX: (312) 422-4796
Toll-free: (800) 424-4301
URL: http://www.aha.org

American Lung Association
1740 Broadway
New York, NY 10019
(212) 315-8700
FAX: (212) 265-5642
Toll-free: (800) 586-4872
E-mail: info@lungusa.org
URL: http://www.lungusa.org

American Medical Association
515 N. State St.
Chicago, IL 60610
(312) 464-5000
FAX: (312) 464-4184
URL: http://www.ama-assn.org

American Parkinson Disease Association
1250 Hylan Blvd., Suite 4B
Staten Island, NY 10305-1946
(718) 981-8001
FAX: (718) 981-4399
Toll-free: (800) 223-2732
E-mail: info@apdaparkinson.com
URL: http://www.apdaparkinson.com

Arthritis Foundation
1330 W. Peachtree St.
Atlanta, GA 30309
(404) 872-7100
FAX: (404) 872-0457
Toll-free: (800) 283-7800
E-mail: help@arthritis.org
URL: http://www.arthritis.org

Centers for Disease Control and Prevention
1600 Clifton Rd. NE
Atlanta, GA 30333
(404) 639-3534
Toll-free: (800) 311-3435
URL: http://www.cdc.gov

Children's Defense Fund
25 E St. NW
Washington, D.C. 20001

(202) 628-8787
FAX: (202) 662-3510
E-mail: cdfinfo@childrensdefense.org
URL: http://www.childrensdefense.org

Cystic Fibrosis Foundation
6931 Arlington Rd.
Bethesda, MD 20814
(301) 951-4422
FAX: (301) 951-6378
Toll-free: (800) FIGHT-CF
E-mail: info@cff.org
URL: http://www.cff.org

Epilepsy Foundation of America
4351 Garden City Dr.
Landover, MD 20785
(301) 459-3700
FAX: (301) 577-2684
Toll-free: (800) 332-1000
URL: http://www.epilepsyfoundation.org

Health Care Financing Administration
200 Independence Ave. SW
Washington, D.C. 20201
(202) 690-6113
FAX: (202) 690-6262
URL: http://www.hcfa.gov

Hospice Association of America
228 7th St. SE
Washington, D.C. 20003
(202) 546-4759
FAX: (202) 547-9559
URL: http://www.nahc.org/HAA

Huntington's Disease Society of America
158 W. 29th St., 7th Floor
New York, NY 10001-5300
FAX: (212) 239-3430
Toll-free: (800) 345-HDSA
URL: http://www.hdsa.org

Muscular Dystrophy Association
3300 E. Sunrise Dr.

Tucson, AZ 85718
(520) 529-2000
FAX: (520) 529-5300
Toll-free: (800) 572-1717
URL: http://www.mdausa.org

National Association of Public Hospitals and Health Systems
1301 Pennsylvania Ave. NW, Suite 950
Washington, D.C. 20004
(202) 585-0100
FAX: (202) 585-0101
URL: http://www.naph.org

National Center for Health Statistics
U.S. Department of Health and
Human Services
6525 Belcrest Rd.
Hyattsville, MD 20782-2003
(301) 458-4636

FAX: (301) 436-4258
URL: http://www.cdc.gov/nchs

National Multiple Sclerosis Society
733 Third Ave.
New York, NY 10017-3288
(212) 986-3240
FAX: (212) 986-7981
Toll-free: (800) 344-4867
URL: http://www.nmss.org

National Tay-Sachs and Allied Diseases Association
2001 Beacon St., Suite 204
Brighton, MA 02135
FAX: (617) 277-0134
Toll-free: (800) 906-8723
E-mail: NTSAD-Boston@worldnet.att.net
URL: http://www.ntsad.org

Sickle Cell Disease Association of America
200 Corporate Point, Suite 495
Culver City, CA 90230
(310) 216-6363
FAX: (310) 215-3722
Toll-free: (800) 421-8453
E-mail: scdaa@sicklecelldisease.org
URL: http://www.sicklecelldisease.org

United Network for Organ Sharing
1100 Boulders Parkway, Suite 500
P.O. Box 13770
Richmond, VA 23225-8700
(804) 330-8500
FAX: (804) 330-8507
Toll-free: (800) 24-DONOR
URL: http://www.unos.org

RESOURCES

Agencies of the U.S. Department of Health and Human Services publish a wide variety of health statistics. The National Center for Health Statistics (NCHS) provides a complete statistical overview of the nation's health in its annual *Health, United States*. The NCHS periodicals *National Vital Statistics Report* and *Vital and Health Statistics* give detailed information on U.S. birth and death data and trends. The Health Care Financing Administration monitors the nation's health spending. The agency's quarterly *Health Care Financing Review* and annual *Data Compendium* provide complete information on health care spending, particularly allocations of Medicare and Medicaid.

The Centers for Disease Control and Prevention in Atlanta, Georgia, tracks nationwide health trends and reports its findings in several periodicals, especially its *Advance Data* series, *HIV/AIDS Surveillance Reports,* and *Morbidity and Mortality Weekly Reports.*

The Center for Mental Health Services reports data concerning the nation's mental health status and services in its periodic *Mental Health, United States*. The National Institute of Mental Health also publishes periodic studies on mental health issues.

The Bureau of the Census, in its *Current Population Reports* series, details the status of insurance among selected American households. The Bureau's *Fertility of American Women* provides the socioeconomic characteristics of women who give birth. Another publication from the Bureau of the Census, *Population Projections of the United States by Age, Sex, Race, and Hispanic Origin,* gives information on the U.S. population.

The U.S. Department of Education's National Center for Educational Statistics published the *Digest of Educa-tion Statistics,* containing information on medical, dental, and nursing school enrollment. The U.S. General Accounting Office, the investigative arm of Congress, reported on *Alzheimer's Disease: Estimates on Prevalence in the United States.*

The Gale Group thanks the American Cancer Society for permission to use information from its *Cancer Facts & Figures—2000* (Atlanta, GA, 2000). We also thank the American Heart Association for permission to use information from its *2001 Heart and Stroke Statistical Update* (Dallas, TX, 2000). Our thanks also go to the many associations and foundations dedicated to research and education concerning other specific and disabling diseases that provided up-to-date information about these conditions. (See "Important Names and Addresses" for a list of these organizations.)

The Gale Group expresses gratitude to the People-to-People Health Foundation for permission to use information from its quarterly *Health Affairs*, published by Project HOPE. Several issues were used in developing this book.

The Gale Group is grateful for the use of tables from *Navigating the Medication Marketplace: How Consumers Choose and A Look at the Self-Care Movement*, both projects of *Prevention Magazine* (Rodale Press, Emmaus, PA, 1998). These publications considered the ways in which Americans try to maintain good health on their own and other aspects of prevention behavior.

The Employee Benefit Research Institute provided helpful information in its *Annual Health Confidence Survey* (Washington, D.C., 2000). As always, Gale Group thanks the Gallup organization for permission to use its opinion polls.

INDEX